Psychotherapeutics
in Medicine

# Psychotherapeutics in Medicine

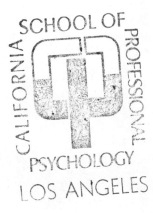

*Edited by*

## Toksoz B. Karasu, M.D.
*Associate Professor of Psychiatry*
*Vice Chairman, Department of Psychiatry*
*Albert Einstein College of Medicine*

*and*

*Director, Department of Psychiatry*
*Bronx Municipal Hospital Center*
*Bronx, New York*

## Robert I. Steinmuller, M.D.
*Assistant Professor of Psychiatry and Medicine*
*Albert Einstein College of Medicine*

*and*

*Director, Department of Psychiatry*
*North Central Bronx Hospital*
*Bronx, New York*

*With the assistance of*
## Betty Meltzer, M.A.

Grune & Stratton
A Subsidiary of Harcourt Brace Jovanovich, Publishers
*New York    San Francisco    London*

Grune & Stratton, Inc.
111 Fifth Avenue
New York, New York 10003

Distributed in the United Kingdom by
Academic Press, Inc. (London) Ltd.
24/28 Oval Road, London NW1

Library of Congress Catalog Number 78-12443
International Standard Book Number 0-8089-1123-6

Printed in the United States of America

# Contents

Toksoz B. Karasu
Robert I. Steinmuller

# Preface

Psychosomatic medicine is receiving increasing attention due to changing emphases in both psychiatry and medical education. It is clear that socioeconomic as well as medical influences will foster the development of health care systems emphasizing comprehensive care by physicians and other primary caregivers, such as physician-associates and nurse-practitioners, working in a multidisciplinary team setting. Psychiatrists will have to develop the knowledge, attitudes, and skills necessary to work effectively and comfortably with nonpsychiatric health care providers as consultants and liaison psychiatrists in a variety of settings with more diverse patients than are usually seen and treated in psychiatrists' offices.

The current explosion of knowledge in psychobiology[1] has also contributed to the resurgence of interest in psychosomatic medicine, following earlier disappointment from the high expectations that flourished during the post-World War II, psychoanalytically oriented era of psychosomatic research and teaching. An integral part of that disillusionment was the failure of psychoanalytic therapy as a treatment technique to match the power of psychoanalytic theory as an explanatory model in psychosomatic medicine.[2] Currently, psychosomatic theorists utilize a variety of conceptual approaches, including psychoanalytical, social-psychological, psychophysiological, ecological, group process, family systems, epidemiological, sociocultural, and general systems theories, in their attempts to understand the biopsychosocial complexities of the medically ill patient in his environment. Although these notions are paid lip service in every area of psychiatry, the liaison psychiatrist observes them daily on a concrete level, in quite specific ways. For this reason, liaison psychiatry has increasingly been seen as an area of paramount educational value not only for psychiatric residents but in undergraduate medical education as well.

Along with this expanding conceptual framework, a broad and diverse repertoire of therapeutic approaches are now available to the psychiatrist and/or nonpsychiatrist for use in those situations where psychoanalytic therapy is unfeasible, unacceptable, unavailable, or possibly ineffectual. These include brief therapy and crisis intervention, a variety of behavior therapies, group and family therapies, psychopharmacology, biofeedback, meditation, and hypnosis.

There is a large and growing literature on each of these treatment approaches and Wolman has recently compiled a comprehensive handbook that reviews them in one volume (including a chapter on the treatment of psychosomatic disorders narrowly defined).[3] This body of literature does not address itself specifically to the treatment of the medically ill patient, however. The psychosomatic and liaison psychiatry literature is also rapidly expanding and now includes a number of excellent monographs and textbooks.[4-14] These books emphasize the historical, theoretical, and conceptual bases of liaison psychiatry. They are generally arranged topically around psychosocial issues pertaining to particular classes of patients or types of health care settings. They emphasize the consultative, liaison, and educational roles of the psychiatrist rather than definitive psychotherapeutic treatment. Generally, discussions of interventions are based on a psychodynamic formulation.

In this book we have attempted to meet the need for a comprehensive and systematic review of the entire spectrum of therapies, specifically applied to medically ill patients. The first three chapters review the field historically and address the process of interviewing the patient and formulating a rational treatment strategy in view of the bewildering plethora of approaches available to the contemporary clinician. Following this is a series of chapters by clinicians who have made authoritative contributions to the development and application of these techniques in the psychosomatic sphere. We have asked each author to describe their method comprehensively, but specifically as it applies to the theme of the book, including indications, contraindications, or modifications needed in the medical setting. Chapters 12, 13, and 14 review treatment by the nonpsychiatric physician, the approach to dying patients and families, and a systems view of therapeutic aspects of the medical ward milieu. The volume ends with a look at research problems in the field.

It is our hope that this book will prove useful to liaison and general psychiatrists, psychologists, psychiatric residents, and others called upon to evaluate and treat medically ill patients. Nevertheless, the internist, pediatrician, or family physician should also find much of value in expanding his awareness of the enlarged armamentarium now available, thus increasing his effectiveness in utilizing a psychiatric consultant. The pluralistic and multimodal approach renders many more patients accessible to psychotherapeutic intervention than ever before, bringing us closer to the goal of being able to provide truly comprehensive care for all.

We are indebted to all of our contributors for their spirit of cooperation. We also wish to thank Norma Brooks for her invaluable administrative and editorial assistance, as well as Rhea Gottlieb and Sandra Quiros for their excellent typing help.

# References

1. *Weiner H:* Psychobiology and Human Disease. *New York, Elsevier-North Holland, 1977*
2. *Reiser MF:* Changing theoretical concepts in psychosomatic medicine. In: *Arieti S (Ed.),* American Handbook of Psychiatry, *2 ed. Vol 4, New York, Basic Books, 1975, p. 477*
3. *Wolman BB (Ed.):* The Therapist's Handbook. Treatment Methods of Mental Disorders. *New York, Van Nostrand Reinhold Company, 1976*
4. *Abram HS (Ed):* Basic Psychiatry for the Primary Care Physician. *Boston, Little, Brown and Company, 1976*
5. *Faguet RP, Fawzy FI, Wellisch DK, Pasnau RO (Eds.):* Contemporary Models in Liaison Psychiatry. *New York, Spectrum Publications, 1978*
6. *Imboden JB, Urbaitis JC:* Practical Psychiatry in Medicine. *New York, Appleton-Century-Crofts, 1978*
7. *Lipowski ZJ, Lipsitt DR, Whybrow PC (Eds.):* Psychosomatic Medicine: Current Trends and Clinical Applications. *New York, Oxford University Press, 1977*
8. *Lipp MR:* Respectful Treatment: The Human Side of Health Care. *Hagerstown, Harper and Row, 1977*
9. *Pasnau RO (Ed.):* Consultation-Liaison Psychiatry. *New York, Grune and Stratton, Inc., 1975*
10. *Reading A, Wise TN (Eds.):* The Medical Clinics of North America, Vol. 61, *Symposium on Psychiatry in Internal Medicine. Philadelphia, Saunders, 1977*
11. *Strain JJ, Grossman S:* Psychological Care of the Medically Ill: A Primer in Liaison Psychiatry. *New York, Appleton-Century-Crofts, 1975*

12. *Strain JJ:* Psychological Interventions in Medical Practice. *New York, Appleton-Century-Crofts, 1978*
13. *Usdin G (Ed.):* Psychiatric Medicine. *New York, Brunner/Mazel, 1977*
14. *Wittkower ED, Warnes H (Eds.):* Psychosomatic Medicine: Its Clinical Applications. *Hagerstown, Harper & Row, 1977*

# Contributors

**Ian Alger, M.D.**
Visiting Associate Professor of Psychiatry
Albert Einstein College of Medicine;
Faculty, Family Studies Section
Bronx Psychiatric Center, New York;
Training and Supervising Psychoanalyst
New York Medical College
New York, New York

**Arthur M. Arkin, M.D.**
Professor of Psychology
Department of Psychology
The City College of the City University of New York
New York, New York

**Peter J. Buckley, M.B., Ch.B.**
Assistant Professor of Psychiatry
Department of Psychiatry
Albert Einstein College of Medicine
Director of Outpatient Services
Department of Psychiatry
Bronx Municipal Hospital Center
Bronx, New York

**Pietro Castelnuovo-Tedesco, M.D.**
James G. Blakemore Professor of Psychiatry
Vanderbilt University School of Medicine
Nashville, Tennessee

**Wilbert E. Fordyce, Ph.D.**
Professor, Department of Rehabilitation Medicine
University of Washington School of Medicine
Seattle, Washington


**Fred H. Frankel, M.B. Ch.B., D.P.M.**
Associate Professor of Psychiatry
Beth Israel Hospital
Harvard Medical School
Boston, Massachusetts


**David J. Greenblatt, M.D.**
Assistant Professor of Medicine
Harvard Medical School
Chief, Clinical Pharmacology Unit,
Massachusetts General Hospital
Boston, Massachusetts


**Marc Hertzman, M.D.**
Director, Inpatient Services
Department of Psychiatry & Behavioral Sciences
George Washington University Medical Center
Washington, D.C.


**Toksoz B. Karasu, M.D.**
Associate Professor of Psychiatry
Vice Chairman, Department of Psychiatry
Albert Einstein College of Medicine
and Director, Department of Psychiatry
Bronx Municipal Hospital Center
Bronx, New York


**Chase Patterson Kimball, M.D.**
Professor of Psychiatry and Medicine
Division of Biological Sciences and in the College
University of Chicago
Chicago, Illinois

**Robert Plutchik, Ph.D.**
Professor of Psychiatry
Department of Psychiatry
Albert Einstein College of Medicine
Department of Psychiatry
Director of Program Development and Clinical Research
Department of Psychiatry
Bronx Municipal Hospital Center
Bronx, New York

**Morton F. Reiser, M.D.**
Professor and Chairman
Department of Psychiatry
Yale University School of Medicine
New Haven, Connecticut

**Richard I. Shader, M.D.**
Director, Psychopharmacology Research Laboratory
Massachusetts Mental Health Center
Boston, Massachusetts

**Aaron Stein, M.D.**
Clinical Professor of Psychiatry
The Mount Sinai School of Medicine of the City University of New York;
Attending Psychiatrist and Chief of the Adult Group Therapy Division
Department of Psychiatry
The Mount Sinai Hospital
New York, New York

**Solomon S. Steiner, Ph.D.**
Professor of Psychology
Department of Psychology
The City College of the City University of New York
New York, New York

**Robert I. Steinmuller, M.D.**
Assistant Professor of Psychiatry and Medicine
Albert Einstein College of Medicine;
Director, Department of Psychiatry
North Central Bronx Hospital
Bronx, New York

**Stuart A. Waltzman, M.D.**
Assistant Clinical Professor of Psychiatry
Department of Psychiatry
Albert Einstein College of Medicine
Acting Director, Psychiatric Consultation-Liaison Service
Bronx Municipal Hospital Center
Bronx, New York

**Daniel R. Weinberger, M.D.**
Clinical Fellow in Psychiatry
Harvard Medical School
Chief Resident, Somatic Therapies Unit,
Massachusetts Mental Health Center
Boston, Massachusetts

**Stephen Wiener, M.D.**
Resident in Psychiatry
Department of Psychiatry
The Mount Sinai Hospital
New York, New York

Peter J. Buckley

# 1

# An Historical Perspective on Psychological Treatment of Medical Illnesses

The interaction between the body and the mind has aroused intense philosophical and medical speculation since antiquity, stimulating endless debates concerning the comparative importance of biological versus psychological components in the etiology, predisposition, and perpetuation of human disease.

Lain-Entralgo has suggested that medicine has always been psychosomatic because the therapeutic activity of the physician is inevitably determined by the reality of the human being toward whom it is directed, since the patient's "personal" conditions are always paramount.[1] Though primitive medicine took this holistic approach to the patient, dualism, with its artificial separation of mind from body, emerged in medicine as early as the classical Greek period.

An examination of the history of psychosomatic treatment shows the fallacy of a purely somatic or purely psychological approach to the treatment of illness. When the somatic treatment of the forebears of contemporary Western doctors, the Hippocratic physicians, failed them, the patients of ancient Greece sought out more eclectic, though less "rational," treatments in the healing temples of Asclepius, where a one-sided somatic approach was not practiced. Nonetheless, the "organic" view of human illness has dominated conventional Western medical practice until very recent times.

The development of psychosomatic medicine in this century has been a major factor in opposing the dualistic philosophy by showing the interplay between biological, psychological, and social factors in disease. Only now is the true complexity of the etiology and pathogenesis of human disease being recognized, an awareness that psychosomatic medicine has been instrumental in developing.

## MEDICAL TREATMENT IN PRELITERATE SOCIETIES

Anthropological studies of medical practice in primitive cultures shed light on the origins of medical therapeutics. Medical treatment in these cultures takes place under religious auspices where the shaman is the prototype of the modern physician. Both the shaman and his patient often enter trance states during religious healing rituals in primitive societies.[2] The underlying basis of these ceremonies is an animistic view of disease in which the disease is regarded as "sent" from the outside. Disease is often viewed as a punishment that the sick individual has received from the gods for a violation of the moral law. In his healing rituals the shaman becomes "possessed" by the spirits, in the course of which he will symbolically expel the evil cause of disease from the body of the patient.

An example of such a ceremony can be found in northern Peru, where the contemporary curandero or folk-healer uses the San Pedro cactus in his healing rites, both for himself and for his patients.[3] The cactus contains mescaline, and the mutual psychedelic experience evoked by the hallucinogen is the catalyst acting within the healing ceremony. All those present at the ceremony imbibe the hallucinogenic cactus brew and are then ceremonially "cleansed" by the curandero, following which he has a vision of the cause of the patient's illness and exorcises the evil. A final purification closes the ceremony.

No differentiation between organic and functional illnesses takes place in these ceremonies which have a potent psychotherapeutic impact on the participants. This lack of distinction corroborates Lain-Entralgo's view that, in these primitive societies, at least, all medical practice is "psychosomatic." Frank has pointed out that the shaman's cure may involve not only the administration of therapeutic agents such as drugs, but that provision is also made for confession, atonement, intercession with the spirit world, and restoring the patient into the good graces of his family and tribe. "The shaman's role may thus involve aspects of the roles of physician, magician, priest, moral arbiter, representative of the group's world view, and agent of social control. His success may depend more on his ability to mobilize the patient's hopes, restore his morale, and gain his reacceptance by his group, than on his pharmacopoeia."[4]

This therapeutic model undoubtedly preceded Western civilization. Medicine in ancient Egypt was also deistic, with prayers and exorcisms being combined with an extensive pharmacology. Evidence from the Kahun Papyrus of 1600 BC would suggest, however, that the earliest Egyptian medicine was somewhat less concerned with the supernatural. This early Egyptian medicine formed the basis of later Greek Hippocratic medicine, but it too had a religious aspect. Before beginning treatment, the physician offered up prayers to the gods to increase the healing power of his medicine: "I will save him from his enemies, and Thoth shall be his guide, he who lets writing speak and has composed the books; he gives to the physicians who accompany him, skill to cure. The one whom the god loves, him he shall keep alive."[5] Thus the Egyptian physician invoked the psychological power of faith alongside his somatic regimen.

## MODELS OF MENTAL ILLNESS IN CLASSICAL GREECE

An early separation of psychological from biological viewpoints in the understanding of mental illness took place in ancient Greece with the development of the Hippocratic and Platonic models of mental functioning. In their studies of the theories of mental activity and mental illness that evolved in ancient Greece, Simon and Weiner show how the Hippocratic and Platonic models of mind were preceded by the Homeric model of mind.[6, 7] In the Homeric model there is no clear idea of mental structure and, as in many preliterate societies, mental illness is viewed as something "sent" by wrathful gods from the outside. As Simon and Weiner point out, however, one aspect of this theoretical framework continues to beset contemporary medical theory, and that is the trend towards the reification and personification of complex processes. Hence the concept of madness being sent by the gods reifies the cause of madness, just as an attempt to find "the cause" of mental illness through a biochemical lesion alone is a similar form of reification. Complex states such as mental or physical illness are not things, and this trend towards reification has bedevilled medical and psychiatric thinking from ancient times until the present.

The Platonic or philosophical model of mind is shown by Simon to be a precursor of the psychoanalytic model—the mind is split into a part that represents reason and another that represents the instincts, just as the psychoanalytic model of mind has its conscious and unconscious parts and, as a later development, its structural model of ego, id, and superego.[8] This Platonic view is an early conflict model, with mental illness viewed as a consequence of an imbalance whereby the unbridled instinctual part gains the upper hand. Treatment is through the Platonic dialogue, again a precursor of the psychoanalytic dialogue, which brings the conflicting parts of the mind into harmony and reasserts control over the irrational part of man. Simon shows that there are significant differences between Freud and Plato and that the analytic dialogue deals directly with the emotions, while the philosophical dialogue attempts to discard them.

A frank psychotherapy did not arise in ancient Greece, however, because of a failure on the part of the Hippocratic physicians to utilize the power of "the word" in their therapy.[9] The Hippocratic physicians succumbed entirely to a somatic view of illness from which all nonphysical factors had to be excluded. This physiological model of illness was first propounded by Hippocrates most famously in his discourse on epilepsy, *On the Sacred Disease:* "It is thus with regard to the disease called Sacred; it appears to me to be nowise [sic] more divine nor more sacred than other diseases, but has a natural cause from which it originates like other afflictions. Men regard its nature and cause as divine from ignorance and wonder, because it is not at all like other diseases. And this notation of its divinity is kept up by their inability to comprehend it."[10] In the *Corpus Hippocraticum,* the brain was recognized to be the source of the emotions: "And men ought to know that from nothing else but thence come joys, delights, laughter and sports and sorrows, griefs, despondency, and lamentations.—And by the same organ we become mad and delirious, and fears and terrors assail us, some by night, and some by day, and dreams and untimely wanderings, and cares that are not suitable, and ignorance of present circumstances, desuetude and unskillfulness. All these things we endure from the brain when it is not healthy."[11]

This point of view, that all illness, including psychiatric disturbance, is based solely on disordered physiology has dominated Western medicine ever since. While not wrong, such a model is incomplete and does not allow for psychological factors in the etiology or predisposition to illness. Under this theoretical banner, all therapy tends to be somatic. Hence the Hippocratic view is the forerunner of the "medical model," with its emphasis on organic causes and somatic treatments.


## PSYCHOSOMATIC TREATMENT IN THE CLASSICAL WORLD

The "rational" treatment of the Hippocratic physicians, based as it was on somatic manipulations such as diet, purges, and bloodletting, failed to help a large proportion of patients. These patients turned to another venue of treatment, this time to be found in a religious setting—the healing temples of Asclepius. The patients who patronized the Asclepia tended to suffer from illnesses that included a major psychological component, though this was by no means exclusively the case. The temples were dedicated to Asclepius, the god of medicine and the son of Apollo and were numerous in the Greek world, the most famous being at Pergamon, Kos, and Epidaurus. As was generally true of Greek temples, the temples of Asclepius were located in striking natural settings. There was one at Athens under the south cliff of the Acropolis, adjoining the theatre of Dionysus, and it was here that Plutus in Aristophanes's play of the same name was cured of his blindness. Epidaurus was known as "the place of pilgrimage," and to some extent was the Lourdes of ancient Greece. The arduous nature of the journey to the Asclepia undoubtedly heightened the psychotherapeutic potency of these temples.

The extraordinary supernatural curative powers of Asclepius were thought to be transmitted through the priests of his temples who carefully orchestrated the rituals performed by the patient-worshippers. Hence, in a socially sanctioned manner, the priests became transference figures with magical omnipotent powers. Upon arrival at the Asclepian after a journey often marked by hardships and danger, the supplicant would undergo an initial period of fasting, cleansing, and religious ritual, following which he would proceed to "incubation" rooms to await the appearance of the god who would appear to the supplicant in a dream and prescribe the cure. This dream-treatment was a central part of the therapy of the Asclepia and was very much in harmony with the culture of the Greek world which was extremely dream-conscious. It is all the more surprising, therefore, that the Hippocratic physicians were uninterested in the meaning and therapeutic usefulness of dreams. The dreams were interpreted by the temple priests, and this frankly psychological treatment was combined with a regimen of somatic treatments, providing an early example of a combined therapeutic approach.

A detailed account of the Asclepian treatment of psychosomatic disorders has survived in the *Sacred Discourses* of Aelius Aristides who kept a diary of his illness and 10-year treatment at Pergamon in the second century.[12] Aristides was a prominent sophist who seems to have been "wrecked by success," and who developed multiple psychosomatic complaints including asthma, gastrointestinal ailments, and urticaria as a consequence. After unsuccessful treatment by the Hippocratic physicians of Smyrna, Aristides had a dream in which Asclepius appeared directing him to enter his temple at Pergamon. For 10 years Aristides resided there, utterly devoted to the god and to treatments that the god directed through Aristides's dreams.

The divine prescriptions were often confusing, but Aristides never wavered in his devotion:

> Indeed it is the paradoxical which predominates in the cures of the god; for example one drinks chalk, another hemlock, another one strips off his clothes and takes hot baths when it is warmth and not at all cold, that one would think he is in need of. Now myself he has likewise distinguished in this way, stopping catarrhs and colds by bathing in rivers and in the sea, healing me through long walks when I was hopelessly bedridden, administering terrible purgations on top of continuous abstinence from food, prescribing that I should speak and write when I could hardly breathe, so that if any justification for boasting should fall to those who have been healed in such a way, we certainly have our share in this boast.[13]

As Rosen points out, the dream prescriptions were indeed painful, even cruel, and clearly satisfied a deep-seated masochistic tendency in Aristides.[14] Many of his dreams show an inordinate sense of guilt, combined with an unconscious wish for punishment, and were undoubtedly interpreted intuitively as such by the temple priests. For ten years Aristides's life revolved around his illness, the divine messages from the god, and his treatments, until he was ultimately cured of his psychosomatic disorders. The therapeutic milieu, with its theatre, gymnasium, and removal of the sufferer from the pressures of the outside world, was clearly an effective one with a positive expectation of cure and a powerful transference relationship to the god.

Many patients came to the temples in a skeptical frame of mind, and yet were cured, testimony to the power of the Asclepia and the readiness of the temple priests to employ an eclectic therapeutic approach. A number of votive tablets have been recovered at the sites of the Asclepia, and these are usually the written testimonials of grateful and successfully cured patients whose testimony may well have been critical to the success and continued power of the Asclepia:

> A man whose fingers were all paralysed but one came as a suppliant to the god. When he looked at the tables in the precinct he did not believe in the cures, and scoffed at the inscriptions. But when he fell asleep he saw a vision. He thought

he was playing dice beside the temple, and just as he was about to make a throw, the god appeared to him and leaped on his hand, stretching the fingers out. As the god went away he thought that he clenched his hand and then straightened out the fingers one after another. When he had straightened them all, the god asked him whether he still disbelieved the inscription on the tablets about the sanctuary. He said no. "Then" said the god, "because you withheld belief before, though they were true, let Doubter be your name in the future." And when day broke he went out cured.[15]

In their prescriptions, the temple priests took cognizance of both the psychological and somatic aspects of their patients' illnesses. This awareness of the interplay between the psychological and the somatic gave the Asclepia considerable therapeutic efficacy, as their enormous popularity throughout classical times attests. The relationship of healing to religion seen in the cult of Asclepius is a common one; in many cultures, all healing is religious and religion is intimately concerned with health and healing.

Alongside the Asclepia, another religious rite, the festivals of Dionysus, sometimes served a therapeutic purpose in ancient Greece. Though these festivals were primarily religious, many of the participants hoped that the "sacred madness" (or possession states) that occurred during the course of the Dionysian bacchanalia would cure them of their illnesses.[16] The syncretic Voodoo religion of Haiti provides a contemporary parrallel to the Dionysian rite. Many Voodoo ceremonies are designated as healing rites, in the course of which the participants become "possessed" and enter a frank trance-state.[17] Rhythmic drumming and dancing in a highly charged group setting, where there is an expectation of possession, facilitates the frequent appearance of these dramatic trance-states among the Voodoo worshippers. Somatic treatments are often combined with this powerful psychotherapeutic procedure. This combined treatment is often effective, since the hungan, or Voodoo priest, is careful to select patients for his ministrations whose illness will be ameliorated by his psychotherapeutic interventions.

The great physician and teacher of the classical period, Galen of Pergamon, was acutely aware of the interrelationship of body and mind in disease. Veith, in her study on the history of hysteria, quotes a vivid example of Galen's medical acumen. Galen was consulted by a woman who was suffering from sleeplessness, listlessness, and general malaise:

After I had diagnosed that there was no bodily trouble, and that the woman was suffering from some mental uneasiness, it happened that, at the very times I was examining her, this was confirmed. Somebody came from the theater and said he had seen Pylades dancing. Then both her expression and the color of her face changed. Seeing this, I applied my hand to her wrist; I noticed that her pulse had suddenly become extremely irregular. This kind of pulse indicates that the mind is disturbed; thus it occurs also in people who are disputing over any subject. So on the next day I said to one of my followers, that, when I paid a visit to the woman, he was to come a little later and announce to me,

"Morphus is dancing today." When he said this, I found that the pulse was unaffected. Similarly also on the next day, when I had an announcement made about the third member of the troupe, the pulse remained unchanged as before. On the fourth evening I kept very careful watch when it was announced that Pylades was dancing, and I noticed that the pulse was very much disturbed. Thus I found out that the woman was in love with Pylades, and by careful watch on the succeeding days my discovery was confirmed.[18]

During medieval times, religious centers continued to function as healing shrines. For example, pilgrims came to the shrine of St. Almedha in medieval Wales to be cured of sickness, and they invoked a trance-state by frenzied rhythmic dancing much as did the worshippers of Dionysus. During their trance, the supplicants would symbolically reenact the various sins they had committed as an act of confession to be followed by later atonement.

## PSYCHOSOMATIC TREATMENT DURING THE 18TH AND 19TH CENTURIES

With the onset of the European Enlightenment psychological treatment underwent a dramatic shift from a religious to a scientific setting. Ellenberger has shown how this change is embodied in the conflict that took place between Gassner, a religious exorcist, and Mesmer, a physician, in 1775.[19] Gassner was a country priest who became one of the most famous healers of his time. He recognized two types of illness, natural and preternatural. The latter he felt were either an imitation of natural illness caused by the devil, the results of sorcery, or a manifestation of frank diabolical possession. It was to these preternatural illnesses that he turned his attention.

Gassner would demonstrate his power over the demon who was thought to be responsible for the patient's illness by commanding the demon to manifest the symptoms of the disease. This demonstration would establish the diagnosis, and would be followed by Gassner's expelling the demon by his imprecations, thus "curing" the patient. This whole process took place while the patient was in a trance-state induced by Gassner. Gassner's credibility was undermined by Mesmer, who produced similar results but had a "scientific" explanation involving "animal magnetism" for the phenomenon. This explanation was more acceptable to the assumptive world of the eighteenth-century gentry and intelligentsia than was Gassner's more medieval view.

Mesmer's theory has been summarized by Ellenberger:

A subtle physical fluid (animal magnetism) fills the universe and forms a connecting medium between man, the earth, and the heavenly bodies, and also between man and man. Disease originates from the unequal distribution of the fluid in the human body; recovery is achieved when the equilibrium is restored. With the help of certain techniques this fluid can be channelled, stored, and conveyed to other persons. In this manner "crises" can be provoked in patients and diseases cured.[19]

Mesmer felt that the crises reflected the disease, for example, for an asthmatic it would be an attack of asthma. Mesmer was obviously using an abreactive method in his treatment and he had many successes, but he became embroiled in acrimonious disputes with the medical establishment. His more extravagant group techniques ultimately led to his being discredited, but his theories attracted many adherents and led to the foundation of the *Societe de l'harmonie* by his disciples. This organization blossomed throughout France and promulgated Mesmer's central tenet that healing occurs through "crises." Mesmer's theories were further developed by the Marquis de Puysegur, who treated patients both individually and in groups. Puysegur's most significant contribution was his recognition that psychological forces were at work and this led to an irreversible breach with Mesmer, who tenaciously clung to his physicalist doctrine of animal magnetism.

The use of hypnotherapy in the treatment of disease surfaced again in the work of the French country physician August Liébeault who enjoyed considerable therapeutic success, and his work attracted the interest of a prominent academic internist, Hippolyte Bernheim, in 1882. Bernheim used hypnosis to treat many different illnesses and became the leader of the famous school of Nancy, and a bitter antagonist of Charcot's theories of hypnosis. The recognition of the power of psychological forces in the treatment of apparently organic diseases was highlighted by the work of Liébeault and Bernheim, and had considerable impact on the medical world, but, in large part because of the discovery of chemical anaesthesia, hypnosis was destined to become more the province of stage performers and charlatans than of physicians.

The term "psychosomatic" was coined in 1818 by Heinroth, who also conceived of psychological conflict as the basis of mental illness; but his views were not revived until the end of the nineteenth century by the work of Freud. Conventional medical research and therapeutics pursued an almost exclusively biological course during this period.

## PSYCHOSOMATIC MEDICINE IN THE TWENTIETH CENTURY

This century has seen a true flowering of psychosomatic thought and practice. As with all scientific fields, the failures of theoretical models when applied in practice, together with new discoveries, have stimulated fresh avenues of investigation. As Reiser points out, however, it is not yet possible to construct a satisfactory theory of the etiology and pathogenesis of psychosomatic illnesses, a situation that reflects current awareness of the complexity and enigmas inherent in the psychosomatic disorders.[20]

The rise of psychoanalysis both as a theory and a psychological treatment in the twentieth century was to have profound ramifications for the field of psychosomatic medicine. Freud regarded psychoanalytic thought as being firmly rooted in biology,

and his effort to close the gap between the biological and psychological is seen most
clearly in *The Project for a Scientific Psychology,* his failed, but brilliant attempt to
develop a neurophysiological model of mental processes.[21] In his early work on the
"actual" neuroses, he developed a frankly somato-psychic theory of anxiety
hysteria: the damming up of seminal fluids in the man and their equivalent in the
woman was thought to be expressed in anxiety.[22] It is of some interest that Galen,
the great physician of second-century Rome, espoused exactly the same theory as an
explanation for hysteria. He felt that the secretion of a substance similar to semen
was produced in the uterus, and that the retention of this substance led to an
irritation of the uterus and the subsequent hysterical fit. Like Freud, Galen
recognized the existence of male hysteria, which he felt was due to sexual
abstinence and the consequent retention of sperm.[23]

The evolution of Freud's work, and the development of the technique of free
association, seemed to provide clinicians with an opportunity to study in
microscopic detail the role of psychological conflict in the etiology and
pathogenesis of psychosomatic illnesses. One of the central tenets of Freud's
psychological theory, the critical role of unconscious intrapsychic conflict in the
etiology of neurosis, was eagerly embraced and became a central theoretical
formulation of psychosomatic medicine.

Flanders Dunbar was the first investigator to suggest that specific personality
factors with particular underlying unresolved neurotic conflicts were at the root of
psychosomatic illnesses. Alexander and his group in Chicago in the 1940s
concurred with this and elaborated a number of hypotheses concerning the nature of
the underlying conflict in different psychosomatic diseases. Their formulations were
based on the psychoanalytic investigation of a small group of patients suffering from
bronchial asthma, peptic ulcer, essential hypertension, neurodermatitis, and
thyrotoxicosis. Alexander suggested that the patients with peptic ulcers suffered
from conflicts over their oral dependent strivings which were discharged through the
stomach: "To be loved, to be helped, is associated from the beginning of life with
the wish to be fed. When this help-seeking attitude is denied its normal expression
in a give-and-take relationship with others, a psychological regression takes place to
the original form of a wish to ingest food. This regressive desire seems to be
specifically correlated with increased gastric secretion."[24] Separate psychodynamic
formulations were postulated for the other psychosomatic diseases investigated by
Alexander and his group. The presence of both a constitutional vulnerability, called
an X-factor, along with an onset situation, were considered to be additional
necessary elements for the precipitation of the manifest disease.

As Reiser has suggested, this organ-specificity model is a linear psychosomatic
theory that does not take into account the multiplicity of factors involved in the
etiology and pathogenesis of psychosomatic disease.[20] The influence of this model
upon treatment, however, was profound, and clinicians directed their therapeutic
efforts at the resolution of the unconscious conflict through psychological means
based on the psychoanalytic technique.

A number of individual successes with the use of psychotherapy were reported.
In a careful follow-up study of psychotherapeutically treated ulcerative colitis

patients, Karush et al, reporting on 30 patients, found that the longer the duration of treatment the better the result.[25] They discovered that the relationship between the patient's dependency needs and the therapist's responsiveness to this issue was particularly important to the outcome. Interestingly enough, they observed that the highest improvement rate occurred when the therapist's empathy and optimism were combined with the patient's hopefulness. There was a failure in this study, however, to determine the varying medical types of ulcerative colitis under study, or to include a control group of colitis patients treated without psychotherapy, making it difficult to determine whether psychotherapy alone ameliorated the different types of ulcerative colitis.[26]

The overall results of the psychoanalytic treatment of psychosomatic disorders have not been as successful as was originally hoped, highlighting the tremendous complexities inherent in these illnesses and our ignorance concerning their basic pathophysiology. Psychotherapeutic intervention, in fact, appears to be most beneficial in the initial stages of the illness, before irreversible tissue damage occurs.

As the organ-specificity model was seen to be inadequate, broader conceptual frameworks and more eclectic treatments have evolved in psychosomatic medicine. Treatment methods have been extended to include psychopharmacological, somatic, and interpersonal modalities alongside psychotherapy. In an extensive review of the theoretical backgrounds of the field, Reiser has shown how the concentration on intrapsychic mechanisms and peripheral autonomic and humoral mechanisms ignored the role of interpersonal and social factors, nonspecific bodily responses, and the mediating role of the central nervous system itself.[20] For a fully developed theory of disease a broader understanding of biological, social, and psychological factors impinging on the patient is necessary.

As Weiner has observed, medicine may well be the only discipline that still lacks a comprehensive theory. He points out that psychosomatic medicine is the one branch of medicine that attempts to provide a comprehensive view of disease encompassing both functional and historical explanations, and that the unstated goal of the psychosomatic approach is the development of a valid theory of health and disease.[27]

A major contribution of psychosomatics to medicine in this century has been the increasing attention that has been paid to the doctor-patient relationship. An outgrowth of psychoanalytic theory has been the recognition that transference is a potent force that must be taken into account in all medical therapeutics. This is reflected in the growth of liaison psychiatry and the awareness of the important contribution that the psychiatrist can make to all medical management. The positive use of the doctor-patient relationship is a powerful addition to the physician's therapeutic repertoire, a fact that was empirically recognized in antiquity by the temple priests of Asclepius. Psychosomatics's greatest contribution to medicine may well lie in promoting a return to the holistic view of disease that recognizes that all illness is to some extent psychosomatic, and that all medical treatment must take into account the ecology, biology, and psychology of the individual patient.

## References

1. Lain-Entralgo P: Mind and Body. Psychosomatic Pathology: A Short History of the Evolution of Medical Thought. A.M. Espinosa, Jr. (Trans.). London, Harvill, 1955
2. Lewis IM: Ecstatic Religion: An Anthropological Study of Spirit Possession and Shamanism. Baltimore, Penguin Books, 1971
3. Sharon D: The San Pedro cactus in folk healing. In Furst PT (Ed.), The Ritual Use of Hallucinogens. New York, Praeger, 1972, pp 114–135
4. Frank J: Foreword. In Kiev A (Ed.), Magic, Faith and Healing. New York, The Free Press, 1974
5. The Papyrus Ebers. B. Ebbell (Trans.). Copenhagen, Levin and Munksgaard, 1937
6. Simon B, Weiner H: Models of mind and mental illness in ancient Greece, I: the homeric model of mind. J Hist Behav Sci 2:303–314, 1966
7. Simon B: Models of mind and mental illness in ancient Greece, II: the Platonic model. J Hist Behav Sci 8:389–404, 1972
8. Simon B: Plato and Freud. Psychoanal Q 42:91–122, 1973
9. Lain-Entralgo P: The Therapy of the Word in Classical Antiquity Rather LJ, Sharp JM (Trans.) New Haven, Yale University Press, 1970
10. Hippocrates: the sacred disease. In Francis Adams, (Ed.), The Genuine Works of Hippocrates. New York, William Wood, 1929, pp 334–335
11. Ibid, p 344
12. Rosen G: Madness and Society. New York, Harper & Row, 1969, pp 110–121
13. Bruno Keil, (Ed.): Aelii Aristidis Smyrnaei quae supersunt omnia, vol 11, XLII, 8. Quoted in Rosen G.: Ibid, p 117
14. Ibid, pp 110–121
15. Guthrie W: The Greeks and Their Gods. Boston, Beacon Press, 1955, pp 252–253
16. Dodds ER: The Greeks and the Irrational. Berkeley, University of California Press, 1972
17. Kiev A: Folk psychiatry in Haiti. J Nerv Ment Dis 32:260–265, 1961
18. Brock AJ (Trans.): Greek Medicine: Being Abstracts Illustrative of Medical Writers from Hippocrates to Galen. London & Toronto, J. M. Dent & Sons Ltd, 1929 pp 213–14. Quoted in Veith I: Hysteria: the History of a Disease. Chicago, University of Chicago Press, 1965
19. Ellenberger HF: The Discovery of the Unconscious. New York, Basic Books, 1970, pp 53–109
20. Reiser MF: Changing theoretical concepts in psychosomatic medicine. In American Handbook of Psychiatry, Vol V. New York, Basic Books, 1975, pp 447–500
21. Freud S: Project for a Scientific Psychology. In The Standard Edition of the Complete Psychological Works of Sigmund Freud, Vol I. London, The Hogarth Press, 1966, pp 283–387
22. Freud S: On the Grounds for Detaching a Particular Syndrome from Neurasthenia under the Description "Anxiety Neurosis." In: The Standard Edition of the Complete Psychological Work of Sigmund Freud. London, The Hogarth Press, 1966, pp 85–117
23. Veith I: Hysteria: the History of a Disease. University of Chicago Press, Chicago, 1965
24. Alexander F, French TM, Pollock GM: Psychosomatic Specificity. Chicago, University of Chicago Press, 1968, pp 16
25. Karush A, Daniels GE, O'Connor JF, Stern OL: The response to psychotherapy in chronic ulcerative colitis. II. Factors arising from the therapeutic situation. Psychosom Med 31:201–226, 1969.
26. Sachar EJ: Some current issues in psychosomatic research. Psychiatr An 2:8:22–35, 1972
27. Weiner H: Psychobiology and Human Disease. New York, Elsevier, 1977, pp xi–xiii

Chase Patterson Kimball

# 2
# Interviewing and Therapy in the Acute Situation

## THE FLOW OF INTERVIEWING

In interviewing the medically ill patient, the primary maxim of interviewing holds, i.e., to begin with where the person is in his or her concerns, and to evolve from there, following the lead of the patient. The interviewer stays with the patient and his concerns, while channeling the course of the interview toward those directions which are most likely to lead to the requisite data necessary for understanding the patient's illness. The nidus is always with the patient, however, most frequently with the patient's first complaint, from which the interviewer and patient together embark, often returning to this port of embarkment to reembark along different streams of consciousness introduced by the patient. To the extent to which these streams are productive, the interviewer will facilitate the course, attempting to navigate the deeper channels, while avoiding the shallower and murky waters whose debris may prove diverting and deceptive. These early streams may subsequently become abandoned, or may be reexplored and further penetrated at a later time, depending upon the flow and changes in current that occur during the interview, while the navigator with his passenger attempts to attain a topographic overview of the area to be covered. Similar to streams and rivers, the interview courses tortuously into long forgotten, and frequently little explored, inner regions of the patient's mind, producing both immediately pertinent treasures and deposits of minerals whose worth may only subsequently be discovered in a context different and distant from the present one. The navigator steers a wary course, keeping a sharp watch for the hidden rocks and submerged stumps that may capsize his craft with its valuable cargo, while making notes as to where these latent obstacles lay in the event that he should return at some future date to open wider and deeper channels.

## THE BEGINNING OF THE RELATIONSHIP AND THE PATH THROUGH THE HEALTH CARE SYSTEM

Of immediate concern is the comfort of the passenger, whose sojourn will be briefer or longer depending upon the ease of the initial experience. First, one must ascertain the extent to which the patient knows what he is getting into and with whom he is getting into it. What are his expectations of the interviewing process, both explicit and implicit? Most simply and frequently, it concerns having a complaint, a hurt, a pain which bothers, frightens, concerns the individual enough that he reluctantly seeks the assistance of another. This may happen immediately, but it is more likely to come after a time of delay in which various home remedies, based upon the individual's intuitive and past experience, are tried. These are attempts to find causative explanations for the complaint, taken from the folklore of the family history, the culture, past personal experience with symptoms, and, most recently, from the "threats" and admonitions issued from the public media and the preventive medicine industry. While provoking increasing anxiety, these efforts lead to procrastination built upon the defenses of anxiety and fear. The patient may resort to the homespun advice of a neighbor, a fellow-worker, or some other associate in his daily life, resulting in a trial of a number of remedies, frequently with at least transient relief. When relief is not forthcoming, or has at best been transient, our patient turns to a professional acquaintance—the nurse in the apartment upstairs, the druggist at the corner pharmacy, the local health food dispensary and its proprietor, and, in other areas, rootworker, practitioner, voodooism, or other local diviner that the subculture has consecrated as advisor to the ill and infirm. With symptoms persistent and unyielding to these ministrations, and with still greater uncertainty and perhaps despair, he comes to the clinic or dispensary or, more recently, the emergency room to queue in line amidst other equally discomforted persons. In such a situation, it is not unusual for the individual to experience either a heightening of his symptom, relating to anxiety, or a decrease, relating to fear and denial or secondary to competitive sensory extinction. Less frequently, he may be in the office of a home or business neighborhood physician, whom he may or may not have seen before. In these situations, the channels in which he is steered depend on the therapeutic persuasions and subdisciplines of the practitioner he has chosen. Most likely he will have been given a remedy or potion of yet another dimension and an invitation to call or return. If his complaint is suggestive enough of a perplexing or interesting problem, he may find himself in a situation of being observed, frequently in an in-patient environment.[1]

With this admission into the temple of the craft, he assumes patienthood and all of the accoutrements thereof. Whether or not he has held such status previously, and with what designation and distinction, will be among the determinants modifying the sickness behavior he is likely to manifest.[2]


## THE ROLE OF DENIAL

The development of illness in the acutely ill medical patient is often like the above description, except frequently accelerated. The course is often one of minimizing the significance of the pain, explaining it away on the basis of some recent experience (something one ate, an activity in which one has participated, an exposure one has had). When initial attempts to obtain relief have failed (an aspirin, Tums, Alka Seltzer, or Ben-Gay), further advice and remedy is sought and obtained from a key individual in one's social field (beginning with a relative, fellow-worker, professional friend, and subsequently, a druggist, experienced lay-person with personal familiarity with the complaint, self-styled diviner or healer, general clinic-physician-emergency room, and, less rarely, a scheduled visit with a physician in private practice or an emergency room. During this course, as the experience of the symptom has become more intense, anxiety based on this intensity, as well as on the possibilities that have come to mind—either related to organ involvement (heart, stomach, liver), or illness (cardiac, cancer, ulcer)—has heightened, leading to an increase in the defenses. The latter may take the form of outright denial—it's really nothing, it's not as bad, it's gone away—or the rationalizations may get more elaborate in terms of identifying the symptom with one that some friend or relative had once which had not amounted to all that much. Accompanying these intrapsychic mechanisms and verbal behavior is other behavior that serves to express these defenses. Such behavior may attempt to mask the underlying symptom, related aroused fears, and the subsequent emotions generated by these. The extent to which this is done will depend on many factors. These include: (1) the cognitive, the diagnostic repertory available to the patient; (2) the affective, the defenses characteristic of the individual's style of handling emotions; (3) the state of consciousness—including the innate, as well as present, threshold of arousal for experiencing perceptions; and (4) the social field, including not only what is seen as appropriate expression by others, but what has come to be seen as appropriate expression by oneself. In regards to the latter, Zborowski has emphasized ethnic background and one's place in the generational sequence (first, second, third) in one's culture as relating to the determination of how individuals of Old American, Irish, Italian, and Jewish descent react to pain.[3] The pattern of responses of individuals suffering chest pain associated with an evolving myocardial infarction have been described by Olin and Hackett as following this sequence of behavior.[4]

## THE SYMPTOM REAPPEARED

The prelude described above suggests the all-important behavioral repertoire that the acutely ill patient has experienced and manifested prior to his first exposure to the physician in the hospital. Obviously, little of this journey becomes known to the interviewer immediately upon his entrance. An awareness that the patient has experienced some such course on his quest for relief is essential, however, for both the empathic and cognitive relationship ahead, during which the specific log will become known. At this point, the patient's primary concern is about the complaint that he can no longer deny or minimize. His emotions are most acutely emanating directly from the intensity of the symptom—the pain, the feeling of suffocation, the feeling of drowning, the feeling of passing out, and the feeling of not feeling. His only demand is for relief, at almost any price. This sets the stage for the first potential conflict between the patient and the physician. The latter's task frequently enjoins him from proffering treatment leading to relief without first understanding the nature of the complaint. Since a large part of this understanding comes from talking with the patient, and since the patient may not be able to talk or express his symptoms clearly, this first encounter may be one of considerable frustration and stress to both parties. It also will affect future interactions.

## THE ENVIRONMENTS OF ILLNESS

While the obvious necessity of the interviewer is to obtain information relevant to the patient's complaint, this will not be forthcoming until the latter has achieved some degree of comfort, not only from the symptom, but from his concern about the symptom, the ambulance ride to the hospital, and the emergency room or acute care unit setting. Immediately, the interviewer becomes the mediator between the unfamiliar environment and the patient. He is seen as the one sensate component as the patient's perceived disturbance alters his relationship to his usual environment. Amidst all of this confusion, the interviewer may stand out as representing the existence of a solid reality, an island or raft, to which the patient may cling while he attempts to take sights and get a further hold on life. The calmness and deliberateness of the interviewer may be the most soothing balm of all, even if it needs to be maintained while performing essential remedial procedures and investigative interviews. For the interviewer, it is not an easy task.

It is a task that is further compromised by the environment in which such encounters most often occur. For most patients this is an environment of noise and strange visual appearances, in which perceptions, under the duress of pain and sometimes its treatment, become blurred, indistinct, and sometimes distorted. From the outset, it is incumbent on the interviewer to attend continually to the mental status of the patient if he is to maintain a dialogue with the patient and remain attentive to the patient's needs. While assessing the cognitive functions of orientation, memory, concentration, and abstractive ability, and noting labile changes in affect, the interviewer, as a stabilizing influence, can also serve to

physician has made his diagnosis on the basis of assessing the mental status of utmost importance, the patient should not be left alone. In our experience, the most appropriate individual is the aide. Frequently, the aide has the ability to act matter-of-factly and with clarity with the confused patient when given the instructions: (1) keep communication simple; (2) identify who you are, who the patient is, where he is, what has occurred, that everything will be all right, that he is a bit confused at the moment, but this will clear; (3) repeat this orienting statement frequently; (4) do not get involved in discussing, analyzing, or assertively denying the patient's hallucinations or delusions; and (5) keep regular notes as to what the patient's preoccupations are.[11]

The task of the physician is to review all of the notes about the patient's behavior and medication records in an attempt to identify major etiological components that have contributed to the delirium. In our experience, the following in descending order of frequency are frequently present factors: (1) iatrogenic analgesics and/or hypnotic sedatives; (2) other drugs used in treating the illness, e.g., steroids; (3) withdrawal states, e.g., delirium tremens, narcotic; (4) underlying illness factors relating to metabolic and hormonal imbalances; (5) loss of sleep; and (6) anxiety specifically related to the illness and the environment. Of these, withdrawal states is an important consideration, especially in terms of delirium tremens, where the incidence of death is between 15 and 30 percent in large, well-attended hospitals once the process has begun. Failure to obtain a history of alcohol or other substance abuse either from the patient or his relatives constitutes negligent care of the individual. Some analgesics appear to be more frequently associated with delirium, e.g., pentozocine. In reviewing the possible contribution of the underlying illness to delirium, it is useful to check through the organ systems: (1) central nervous system—subarachnoid, subdural, occlusive vascular, edema, tumor, metastasis, degenerative and depositive diseases; (2) cardiovascular—hypoxia, hyperventilation, cardiac output, blood pressure (hypertensive encephalopathy); (3) respiratory—airway, embolus, aspiration, infiltrate, chronic obstructive pulmonary disease, neoplasm; (4) gastrointestinal—esophageal varices, stomach carcinoma, peptic ulcer, pancreatic carcinoma, colonic neoplasm, parasites, malabsorption syndromes, hepatic disease (encephalopathy), hepatitis, cirrhosis, neoplasm, Wilson's disease; (5) hematopoetic—bone marrow, anemia, lymphoma, hemorrhage, intravascular clotting, thrombos, embolus; (6) genitourinary—renal disease, bladder and urethral dysfunction, uremia, neoplasm; (7) endocrine—the hyper- or hypo-function of each hormonal system; (8) neuromuscular—the degenerative neuromuscular diseases affecting brain function, e.g., amyotrophic lateral sclerosis, multiple sclerosis, neoplasm. To the extent that such contributive designations are identified, remedial measures may be undertaken. It may take time to correct these, during which continued attention is imperative. It is not infrequent for postoperative surgical patients, immediately after return from the operating room, to experience hyperventilation of titanic proportions. All concerned treat this as a medical emergency. This hyperventilation may be viewed as a compensatory phenomenon in which the individual is responding to the previous anesthesia; the treatment is, of course, that of having the patient breathe into a bag.

Steroids when given in large amounts to patients with conditions such as dermatological ones, the cerebrovasculitis of disseminated lupus erythematosis, etc., are notorious associates of delirium. Anxiety relating to the illness, loss of sleep, and the effect of environments on disorientation and delirium have previously been considered. When hallucinations and delusions associated with agitation persist despite orienting attempts and efforts to correct specific factors, phenothiazines or haloperidol drugs are useful in diminishing these symptoms. These are used in the smallest amount of that agent with which the physician is most familiar, and it is preferable to give them orally than parenterally. Reassessment of the patient should take place at 30-minute to one-hour intervals, at which time, if the state remains one of agitation with delusions and hallucinations, another dose is administered. Eighty percent of the patients respond after three to four such evaluations and administrations. The cumulative amount is then given at 8-hour intervals. Because of the disturbing effects of hallucinations and delusions—patient recall these as similar to bad nightmares and reexperience some of the emotions relating to them—it is best to maintain the patient on the agent for 10 days. Contraindications to the use of these medications are few at this dosage range. Orthostatic hypertension associated with the phenothiazine is not usually a hazard in patients who are bedridden. Cardiotoxicity is rare at the dosage range suggested above. It is of note that the amount of drug necessary to curtail the extreme symptoms of delirium, which are frequently viewed as those of an acute paranoid schizophrenic reaction, is much less than what the latter reactions require. Another dissimilarity is that most frequently, the patient experiencing delirium views the delusions and hallucinations as ego-alien, as compared to the more usual ego-syntonic view of delusions and hallucinations held by the individual suffering an acute schizophrenic reaction. One explanation for this may be the suddenness of the experience in the patient with delirium; whereas in the patient with a schizophrenic reaction, the delusions and hallucinations have been held for some time prior to being expressed and have become ego-syntonic secondary to having been ego-alien. Nevertheless, the similarities between acute delirium and an acute schizophrenic reaction recalls the work of McGhie and Chapman, who noted inattention and perceptual distortions as characterizing the earliest stages of the schizophrenic reaction.[12] Attention to these factors is a necessary part of the interviewer's work inasmuch as they appear to be so frequently ignored by the team directly caring for the patient, even though pertinent observations have been made and recorded in the chart. Until the patient's sensorium has cleared, the interviewing process needs to be limited and brief. Patients fatigue easily and become more confused and disoriented. They are hypersensitive to questions demonstrating emotional lability. Their verbalizations may border on the inarticulate, and their conversations may alternate between relative muteness and monosyllabic to tangential expostulations on the state of the world. The order of the day is to keep the interview simple and brief, returning several times during the day in order to augment the information previously obtained, to make new observations, and to further the relationship that has been established with the patient. In each of these transactions, the comfort of the patient is first and paramount. It can best be ascertained by the simple question, "How are you?" Each transaction is a mini-interview, having such an opening, a middle related to obtaining specific new present and historical data as to the current condition of the patient, and an ending. The ending is important in that it can be a simple communication to the patient as to where the interviewer thinks he is at in his ongoing assessment, what he plans next, and when he plans to see the patient again. Such markers are the buoys to which a patient may cling in the turbulent and oftentimes silent intervals between visits.

## SEQUENTIAL PROCESSES IN THE INTENSIVE CARE UNIT (ICU) AFFECTING PHYSICIAN-PATIENT INTERACTION

The ICU-phase of illness is that period in which the acuteness of the illness episode stabilizes. It is one in which the patient gradually comes into an awareness of his changed state of health. This process is a slow and evolutionary one characterized by progressive stages that vary from one individual to another depending upon underlying personality characteristics.[13] During the earliest period, the dominant affect of the patient in the coronary care unit is that of anxiety. This anxiety is directly related to the severity of the patient's discomfort. His preoccupation is to the pain, the diagnostic and therapeutic procedures. The experience of pain is of greater urgency than the fear of death. Indeed, death at this point may only be thought of as a desire to be free of pain. For most patients, this is not a time to speak about death and dying with them. Relief is what is desired. Response to their immediate discomfort is what is demanded. The demands are plaintive ones. While the individual needs reassurance, this needs to be direct, simple, concrete. While he needs didactic instruction, these need to be direct, nontechnical, and clear.

This anxiety, related to discomfort, is accompanied most frequently by a denial of what has occurred, what is occurring, and what the consequences of the occurrence may be. Part of this denial may be related to a failure to perceive or assimilate what has occurred secondary to an altered state of consciousness, anxiety, and/or extinction. Denial *per se* is neither desirable nor undesirable; it depends on the consequences. When it leads to a failure to acknowledge illness, it may result in noncompliance by the patient in necessary diagnostic and therapeutic procedures. In this situation, it is necessary to overcome the denial, using the method that best succeeds in getting the individual to comply. This sometimes may be direct confrontation, but it is usually preferable, when there is time, to assess the basis for the denial and then attempt to remove it. If the denial is on the basis of an altered state of consciousness, obviously it will be necessary to investigate the contributing factors to this condition. If it is on the basis of anxiety, then the need will be for the interviewer to form or extend his therapeutic relationship in order to reduce the defenses sufficiently to allow the patient to ventilate his anxiety. This may need to be a gradual and stepwise progress, repeated several times during the course of a day or over several days.[14] Later during this acute phase, the denial may be of the consequences of illness and interfere with the patient becoming acclimated to a changed state. In this situation, didactic instruction given in a group therapeutic setting with other patients sustaining the same problem may be helpful.[15] The group therapeutic process may reduce the patient's feelings of being singled out for this affliction by providing a setting in which he can identify with other victims and share coping efforts. Such groups help individuals to open up and work through grieving responses, especially during the convalescent phase of illness.

Following anxiety, as stabilization and familiarization have occurred, the dominant affect, anxiety, is replaced by a sadness or depression which lasts for varying periods of time. Cassem and Hackett observe this as peaking by the fourth day and receding thereafter.[13] Others of us feel that this most frequently extends into the convalescent phase of illness, and in some individuals into the rehabilitative phase. In the acute situation, the depression may be expressed in terms of the individual's characterological traits. Responses may range from denial of feeling depressed to expressions of plaintiveness and demandingness. Anger and crying are often present. In the convalescent phase, the manifestation of depression may be one of withdrawal, increased sleeping, and reduced cooperation. At times, this can be explained as a conservation-withdrawal process in which the stressed individual, having survived the acute period with the expenditure of much energy, attempts to restore his strength through reduced interactions with the environment.[16] When limited, this may be viewed as a usual postcrisis phenomenon. For the interviewer, it becomes a task of assessing whether this is the case or whether there are other factors associated with this behavior. When the former explanation prevails, it is reasonable for the interviewer to desist from lengthy interactions until the patient has recovered. This is usually a matter of three to five days.

## CONVALESCENCE AS A GRIEF PROCESS

Whereas self-grieving for the injury or loss of health and function that has been experienced commences during the acute phase, it becomes the dominant natural psychological process of the convalescent phase. As we have noted, the earliest manifestations of grieving are the denial of illness and of feelings about illness and its consequences.[17] We have already discussed the protective aspects as well as the hazards of this usual response in terms of adaption and maladaption. When it persists, it may have increasing maladaptive consequences for the individual that need to be handled through the interview process. Individuals may develop symptoms which are modeled after those of the underlying illness or those of key individuals. The interviewer may become alerted to these through the quality of the description. It may be bizarre, as in the case of a patient who described her headache as "like seven little dwarfs inside my head banging to get out." The precise description of the pain may vary greatly from that of the one after which it is modeled, such as in the case of the individual who has had a myocardial infarction and describes a new pain as over his heart while pointing precisely to his left nipple. The disentanglement of a conversion symptom based on one of an underlying illness process is one of the most difficult and time-consuming in consultation work, and may require intensive investigation over a short period of time. A bizarre or atypical presentation may be accompanied by either exaggeration or an understatement of affect *(la belle indifference)*. The development of the conversion phenomenon may relate directly to the immediate crisis of illness or to another proximate situation in the patient's life which has gone unnoted in the interviews to date with the patient. Closer attention to the illness onset situation at this point in the evolving interview process may serve to identify other stressful occurrences concurrent with that of illness. These may be in the areas of marital, social, or professional life, and reflect real, threatened, or fantasied loss.[18] Specific attention will need to be focused on the times at which the symptom occurs, what has preceded it, the behavior of the patient during it, the reactions of others—and especially significant others—to the patient during it, and the state of affairs following it. A reevaluation of the patient's emotional state may suggest the presence of considerable anxiety, fear, or depression, which the symptom serves to both mask and to allay in terms of drawing the attention of others in the environment to minister to his concern.

Denial usually gradually gives way to a ventilation of affect which also usually raises affect in others, i.e., the staff and interviewer, leading the latter to fend off the affect by repressive defenses of their own which are communicated to the patient. This leads to the suppression of affect and reinforces the mechanisms of defense that the patient has utilized in fending off the assaults that the illness has on his self. The interviewer's job is to walk the tightrope between permitting the expression of affect without it becoming of such proportion and momentum as to unleash even more inappropriate defenses and behavior. The communication of anxiety, sadness (crying), and anger is a natural process in the course of illness, which for many of us can only be done within the context of the physician-patient interaction. When the interviewer has been successful in facilitating such expressions, he should not deprive himself of the fruits of this work. As the patient externalizes his feelings he begins to accept this illness, meaning his changed self, and examine the usefulness of the defenses which he has used in containing these emotions, the unacknowledged thoughts about his illness, and its potential consequences to his self.

The assessment of defenses is a mutual task for the interviewer and the patient, constituting the third stage of the grieving process. This occurs over an indefinite period and traverses the same terrain in subsequent interviews, marching, as it were, up and down the inclined plane of the defenses from the primitive to the most sophisticated, and usually retreating toward the end of a session to the earlier covering defenses. In each session, however, inroads toward insight are made and will be more easily and quickly reached in an ensuing encounter. At times, subtle progress is made, while at others, cataclysmic abreactions may erupt resulting in great leaps forward. In these situations as in other therapeutic situations, it is judicious to allow for some covering toward the end of a session. The ground lost is easily recovered in the next session. As more sophisticated defenses take the place of the earlier ones, the individual begins to take active conative steps toward effective coping and, in time, mastery of his previously compromised situation. At these times, the therapist serves as a reflector of these forward steps, mirroring tacit approbation and supporting refinements in the actions contemplated and tested.

In the rehabilitative stage the effective reinstitution of a sophisticated repertoire of defenses will become increasingly translated into deliberative coping devices serving to compensate for the deficiencies residual to the disease process. Such a repertoire will be of greater depth and sometimes of a different tune, however, as a result of the changes in attitudes toward living that lead to new orientations about oneself and the world that serious illness occasions. For most of us, the illness or its effects will remain, quiescent and/or with exacerbation. The challenge for therapist and patient is to study through asking the appropriate questions and recording observations of those factors that affect the course of the process. This task may need to be done with the cooperation of significant others: parents, spouses, children, and close friends and associates in addition to the physician. The latter will need to keep in close and frequent contact with the patient, monitoring not only the biological correlates of the illness, but the psychological and social ones as well. Identifying whatever correlations occur will allow the physician to choose the appropriate resources in the community, home, and professional environment that may be instrumental in smoothing the course of the illness.

## MORE SPECIFIC SITUATIONS AFFECTING THE INTERVIEWING PROCESS IN ACUTE ILLNESS

Up until now, we have considered the more or less usual course of the severely and acutely ill patient within the hospital environment. In this, we have noted how the illness itself—especially the pain associated with it, the environment in which the patient is treated, his emotional reactions (anxiety, fear, sadness, anger), the not infrequent alterations in consciousness associated with these, and the accompanying and succeeding grief processes leading up to the rehabilitative and posthospital phase of illness—all affect the interview process and the therapeutic process intrinsic to it.

In addition to this common course and the factors that we have discussed so far, there are specific and less frequent situations that affect interviewing and that occasion the need for specific therapeutic interventions. These specific factors relate to the state of the patient and his specific disease, as well as to his personality and behavioral patterns. The factors associated with specific pathophysiologic problems can only be addressed in brevity in this chapter. High among these are those diseases relating to central nervous system processes that directly result in communicative difficulties. These include the receptive and expressive aphasias, as well as those processes interfering with vocalization such as the paralyses of tongue, facial, larynx, and respiratory musculatures. In these situations, the interviewer will need to establish a common ground of communication that will be effective with the patient. At first, the intermediary of a parent, spouse, or child may assist in making the patient's wishes, needs, and feelings known. The use of graphic charts and pointers may serve to identify locations of pains, needs, and concerns. The presence of a committed and sensitive aide or attendant can help to establish a communication system that works. Delegating responsibility will help the busy physician and psychiatrist avoid or diminish the problem of coping with his or her own failure and resulting frustration attending the impediments to communication. With patience and time, communication processes can be established with any alert patient which will be satisfactory for not only the communication of need affecting specific diagnostic and therapeutic tasks but in transmitting the all-important feelings relating to this task. In effecting this, the physician will need to convey a sense of his sincerity, patience, and comfort in working this through with the patient. At the same time, he will need to measure the extent and intensity of these contacts to conform with the patient's tolerance for frustration and fatigue. This usually means seeing the patient more frequently for shorter intervals. While initially, the efforts to communicate over these handicaps appear insurmountable to both bodies, with practice both can make use of nonverbal communications with considerable facility, frequently reaching greater empathy than often prevails in verbal exchanges. Similar communicative skills need to be developed when patient and physician attempt to communicate over language and cultural barriers. It cannot be ignored that even when both parties claim English as their primary tongue, there may occur such discrepancy between the level of sophistication, including technical jargon, that little is transmitted. Interpreters prove a poor substitute because of their usual lack of familiarity with medicine and the absence of a direct relationship with the physician, resulting in little emotional communication. When an interpreter is utilized, it behooves the interviewer to observe the patient rather than the interpreter during the interview. He may pick up valuable clues on the basis of the patient's nonverbal response which are not registered or reported by the interviewer.

Patients with specific illness problems have a number of responses in common.[19] Patients with severe burns will have different problems than those with lymphoma; victims of polio will differ from patients on chronic renal dialysis. In working with patients with these afflictions, the physician will need to gain familiarity with the common problems relating to an illness process. Specific studies have been made regarding the psychosocial aspects of many disease processes.[20] Although for the most part, these are in need of further refinement and definition, some greater understanding of an individual's response can be gleaned from referring to the specific studies.

I have referred to the individual differences in responding to acute and catastrophic illness. Although these relate to such variables as age, severity of illness, social support systems and resources available to the individual, and previous experience with illness, they also relate to temperament, basic personality characteristics, and behavioral patterns of the individual.

Various investigators have characterized these using a number of approaches. Kahana and Bibring have used a nomenclature based on phenomenological observation of medical patients, e.g., the demanding patient, the hostile patient, etc.[21] Others have used more classical classifications, stressing the defenses used to bind emotions evoked by the stress of illness, e.g., obsessive-compulsive, hysterical, etc.[22-25] Regardless of the scheme adopted, some identification of the kind of individual one is working with will lead the interviewer to identify him as falling more toward one category or another, and will alert him to the possibility of a specific behavioral response as a way of coping with the present illness. The extent to which the interviewer is prepared for these reactions, he will be able to address them. Included below is a sketch of six personality classifications that may be useful to the interviewer in responding to the heightened defenses occasioned by acute and severe illness.[26]

## Obsessive-Compulsive

The individual with an obsessive-compulsive personality is frequently hard-working, conscientious, industrious, and a perfectionist. His habits are marked by orderliness and stereotypy; his work, by rigidity and inflexibility. He cannot accept change, which in the face of his patterns may become even more rigid and stereotyped. Things have to be just so. There needs to be a place for everything and everything needs to be in its place. Until this is so, he cannot sit back and rest. Since things are never just right, because the obsessive is always thinking about something that needs doing, he is always busy. Even when he is sitting still, he needs to somehow be doing two things at once. If he is looking at television, he is also doing something with his hands. When he listens to music, his thoughts are far afield "worrying" about something that he is planning or that needs doing. In all that he does there is a sense of urgency, a driven need to get things done and over with, while at the same time his perfectionism may drive him to exact repetition until things are the way they should be. There is only one way, one method, one perfection, not so much dictated by the individual but by his conscience or superego, dominating and directing his every action. On the one hand, such emphasis on an idealized perfection frequently interferes with productivity; the inflexibility and inability to deviate prevents innovation. On the other hand, this individual may do extremely well performing technical tasks requiring unswerving attention to detail and rigid adherence to procedure. As long as there is work to be done, a task, anything that will provide a structure for him to organize and direct his activities, he is able to bind his underlying anxieties by compulsive activity. His style of thinking is stimulus-bound, dogmatic, opinionated, and appears unresponsive to anything anyone else may say. This is not necessarily because it is disagreed with, but more likely to be because of an inability to countenance or hear anything that will distract the thought sequence set in motion; such an interference would upset everything, resulting in chaos and anxiety. When not in absolute control of his environment, i.e., when not at home or in a familiar and secure work situation, a pervasive sense of uneasiness is experienced that leads to a stilted social manner and posture, lacking in spontaneity, and burdened with perfunctoriness which is made only more acute by the individual's self-awareness. While often opinionated and dogmatic in responding to peripheral issues, the individual, when confronted by a problem central to his own life, is plagued by doubts, reservations, and deliberateness that leads to indecisiveness, failure to act, frustration, and finally, to anxiety or depression with the awareness of one's inadequacy, missed opportunity, and resulting loss. The lack of a sense of self is everywhere apparent as this person attempts always unsuccessfully to adopt one role and then another which, in his continual search for absolute perfection, he disregards because of their failure to satisfy his superego demands. He never does anything exactly because he wants to, but rather because he should. This style serves to weave a web in which the individual is eternally entrapped and which prevents the individual from ever doing anything of his own in his own right, and hence assures that he will never achieve any real satisfaction or gratification.

The more entrenched and formidable these patterns become, the more maladaptive they are, tending to result in increasing purposeless and goalless activity. The importance of recognizing these styles is their prevalence in a general medical population. At a time of illness and the resulting increased anxiety, such patterns usually become exaggerated. The physician realizing this can assist his patient in overcoming the anxiety by working with him in structuring his illness experience in ways which reinforce the patient's need for control. A precise outline of what is wrong, what needs to be done, and when it will be done, frequently accomplishes this with gratifying results for both patient and physician. When these patterns become so formidable as to interfere seriously with the social and domestic functioning of the individual, there is generally a need for further exploration and treatment by a psychiatrist. At times of increased stress, these patients may exaggerate latent phobias that may respond to conditioning therapies, if treated early.

### Paranoid

The paranoid individual is best characterized by the single word "suspicious." He is at every moment on the watch for the overt or covert insult, slight, or potential threat to himself and the world that he has built around him. Such a style attempts to protect him from his sense of vulnerability and penetration. His fear of violation demands that he be ever on alert and guard against all manner of attacks on all sides, at all times. To this end, he scans word and picture, deed and talk, the slightest movement or sound in his perceptual sphere for the personal message that it may have for him. The fear and its underlying wish that he might be slighted or otherwise selected for vulnerability or honor is projected outward on to the environment, which is always viewed as menacing and hostile. At the same time as there is an omnipresent fear of external control, the paranoid individual exercises intense internal control. There is a lack of spontaneity in his behavior which leads to a loss of affective expression. Constant preoccupation with autonomy leads to a constriction and narrowing of behavior. Rigidity and intentionality characterize external behavior, which is always calculated and frequently gives the impression of being feigned or imitative. Whether the individual gives an external appearance of furtiveness, constriction, and suspicious apprehensiveness, or of aggressive edginess and arrogance bordering on the megalomanic, or of rigid preoccupation, the quality of hypervigilance is ever-present. Beneath these facades, almost always hidden from public view, is extreme hypersensitivity and feelings of shame and inadequacy, which the externalized projections have been erected to shield. The paranoid position is both a psychological and a physical one. The individual is in a continuous state of mobilization in preparation for an emergency. In this defensive vigilance, there is continual muscular tension. In situations in which the predisposed individual is threatened with real or fantasied injury, these usual modes of perception are exaggerated, leading to the loss of a sense of proportion and to behavior out of context with the social situation. Delusions may occur which dramatize the internal fears of the individual. At the same time, there is a frightening intactness and internal logic to the delusion that may escape the unsuspecting physician and may only be detected after talking with the patient's relatives and family. When threatened by physical injury or discomfort, the paranoid patient's anxieties and defenses against these are at a high level. At such times, he will view the environment with even more than his usual suspicion, and will need very simple, direct explanations of all those working with him about what is wrong, what is to be done, and how it will be done. Even then, the physician and staff should be prepared for constant criticism and antagonism by the patient. Understanding that an acutely anxious and sensitive individual exists beneath this facade will tend to alleviate the counter-transference and passive-aggressive tendencies aroused in the staff in response to these projections.

### Hysterical

The basic mechanism of the hysterical personality is repression of underlying conflicts resulting in emotions that are often out of context and always out of proportion to the environmental or social stimulus. The hysteric lives his life by reacting to stimuli with affect, projecting theatrical, seductive (promising more than what is delivered), and exhibitionistic presentations of himself. A single affect is rarely sustained, however, and the general mood is one characterized by a fleetingness and lability. At times, especially around issues or incidences likely to give rise to affects of displeasure, the hysteric appears unconcerned. This style, the affectual facade, the lack of sustained presentation has caused investigators to note the apparent shallowness of the hysteric's behavior and to suggest an underlying sense of inadequacy and core of depression or emptiness. The affectual style is matched by an equally superficial cognitive style. This is one characterized by a global approach to events, which are grasped in their totality by visual impressions rather than by careful and detailed analysis. There is an incapacity for intense or persistent intellectual activity, but rather an exaggerated tendency for distraction, vagueness, and suggestibility. There is an obliviousness to factual detail and an inability to describe things with sharp definition and precision which contribute to an impression of naiveté, incredulity, and deficient intelligence. Ideas are not developed, but are seemingly pulled out of the air, or materialize as hunches, and are presented in their initial form as accomplished fact. The hysteric appears to be unable to work through any thought or problem according to traditional logic. It is suggested that the purpose of this mode of behavior and cognition is to deliberately prevent the individual from taking a look at himself and to shield him from an awareness of the underlying emptiness and uncertainty which he only vaguely feels. Such an individual, confronted with catastrophic environmental situations or physical difficulties, reacts in characteristic dramatic ways, often marked either by exhibitionism or indifference. The hysteric may not be able to summon the necessary attitudes for the remediation of problems. The hysteric may need the reassuring guidance of the physician. This is best done in a matter-of-fact manner suggesting certainty and allowing for the dramatic, though medically irrelevant, productions of the patient. These patients do not require precise and detailed descriptions of their illness. In fact, they may often become extremely uncomfortable when such descriptions are offered. The physician's plight may need to be diverted more at confronting the denial utilized by the patient in regard to his illness which may interfere with diagnostic procedures or therapy. This denial may require the ingenious efforts of the physician to convince the patient through processes that defy logical explanation.

## Impulsive

The impulsive style is one in which there is an impairment of normal feelings of deliberateness and intention. Individuals with this handicap seem to act on impulse, whim, or urge. Action is unplanned and instantaneous, abrupt, and discontinuous. It is as though there is a short circuit between stimulus, whether arising internally or externally, and response. Impulsive activity is not limited to the small and inconsequential acts of life but is involved in monumental and frequently catastrophic ones, such as robbing a bank. The incriminated individual may offer the seemingly shallow, but matter-of-fact, explanation, "I just felt like it," without any show of affect. It would seem on closer scrutiny, however, as if the act itself may be a way of handling an affect that is only dimly perceived, never documented. It would appear also that these persons have a low tolerance for frustration or tension. It may be hypothesized that these individuals lack a discriminatory perception of a range of emotions, but rather at the time of feeling a vague discomfort, strike out in a way often appearing antisocial. This hypothesis has led many to view the impulsive individual as lacking in development of super-ego or conscience; but on closer scrutiny, one is struck with the professed rigidity and conformity to the prevailing moral and social code, even in the face of contradictory behavior. This pattern is also reflected in the concrete and passive thinking that is manifested. Behavior is explained in terms of having been made to do the inappropriate act by the simple mechanism of projection; because an urge to do something has been felt, this is offered as the complete explanation for the act. An impulsive's concerns rarely extend beyond the immediate boundaries of his own existence. There appears to be either an absence of or intolerance for imagination or speculation. Thought is devalued and sacrificed for the physical act, in which there appears to be more compulsion than pleasure. Because of this, the impulsive appears to be lacking in his ability to have meaningful and empathic relationships with others. Other people are viewed in terms of their use or compliance in some immediate action at hand. The impulsive's inability to take distance from himself assures that reflectiveness and revision are not a part of his style. Individuals with impulsive disorders may become sociopaths, alcoholics, and drug addicts because of perceptual and cognitive styles that lead to indiscriminatory behavior and dependency on objects outside of themselves. When confronted by physical difficulties, both of these may become exaggerated in the face of rising anxiety and frustration. The physician cognizant of the predilection of his patient to such actions may allay some untoward, precipitous, and catastrophic behavior by attempting to anticipate the anxiety. This may be done simply by simple formulations of what the difficulty is, how it will be investigated and treated, and what the prognosis is. The physician may be able to prevent acting-out by matter-of-fact limit-setting in terms of his own or the hospital's authority. Long-term care may require frequent brief reinforcement of the terms of the initial contract between patient and physician.

## Depressive

A basic depressive life or neurotic style is characterized by reacting to internal or external events less with anxiety than depression and less with an active response, but rather one of withdrawal. It is a style marked by passivity, and one that is easily and readily vulnerable to environmental manipulation. While it contains characteristics to be found among the hysteric and impulsive styles, it is less ritualized, less structured, and in many ways more primitive. While many individuals may, in the face of insurmountable catastrophes, react by giving-up, the depressive is always so predisposed. The precipitating stimulus is frequently mild and sometimes merely imagined. A psychological and physical withdrawal immediately ensues. The psychological stance includes ideations of inadequacy and emptiness, sometimes proceeding to more aggressive self-condemnation. Expression is more often given to fears of being left, abandoned, or ignored, and to attitudes of helplessness or hopelessness. These individuals are inordinately dependent on external supplies coming from others in the environment and seem to have an omnipresent fear that these will be denied them for one reason or another, usually because they feel undeserving. Their whole life-style appears to be one of assuming an ever-present supply, and their behavior is a manipulative attempt to achieve this. Their behavior is marked by a passive-aggression that defies the environment to deny them of their just but undeserved due. Since they are always fearful that external resources will be withdrawn and that they will come face to face with their own emptiness, much of their cognitive style is aimed at achieving involved and symbiotic relationships with others. When there are not others around with whom to make these involvements, refuge against the internal feelings of displeasure may lead to dependence on drugs or alcohol. When there is a sense of total abandonment, the characteristic posture is one of helplessness; and when this is not effective in securing the attention and needs of others, hopelessness may ensue which defies help. The passivity of this state is not without aggressive manipulation, which is directed both at the self and others. The individual entrapped in this state is vulnerable both to his own destructive acts, as well as prey to those who would take advantage of him for their own purposes. It is more than likely that this state itself has correlative and analogous biological aspects that make the individual more vulnerable to the environment. At times of physical illness, the patient with this predilection gives up and becomes entirely dependent on the environment. He may do this, even while maintaining the semblance of independence through defiance. This calls for a reassuring, sympathetic, nurturing attitude on the part of the physician and nursing staff, who may also have to decide to what extent regression is to be allowed. The description presented here should not suggest that these individuals lack perception, or even great capability at times, when they are not faced with or experiencing the threat of diminished external supplies.

### Infantile

The infantile personality described by Ruesch[23] is mentioned here because it contains characteristics that have been mentioned for the preceding five. In this way, this style is more amorphous, and has resulted in less rigid, formalized, and consistent patterns of cognition and behavior. Ruesch identified an infantile personality as the core problem in psychosomatic medicine, with the following characteristics: (1) arrested or faulty social learning; (2) impaired self-expression channel through either direct physical action or organ expression; (3) persistence of childhood patterns of thinking and ideation; (4) dependency and passivity; (5) rigid and punitive conscience; (6) overextended ideals; and (7) absence of ability to integrate experience. Ruesch, less concerned with specificity factors, did not offer an explanation of why one organ system rather than another was chosen for the expression of conflict; rather, he outlined a therapeutic approach, rare in the history of psychosomatic medicine, for physicians working with patients having infantile or immature personalities which included: (1) reeducation through benevolent firmness; (2) instructing the patient as to the manipulative and implicit content of his complaint; (3) the reduction of long verbal productions to single words or sentences concerning problems; (4) the externalization of feelings and emotions as objectifications in their own right, rather than via organ expressions and complaints; (5) the acceptance of the patient himself as a psychologic and biologic entity distinct from others; and (6) the model of the physician as a consistent, accepting, available, and self-expressive person.

## Pharmacotherapy

In addition to the brief discussion of measures that is suggested above that the physician assumes in response to patients with specific characteristics, pharmacological agents may often serve as useful adjuncts in helping the individual adjust to the present emotional or physical problems for which he seeks assistance. The use of psychopharmacological agents in individuals with the various styles described above should be directed at the prevailing affect. Where anxiety appears to be the motivating force, then temporary use of short-to-intermediate-acting barbiturates in nonaddictive individuals, or phenothiazines in small amounts are suggested. Where depression appears as the predominant affect, the use of the tricyclic antidepressants may modulate the experience of the patient to the extent that psychotherapeutic intervention becomes more feasible. Some patients with both anxiety and depression will benefit from a combination of an antianxiety and an antidepressant medication.

## INTERVIEWING AND THERAPY

In this chapter, little distinction has been made between interviewing and therapy. Therapy here is addressed as the process of knowing the patient, obtaining the necessary information about him in order to address his needs by assessment and treatment. As in all patient-physician contacts, the development of an effective relationship is fundamental to this process. Within this relationship the process of therapy will ensue. There will be an exchange of information, an opportunity for reassurance and didactic instruction, the development of mutual empathy, and the permission to give expression to feeling, all fundamental to the therapeutic process. Within the course of this process over time, there will develop an opportunity for insight leading to a greater awareness and experience of self for both of the individuals involved.

## References

1. White K, Williams T, Greenberg B: The ecology of medical care. N Engl J Med 265-885–892, 1961
2. Mechanic D: The concept of illness behavior. J Chronic Dis 15:189–194, 1961
3. Zborowski M: Cultural components in response to pain. In Apple D (Ed.), Sociological Studies of Health and Sickness. New York, McGraw-Hill, 1960, pp 118–133
4. Olin HS, Hackett T: The denial of chest pain in 32 patients with acute myocardial infarction. JAMA 190:977–981, 1964
5. Kornfeld D, Zimberg S, Malm J: Psychiatric complications of open-heart surgery. N Eng J Med 273:287–292, 1965
6. Kimball CP: Intensive Care Unit (ICU). In Arieti S (Ed.), American Handbook of Psychiatry, IV, 2nd Ed. New York, Basic Books, 1976
7. Engel GL, Romano J: Delirium, a syndrome of cerebral insufficiency. J Chronic Dis 9:260–277, 1959
8. Ludwig A: Altered States of Consciousness. Arch Gen Psychiat 15:225–234, 1966.

9. Lipowski ZJ: Physical illness, the individual and the coping process. Psychiatry Med 1:91–102, 1970

10. Quinlan D, Kimball C, Osborne F, Woodward B: The experience of cardiac surgery. V. Psychother Psychosom 22:310–319, 1973

11. Kimball CP: Delirium. In Conn HF (Ed.), Current Therapy 1974. Philadelphia, WB Saunders Co, 1974, pp 833–835

12. McGhie A, Chapman J: Disorders of attention and perception in early schizophrenia. Br J Med Psychol 34:103–116, 1961

13. Cassem NH, Hackett TP: Psychiatric consultation in a coronary care unit. Ann Intern Med 75:9–14, 1971

14. Kimball CP: Clinical case method in teaching comprehensive approaches to illness behavior. Psychosom Med 37:454–467, 1975

15. Bilodeau CB, Hackett TP: Issues raised in a group setting by patients recovering from myocardial infarction. Am J Psychiatry 128:105–110, 1971

16. Kimball CP: Psychological responses to the experience of open heart surgery. I. Am J Psychiatry 125:348–359, 1969

17. Lindemann E: Symptomatology and management of acute grief. Am J Psychiatry 101:141–148, 1944

18. Engel GL, Schmale A: Psychoanalytic theory of somatic disorder: conversion, specificity and the disease-onset situation. J Am Psychoanal Assoc 15:344–365, 1967.

19. Kimball CP: Psychosomatic theories and their contribution to chronic illness. In Usden G (ed.): Psychiatric Medicine. New York, Brunner/Mazel, 1977, pp 259–333

20. Kimball CP: Conceptual developments in psychosomatic medicine: 1939–1969. Ann Intern Med 73:307–316, 1970

21. Kahana RJ, Bibring GL: Personality types in medical management. In Zinberg N (Ed.), Psychiatry and Medical Practice in a General Hospital. New York, International University Press, 1964, pp 108–123

22. Shapiro D: Neurotic Styles. New York, Basic Books, 1965

23. Ruesch J: The infantile personality: the core problem of psychosomatic medicine. Psychosom Med 10:134–144, 1948

24. Nemiah J, Sifneos P: Affect and fantasy in patients with psychosomatic disorders. In Hill OW (Ed.), Modern Trends in Psychosomatic Medicine, II. London, Butterworths, 1970, pp 26–34

25. Marty P, de'Uzan M: La "pensée opératoire." Rev Fr Psychanal 27:(Suppl.) 1345, 1963

26. Kimball CP: Techniques of interviewing. III: the patient's personality and the interview process. Med Insight 4:26–40, 1972

Robert I. Steinmuller

# 3
# Psychotherapeutic Treatment Planning for the Medically Ill

## INTRODUCTION[1-7]

Psychosomatic medicine was nourished, and flourished, under the aegis of psychoanalysis. In the post-World War II decades, consultation liaison services developed in general hospitals, operating primarily in a patient-centered psychodynamic frame of reference. Sophisticated internists and other non-psychiatric physicians, influenced by the teaching of the psychosomaticist, and often by their own personal experiences in psychoanalysis, began referring some of their patients for psychiatric consultation. Often the explicit, or implicit, request was not for assistance in their own management of the patient, but rather for the psychiatrist to evaluate the patient for "therapy." The psychiatrists, in the full bloom of their own optimistic enthusiasm were delighted to comply. For the most part, the therapy that was offered was either psychoanalysis or a form of psychoanalytically oriented intensive psychotherapy. The results paralleled those in general psychiatry. In many ways, psychoanalytic methods were more powerful as investigative tools than as therapies. A vast body of valuable information was accumulated regarding the psychodynamics of physical illness, the nuances of the doctor-patient relationship, and the relationship of personality type, intrapsychic conflict, ego mechanisms of defense and adaptation, and life stress, to the predisposition, precipitation, maintenance, or alleviation of somatic illness. Many patients were clinically improved, some dramatically. The inflated expectations of wholesale "cures" of patients were not realized however,—even for the "holy seven" diseases stamped with the imprimatur of "psychosomatic disorders." Psychosomatic medicine, like psychoanalysis, had oversold itself.

Workers in the field went back to the drawing board and spawned the present era of vigorous, rigorous, experimental, controlled research into the mechanisms

35

entailed in psychophysiological interrelationships;[7] eschewing for the while grand attempts at synthesizing a comprehensive psychobiological theory of illness and health. In an ironic perversion of the original credo of a holistic comprehensive view of all diseases, psychosomatic medicine became increasingly viewed as a new specialty, of dubious legitimacy, concerned with a small group of "Psychosomatic Diseases" (implicitly distinguished from the "real" diseases). This, plus the therapeutic disillusionment, culminated in a rapid decline in the status enjoyed by the field. Anxious to avoid the latterly acquired narrow connotations of the psychosomatic concept, psychiatrists in the general hospitals, committed to a comprehensive bio-psycho-social approach to all medically ill patients, embraced the rubric of "Consultation-Liaison Psychiatry" for their clinical and teaching activities, viewing psychosomatic medicine as their "basic science."[8-14]

Meanwhile, several "revolutions" were occurring in psychiatry proper: psycho-pharmacology, with its explosive impact on practice and theory, leading to a rebirth of biological psychiatry; social and community psychiatry, with its emphasis on an ecological viewpoint, the importance of social support systems, crisis theory and crisis intervention, and group and family therapy approaches; behavioral psychology, with its claims to rapid, specific, and effective therapy, as well as a radically different way of understanding normal and pathological behavior; and humanistic-existential approaches emphasizing the natural healing and self-regulatory forces within the human organism, merging inperceptibly into the mystical antiintellectual, antiprofessional fads and cults currently in vogue. All of these currents have influenced the approach of the liaison psychiatrist, who must deal with all levels of behavior from molecules to social systems.

The bewildering plethora of therapies currently available renders the job of formulating intervention strategies that much more complex, however. It is no longer enough to assess the suitability of the patient for psychoanalytic therapy. Declining to throw the baby out with the bath water, most liaison psychiatrists retain a fundamentally psychodynamic point of view, recognizing the crucial significance of unconscious mental processes; of intrapsychic conflict and modes of defense and adaptation; of symbolic meaning; and of historic determinism. Nonetheless, their approach and treatment planning must be eclectic.

The term "eclectic" has acquired pejorative connotations—justified if it is taken to mean either a mindless sequential embracing of every new therapeutic fad or an unthinking admixture of bits and pieces of disparate approaches without regard to whether they are complementary or contradictory, and without any rational basis for selection or timing. Few proudly claim to be eclectic, preferring euphemisms such as "pluralistic." Nonetheless, whatever the name, some attempt must be made to order and integrate these viewpoints and therapies so that rational treatment planning can take place.

Rational treatment planning would presume a comprehensive theory of the psychosocial aspects of somatic illness. At present, there is no one universally applicable model, although a psychodynamic, ego psychological, adaptational approach seems most useful. One such comprehensive theory has been adumbrated recently by Lipowski.[15-18] Although not a psychosocial theory in itself, General Systems Theory provides another useful approach to organizing the multiplicity of levels of exploratory models; and has been applied to the consultation-liaison setting by Miller.[19, 20] Working from these formulations, we can begin to rationally devise a flexible and eclectic strategy for treatment planning.

## FORMULATION OF THE TREATMENT STRATEGY

The therapeutic strategy depends on the nature of the problem, the nature of the patient, and the nature of the therapist.

The formulation of the problem will both influence and be influenced by the treatment strategies available to the practitioner. Unfortunately, all too often the therapist's usual mode of conceptualization and treatment will dictate his understanding of the problem, and the patient will be deemed either suitable or unsuitable for the treatment the therapist is prepared to offer, rather than his assessing what therapeutic approach is most suitable for the given patient, making an appropriate referral if necessary. Therefore, a successful outcome depends strongly on the adequacy of the consultative process and a precise formulation of the nature of the problem. Consultations with medically ill patients are frequently unusually difficult situations, especially for the psychiatrist not experienced in liaison-consultation work.[21-24] Medically ill patients rarely initiate a psychiatric consultation themselves. Generally, they are poorly prepared for the consultation by the referring physician and may (sometimes correctly) interpret it as rejection and abandonment by their physician. The validity of the patients' complaints may be called into question and the patients' need to vindicate themselves from the tainted labels of "crock," "malingerer," "hypochondriac," etc, frequently interferes with an open acknowledgement of emotional conflict, stressful life situations, or other psychological data which they fear will be "self-incriminating." The consultant is placed in the difficult position of having to provide some education and explanation before a comprehensive understanding of the patient is achieved in order to obtain the very data on which such an understanding hinges, running the risk of thereby skewing and contaminating the data.

MacKinnon and Michels[25] and Kimball[26] have reviewed the techniques of interviewing in such situations. The reduction of the patient's defensiveness, development of rapport and trust, and establishment of what might be called a "consultative alliance" may well require an extended series of interviews. The therapist must eschew reductionistic, either-or, dichotomous thinking in regard to both diagnosis and therapy. The maintenance and communication of an open-ended, multicausal, comprehensive approach facilitates a more open acknowledgement of psychosocial difficulties by the patient, and a greater willingness to accept therapeutic recommendations. In line with the multifactorial, nonlinear model of somato-psycho-somatic interrelationships, the therapeutic approach itself can and should be multimodal in most cases. It should be underscored that it is not necessary to be able to reverse or neutralize the primary etiological factor in a disorder in order to ameliorate the clinical illness. An example in the somatic realm is the use of diuretics in the treatment of congestive heart failure. What is needed is an alteration in the net balance of forces that will facilitate the restoration of physical and/or psychological homeostasis. Modification of any component of a system will have effects on all other components of the system. This accounts for the sometimes dramatically powerful effects of rather nonspecific therapeutic interventions despite their derogation by proponents of various "schools" of therapy.[27, 28] It is a mistake to consider the different therapies in molar fashion. Ideally, the consultant should not decide to send the patient to a behaviorist or psychoanalyst or family therapist; rather he should be considering the component processes of the various therapies that may be integrated into a meaningful "treatment package" designed to fit into the analysis of the psychopathological processes. In most instances, there is more than one way of "skinning the cat," and little or no empirical data to indicate the superiority of one approach over the other.[29] The critical decision will be dictated by various factors related to the patient, the therapist, and their environments.

## TREATMENT OF STRESS-RELATED "PSYCHOSOMATIC" DISORDERS

Various kinds of psychotherapeutic interventions have been shown to aid patients with stress-related disorders: psychoanalysis, behavior therapy, group therapy.[29-31] Psychophysiological mediating mechanisms for most of these disorders are not established at present time, but heightened psychophysiologic arousal with activation of central nervous system (CNS), autonomic, and endocrine pathways, and alteration in the immune systems, is probably the trigger for altered visceral function, which, together with other necessary factors (i.e., allergies, virus) leads to clinical activation of disease.[1] A variety of approaches may be used singly or together to restore psychological and physiological homeostasis.

In some patients a repetitive psychodynamic conflict-constellation can be identified as precipitating episodes of illness which may or may not be identical with the formulations proposed as specific by the Alexander group in Chicago.[31a] It would seem in such instances that insight-oriented psychotherapy or psychoanalysis would be the treatment of choice. This is not always the case. The presence of neurotic conflict is not a sufficient indicator of good prognosis for psychoanalytic therapy. There is a vast literature on the indicators of suitability for psychoanalysis. Dewald has reviewed those factors prognostic of good outcome with psychoanalytic psychotherapy: general ego strength, object relationships, motivation, psychological-mindedness, ego defensive organization and style, intelligence, tolerance of anxiety and frustration, alloplastic vs autoplastic ratio, and others, including the nature of the illness, reality factors, and therapist factors.[32]

For those patients who meet these requirements, and in whom specific unconscious conflicts are of central importance, psychoanalysis or psychoanalytically oriented therapy are the treatments of choice.[33]

The French psychoanalysts Marty and de M'uzan, however, have described a specific cognitive style in psychosomatic patients which they labeled "pensee operatoire."[34] This refers to a literal, concrete, externally oriented, rather rigid and restricted form of thinking, bound to the factual minutiae of the "real world." Nemiah and Sifneos have extended these observations and cite a lack of representation of affect and fantasy and a poverty of inner mental life in striking contrast to that of the classical psychoneurotic patient, even after periods of psychoanalytic treatment. They postulate that this "alexithymia" is not the result of ego defenses such as repression, denial, and isolation, but has a neurophysiologic basis, and is therefore not amenable to correction by analytic means. Furthermore, they propose that this inability to interpose a level of fantasy and psychic elaboration may be responsible for the somatic hyperreactivity of these patients to life stress.[35, 36] Patients who descriptively fall into the alexithymia category present formidable difficulties in psychoanalytic treatment, regardless of the correctness of the explanatory concepts. It is this writer's experience that some such patients, after lengthy preparatory psychotherapy, can "learn" to become analytic patients, and subsequently benefit from analytic treatment; however, for many, treatment becomes a frustrating, difficult, unsatisfactory process with results disappointing to patient and therapist alike. Fortunately, many patients with psychosomatic illness are not alexithymic, and are analyzable as attested to in the case reports of analysts such as Schur[37] and Sperling.[37a] For those who are not analyzable, and/or where nonspecific external life stresses are the major problem, other forms of therapeutic intervention are suitable.

NONSPECIFIC SUPPORTIVE MEASURES

All psychotherapies offer (or should offer) an emotionally charged relationship with an expert who provides competence, caring, concern, empathy, compassion, confidentiality, and the opportunity for ventilation, clarification, and reassurance. Such "relationship therapy" mobilizes and gratifies strong transference feelings, and frequently suffices to restore psychic equilibrium with physiological improvement.[27] Hospitalization on a medical ward may intensify these beneficial effects and lead to the rapid disappearance of symptoms. Such "transference cures" are not to be derided or lightly dismissed. They are not necessarily transient and do not require intensive involvement with the therapist. Frequently, brief and widely spaced sessions, phone contacts, even postcards, suffice to maintain the power of the relationship for years and across continents.[38]

Since issues of separation and object-loss seem, in a nonspecific way, to be important factors in the onset of illness,[39, 40] the provision of a substitute relationship can be seen to have potent compensatory benefits. The benefits of the relationship accrue to patients in all forms of therapy, and may outweigh the contributions of more specific component processes, contributing to the difficulty in establishing the superiority of one form of psychotherapy over another. This therapeutic use of the relationship should not only, or always, be left to the psychotherapist. Very valuable gains can be made by educating the primary physician in the judicious use of the drug "Doctor."[41, 42]

FAMILY THERAPY

When psychophysiological symptoms are manifest in the context of family conflict or turmoil, especially in children or adolescents, family therapy may be the treatment of choice.[43-46] Minuchin and co-workers have developed an open systems model that describes three necessary, but not sufficient, conditions for the development of severe psychosomatic problems in children: (1) a specific type of family organization that encourages somatization; (2) involvement of the child in parental conflict; and (3) physiological vulnerability. Children's psychosomatic symptoms are seen as not only responses to stress within the family, but also importantly, as playing a major role in maintaining family homeostasis. Therapy then must be directed at not only changing family processes that trigger symptoms, but also the reinforcement the symptoms receive by allowing the child to be an "avoidance circuit" as the "symptom bearer" of the family. The model applies as well to many situations in which an adult member of the family is the identified patient.[47, 48]

CONJOINT MARITAL THERAPY AND/OR SEX THERAPY

When marital and/or sexual difficulties lie behind the presentation of psychosomatic symptoms, conjoint marital therapy and/or sex therapy may be the treatment of choice; particularly in cases of dyspareunia, chronic pelvic pain, recurrent sterile "cystitis," nonspecific vaginitis, some cases of back pain and headache, psychogenic impotence, and vaginismus.[49, 50]

OTHER "ACTIVE INGREDIENTS"

Psychophysiological symptoms may appear at times of developmental or other transitional life crises such as marriage, childbearing, career change, and geographic relocation. Although vulnerability to such crises may be enhanced by residues of earlier unresolved, unconscious conflicts, nonetheless an active reality-oriented, problem-solving counseling approach in a time-limited frame may suffice. In other situations, where mobilization and some resolution of the underlying neurotic conflict is advisable, the type of time-limited, insight-oriented brief therapy described by Sifneos, Castelnouvo-Tedesco, Levin and Ornstein and others is appropriate.[51-59] Here too, features pertaining to the patient's personality structure, rather than the type of symptom or type of precipitating situation, would determine which strategy to adopt.

BEHAVIORAL APPROACHES

If it is ascertained that the symptoms reflect inadequate coping with difficult work, family, and social situations due to behavioral deficits rather than intrapsychic conflict, a variety of behavioral modification techniques may be utilized. These include assertion training and social skills training, and use procedures such as behavioral rehearsal and role-playing, role reversal, coaching, modeling, video feedback, behavioral homework assignments, etc. Such procedures are conducted advantageously in a group format.[60-63] Relaxation and desensitization procedures may be necessary if anxiety interferes with the learning or implementation of the relevant behavior in the real-life situation.

SELF-MANAGEMENT TECHNIQUES

Finally, regardless of the underlying causes, a variety of stress-management techniques may be implemented to deal directly with stress and/or to buffer or neutralize its physiological consequences. Such techniques include the "stress inoculation" techniques of Meichenbaum,[64] the "anxiety management techniques" of Suinn and Richardson,[63, 66] and a variety of relaxation techniques, including progressive relaxation, autogenic training, hypnosis, transcendental meditation, Benson's "relaxation response",[67, 68] biofeedback training, and combinations such as autogenic feedback training.[69]

In addition to their use as general relaxation methods, biofeedback techniques can be utilized more specifically for the control of psychophysiological symptoms such as palpitations, arrhythmias, hypertension, vascular headaches, neuromuscular symptoms, etc. There is doubt as to the generalizability and transferability of the learned effects from the treatment situations into the 24-hour real-life-space of the patient, however, and such methods cannot at the present time be viewed as substitutes for standard medical management of hypertension and cardiac arrhythmias, but rather as an adjunct.[70-77]

These techniques are particularly useful for certain patients otherwise extremely resistant to psychotherapeutic approaches. Their physiological emphasis fits in with the patient's defensive use of denial, and can support such defenses when this is indicated. (When such defensive distortions are undesirable they can be counteracted by appropriate interpretations and clarification.) Furthermore, they do not require a capacity for introspection, psychological mindedness, or the verbal communication of inner mental life. Presenting them as self-management, self-control, and self-regulatory techniques, reduces the threats of passivity, dependence, and loss of autonomy that some patients fear in psychothearapy.

PSYCHOPHARMACOLOGICAL APPROACHES[78-83]

Although anxiety is presumed to be a central aspect of these disorders, neither major nor minor tranquilizers have been reliably shown to be useful in their management, and the latter are liable to abuse and habituation. When patients are confronted with self-limited short-term crises, brief, limited courses of benzodiazepines may be helpful, but chronic administration should be avoided. Masked depression and depressive equivalents will be discussed later. If careful scrutiny suggests that the psychophysiological disorder represents such a depressive equivalent (especially likely in headaches, other pain syndromes, and some cases of ulcerative colitis, asthma, and dermatoses) then tricyclic antidepressants may be an important component of the treatment program.

My intent is not to present seven alternative treatment strategies, but rather a variety of tactics which may be systematically combined and implemented in accordance with a psychodynamic assessment of the relative contribution of the various pathogenic vectors and the relevant parameters of the patient's intrapsychic and interpersonal resources and difficulties. An eclectic, active, flexible, psychotherapeutic approach ensues,[84] in which, for example, the patient may be seen individually one or more times per week, and together with his or her spouse once a week. A positive transference is preserved and usually uninterpreted, with early and vigorous interpretations made of negative transferences. The therapy sessions may include superficial and inexact interpretation of preconscious derivatives of relevant conflict material, as well as variable admixtures of supportive, educative, and behavioral techniques as described below. In addition, the patient may be directed to practice a relaxation technique on a daily basis at home. A given therapist may not be competent in all these techniques, and may selectively refer the patient for some aspects of the treatment. In such cases, close communication and cooperation between the therapists is required, as is true of the relationship with the primary medical practitioner.

## Psychopathological Reactions To Physical Illness

The encyclopedic reviews of Lipowski deserve close, sustained, and repeated reading for a thorough grasp of the complicated interrelation of psychological, biological, and social factors. I will review here selected aspects of Lipowski's multifactorial schema pertinent to the formulation of rational therapeutic strategies.[15-18]

It must be stated at the outset that the arbitrary contraposition, adopted here for ease of presentation, of physical illness precipitated or aggravated by psychosocial stress versus psychopathology precipitated or aggravated by physical illness, does violence to the complexity of a holistic nonlinear model of human illness and health.[85-92] Not only do psychosocial factors contribute to the onset of disease; bodily injury or illness itself constitutes a major source of psychological stress, which in turn may influence the course and outcome of the illness by impairing the host's capacity to cope with it physiologically and psychologically. Regardless of its etiology, physical illness may (1) make manifest a latent psychiatric disorder; (2) aggravate a preexisting syndrome; or (3) give rise to psychopathology denovo.[93] The following pathogenetic mechanisms may be implicated:

1. Direct impairment of brain functioning
2. The disturbing conscious or unconscious personal meaning of the illness
3. Impairment of one's capacity to cope with needs, secure valued gratifications, and defend against inner conflicts

4. Aggravated unresolved intrapsychic conflicts
5. Impaired performance of sexual, social, and economic roles, and thus, weakened self-esteem, identity, and sense of competence and security
6. Altered internal and external sensory inputs and feedback
7. Changed body image
8. Disrupted sleep-wake cycle

These are all moderated by other variables such as psychological predispositions of the patient, his emotional state prior to the onset of illness, the availability of social supports, timely therapy, and features of the physical environment.

Aside from direct impairment of cerebral functioning, the most important consideration is the subjective meaning for the patient of illness-related information. Lipowski[18] describes three broad categories of such meanings: (1) threat; (2) loss; and (3) gain or relief. In some instances, there is a fourth meaning, of "insignificance." The crucial point is how the type of illness and somatic dysfunction fits with the patient's selective vulnerability to its personal meaning for him.

Body parts and functions achieve special personal significance if they play one or more functions in the psychic economy:

1. To provide gratification, pleasure, pride, self-esteem, competence
2. To help maintain satisfying object-relations and effective coping with the environment
3. To help resolve or avoid intrapsychic conflict and painful affects
4. To enhance self-concept, body image, and personal, sexual identity
5. To enable maintenance of sexual, social, and occupational roles
6. To have unconscious symbolic significance of great value

Thus physical illness may disrupt psychological equilibrium if it (1) means threat or loss; (2) interferes with major sources of gratification; or (3) intensifies intrapsychic conflict by facilitating the emergence of repudiated wishes, by weakening ego controls, or by signifying punishment for real or neurotic guilt. A different kind of pathological equilibrium may become established when the illness signifies a gain or relief, and the disability or symptoms have become an essential part of the person's self-image or transactions with his environment. Assessment of the relative contribution of each of these mechanisms, as well as the previously mentioned modifiers, offers an opportunity for planning specific therapeutic strategies and tactics along a variety of dimensions.

The main psychopathological reactions observed are depression, anxiety reactions, conversion reactions, psychotic reactions, and personality disorders. Each of these will be discussed in terms of therapeutic planning.

DEPRESSION

For many, physical illness has the personal meaning of punishment, weakness, or damage. It always means the loss of one's concept of the self as a healthy, whole human being. There are losses of bodily parts, functions, accustomed roles, sources of gratification, and valued modes of coping and adaptation; frequently loss of independence, autonomy, and economic status and security. In addition to these narcissistic injuries, there may be real or threatened object-loss. There may also be identification with ambivalently regarded lost objects, envy (of well persons), guilt, shame, inferiority feelings, resentment, and anger, directed both outwardly and inwardly. Add to this the common ingredients of pain, fatigue, lassitude, weakness, poor appetite, and feelings of helplessness, hopelessness, and abandonment; and it is surprising that every chronically ill person is not depressed. In fact, depression of various types is exceedingly common in chronic illness and plays a major role in the associated morbidity, disability, and invalidism.[94]

A "healthy" grief reaction is appropriate in such circumstances. All too often, however, fairly severe depressive reactions are either not taken note of or are dismissed as "natural and inevitable, given the situation."[95, 96] It is a mistake to assume that a patient's emotional reaction is based on a realistic appraisal of the clinical situation, or that they are reacting to the elements of the situation which seem most obviously distressful to the observer. Patient's fantasies are frequently even worse than the reality, and there usually are many unrealistic and distorted fears and expectations which can be clarified and ameliorated if only one takes the trouble to first find out what is bothering the patient. The personal, distressing significance of the illness may be idiosyncratic and revolve around a rather peripheral, superficial, or remediable aspect of the total situation, which is *not* hopeless, and which can provide a useful focus for therapeutic activity counteracting the felt helplessness of both patient and physician.[97] One frequent source of depression is the emotional abandonment of the patient by the physician who feels impotent to "cure" the disease. In such situations, active intervention is indicated to help remind the physician that, while he can't always cure, he can always care for the patients, and that his ongoing support and relationship are valid and potent therapeutic activities.

Zealous and active medical therapeutic involvement in the care and treatment of associated "minor disorders"; attention to pain relief; palliation of other discomforts, concern over nourishment, sleep and bowel habits; all help maintain the patient's hope, morale, and self-esteem. When the total reality-picture is very dismal—even apparently trivial—superficial gains loom large and yield surprisingly high dividends.

So the first step in both diagnosis and treatment of depression in medically ill patients involves an unhurried, patient exploration of the patient's personal, subjective appraisal of the meaning and portent of his illness, as well as an assessment of his relationship with his primary physician, followed by repeated doses of clear, unambiguous, realistic information about the illness, and reassurance that the physician will continue to actively care for him regardless of the possibility of definitive cure. These "simple" measures are frequently overlooked, and the patient is instead referred for psychotherapy (if he isn't simply left alone), or even worse, started on a course of antidepressant medication (usually in inadequate and inappropriate doses, to boot).

The chronically ill or disabled person may also be aware of real or impending object-loss within his family system. Caring for the ill patient may be an immense burden, taxing the resources of the spouse or parent to the limit. There may be covert (or even overt) messages that everyone would be better off if the patient were dead or gone, adding guilt to the feelings of abandonment. In these situations, the most strategic deployment of therapeutic resources might be to support the support system. Provision of homemakers, visiting nurse service; obtaining help from other family members, and similar environmental manipulations, should be tried before undertaking more formal psychotherapeutic intervention. When it is clear that there is serious marital or family pathology, perhaps preceding the illness, and now exacerbated by it; or when the spouse has a neurotic need to maintain the patient in a passive, helpless role; then marital or family therapy is indicated.[45] Similarly, when sexual difficulties are both contributing to and being exacerbated by depression, sexual counseling or sex therapy should be implemented.[49, 50] Even in situations with organic impairments such as diabetes, it is not infrequent to find a large psychological component contributing importantly to the overall difficulty. When the sexual dysfunction is irreversible, counseling can often still help the couple achieve a mutually pleasurable erotic relationship, thus maintaining self-esteem and sexual identity as well as libidinal gratification of the patient.

Patient self-help peer groups such as Ostomy Clubs, Mended Heart Clubs, National Association of Patients on Hemodialysis and Transplantation (NAPHT), and Reach for Recovery, are immensely useful. They provide role models of other patients with the same illness who lead active, competent, gratifying lives. Through their meetings and newsletters they provide information on coping techniques, job and recreational opportunities, "tricks of the trade" that make life easier or more comfortable, and information about the illness. More formal groups, often led by nurses or social workers, along supportive and educational lines, are frequently useful. These are sometimes run as couples-groups involving the spouse.[98-101]

It is important to seek out and capitalize on the patients' remaining assets, competencies, and adaptive capacities. Vocational rehabilitation with retraining if necessary, is more valuable than disability retirement for most patients, psychologically as well as financially. Favored social and recreational activities should be resumed if possible, or suitable substitutes sought. Exercise programs, such as jogging (and even marathon running for selected patients) have proved useful in the rehabilitation of cardiac patients; helping to maintain their sense of physical vitality, masculine identity, and self-esteem, as well as providing physiological benefits.[102-106]

Patients with myocardial infarction exemplify many of the above points. Hackett and Cassem have demonstrated that after an initial period of anxiety, most such patients go through a depressed phase.[107] The heart has powerful emotional significance—representing life itself, strength, courage, manliness, love, emotionality, and other valued qualities. Men in particular after a heart attack frequently feel "all washed up," "no longer a man." Afraid he will no longer be able to "pull his weight," both literally and figuratively, at work, at home, and in bed; he sustains an enormous sense of damage, vulnerability, and fragility, with concomitant narcissistic mortification and loss of self-esteem, disturbance in his body concept, and impairment in his sense of masculinity. All too often he receives vague, ambiguous, and inconsistent messages from his doctor regarding work, recreation, and sexual activity. Such statements as "take it easy" and "use moderation" lend themselves to subjective interpretations by the patient. Sometimes, sweeping injunctions to "give up working," "move," or make similar wholesale changes in the patient's life are arbitrarily and capriciously made without real regard for either the patient's actual functional capacities and the actual demands of his job, or the devastating and deleterious impact such changes would have on the patient and his family's overall adaptation and functioning. Frequently the depression hits after returning home from the hospital, when the patient, suddenly aware of massive weakness (really due to deconditioning rather than cardiac insufficiency) erroneously concludes he has been severely and permanently damaged. An anxious spouse's overprotectiveness and infantilization may also contribute to the overall picture. In this context appropriate interventions include optimistically toned educational programs, individually and in group, as to the nature of coronary artery disease, the probability of good functional recovery, the possibilities of active preventive measures, and a realistic timetable for resumption of work, sex, and recreational activities. The spouse should be incorporated into these programs. Referral to a cardiac rehabilitation unit is useful in complicated cases. Stress testing allows for accurate estimation of work capacity which can be matched with the known energy costs of most occupational and recreational activities, enabling the physician to give the patient "scientific," objective, concrete, and rather precise guidelines as to his present and potential capabilities. Exercise programs such as running, swimming, or cycling, aside from contributing to a reduction of coronary risk factors, have potent antidepressant benefits as well, for reasons alluded to above. Couples groups, and "Mended Hearts Clubs" provide useful support.[100] The majority of depressed patients will respond well to an active, directive, reality-oriented therapy incorporating some or all of the above components.[103]

There are two groups of patients for whom further psychiatric intervention is necessary. Some patients will have features of an "endogenomorphic" type of depression. These include the classic vegetative signs of appetite, sleep, and bowel disturbances; diurnal mood variations; loss of all pleasure, gratifications, and interests; as well as a lack of responsiveness to ordinary reassurances or gratifying inputs from the environment. In such cases antidepressant medication should be used in adequate doses for an adequate period of time. The more the clinical picture approaches that of the classic endogenous type, especially with a positive family history or previous history of affective episodes, the more likely there will be beneficial response to the medication. Even in those cases which are not typical (and therefore less likely to respond), however, if the depression is not ameliorated by other means, a therapeutic trial is indicated. The second group consists of patients in whom unresolved intrapsychic neurotic conflicts regarding passivity, dependency, power, castration, guilt, or death have been mobilized and activated by the illness, but where the neurotic process more than the external reality maintains and prolongs the depression. These patients require individual psychotherapy. If they meet the requirements cited earlier, they may be accessible to a psychoanalytic long- or short-term therapy, which would be the treatment of choice.

For patients more in the alexithymic mode, a preferred approach would be cognitive therapy as described by Beck and Mahoney.[109, 110] Even in these patients, however, the use of psychotropic drugs and/or exploratory psychotherapy must supplement, not replace, the reality interventions and environmental manipulations described above. The grave risk is of therapist and patient solipsistically ignoring the ineluctable and pervasive external reality of the physical illness and the patient's relationship with his health care, family, and occupational environments. Study of patients who do not become or remain depressed usually reveals: (1) an ongoing relationship with a physician who remains therapeutically engaged with the patient; (2) object-relations—a continuing social support system, usually the family; and (3) maintenance of valued roles or substitution of some new sources of gratification and esteem. The therapeutic strategy should incorporate tactics designed to achieve each of those three goals whenever possible. The importance of the primary physician's communication with patient and family cannot be overstressed.

Certain illnesses seem to lead to depression or depression-like syndromes in a more direct way. Depression may accompany, or even be a presenting symptom, in retroperitoneal carcinomas, certain viral infections, liver disease—especially hepatitis, infectious mononucleosis, and endocrine disorders such as hypo- or hyper-thyroidism, hyperparathyroidism, or other hypercalcemic states.[111] Telling the patient that this is a known, expectable reaction, based on physiological causes, and usually either correctable or self-limited, allows him to deal with the situation adequately and avoids secondary vicious feedback cycles. It is not clear whether antidepressant medication is of any value in these instances. Primary therapeutic attention should be directed at the underlying cause.

Medication, including reserpine, aldomet, adrenal steroids, and oral contraceptives, may induce depressive reactions. Discontinuation or substitution when possible usually alleviates the problem. With reserpine, however, certain individuals (perhaps with genetic predisposition to primary affective disorders) develop endogenomorphic depressions which persist after the reserpine is discontinued and require treatment with antidepressant medication.

In considering the relationship of depression to somatic illness, the concepts of masked depression and depressive equivalents should be mentioned. Certain patients display the behavioral, psychomotor, cognitive, and somatic components of the depression syndrome without acknowledging a depressed mood; or they attribute whatever depressed mood they are aware of to somatic symptoms. In addition to the usual vegetative, depressive symptoms, they frequently have other poorly defined somatic complaints. They suffer intensely, and complain of pain (headaches, backaches, pelvic and/or abdominal pains, or "it hurts all over doctor"). Hypochondriacal concerns are frequent. Some of these patients can be brought to an awareness of their underlying depression and deal with it in a psychotherapeutic setting.[112-114] For many others, the defenses of somatization, denial, and displacement are unbreachable, but they frequently respond impressively to tricyclic antidepressants.[115]

It is essential that the physician pick up on the depressive thinking, vegetative signs, nonverbal cues, and other indicators of depression. Here again it is useful to avoid arguments with the patient regarding chicken and egg sequences. Most patients will accept that depression could develop in a setting of physical suffering and thereby make them feel even worse, and that treatment of their depression could prove helpful.

A cautionary note to the physician: as indicated above, some of these patients *will* turn out to have serious physical illness if followed. Don't think dichotomously!

Pain syndromes will be discussed further below.

ANXIETY REACTIONS

Fear, like pain, is a necessary and useful aspect of mental life, possessing the highest adaptive value in survival of the organism. Both are signal affects warning of the threat of damage to the physical or psychological integrity of the organism. In anticipation of threatening situations such as impending hospitalization or surgery, an optimal degree of anxiety mobilizes coping and adaptive techniques such as increased vigilance, information-seeking, anticipatory rehearsal in fantasy, etc, and leads to greater mastery of the psychological stress than where no anticipatory anxiety existed.[116] Persistent, excessive, displaced, or free-floating anxiety, however, is maladaptive; may be disorganizing; can lead to more functional disability and invalidism than the somatic illness itself; and can even be life-threatening (as for the patient with acute myocardial infarction). Here again, the importance of adequate and repeated communication of information and reassurance by the physician cannot be overemphasized. Illness or injury poses threats of all the losses discussed in the section on depression. Usually, many of the fears are unrealistic and exaggerated. Pat reassurances ("don't worry everything is alright") frequently fail to reassure, however. The provision of concrete information, as unambiguously as possible, in plain language understandable to the patient (this may require an interpreter in some cases), accompanied by simple drawings and diagrams, is of inestimable help. No matter how grim the reality, it is usually easier to deal with than vague or florid fantasies. It should not be assumed that even well-educated patients have an accurate understanding of anatomical relations, pathological processes, and diagnostic and therapeutic procedures. Providing realistic expectations and helping patients anticipate predictable difficulties, (e.g., telling a child the injection will hurt) leads to better coping, less anxiety, and a more trusting doctor-patient relationship. Even telling patients that their anxious and depressive reactions are commonplace, expectable, and understandable, is reassuring ("You mean everyone feels that way?").[117-121]

Anxiety in the hospital setting frequently has less to do with the illness itself than with separation, enforced passivity, being stripped of one's usual roles and identity, not being in control of one's life, not knowing what to expect, exposure to strange equipment, jargon, bedside rounds, etc. The appropriate environmental manipulations are obvious but not always implementable by the psychiatric consultant.[122]

The provision of realistic information fosters intellectual mastery and active coping, and is a keystone to the management of anxious reactions to illness.[108, 123-131] The role of the primary physicians is paramount. Patient-education, in group or individual format, by nurses, health educators, and dietitions, is immensely valuable, however, as is the excellent reading material provided for patients by associations and foundations in the fields of heart disease, diabetes, hemophilia, renal and lung disease, cancer, etc. Biblio-therapy with carefully chosen material is very useful. Anxious patients usually can't clearly hear and remember what the doctor said, but will return again and again to the pamphlet he gave them. (Of course, at a deeper level the pamphlet can serve as a transitional object, and the giving represents a transference gratification.) When the anxiety is severely disorganizing, or life-threatening, as in the Coronary Care Unit (CCU), benxodiazepine therapy is indicated. In the latter instance, Hackett believes it should be routine. It should not be given as a substitute for the supportive measures indicated above, however; nor should chronic use be prescribed. Hypnotic relaxation is an underutilized technique quite effective in the CCU, Burn Unit, and other hospital settings. When used for this purpose, high hypnotizability is not necessary.[132, 133] The majority of patients do well with the above measures.

When the anxiety becomes persistent, severe, and especially when it becomes transformed into free-floating anxiety with nameless dreads and generalized apprehension of impending doom, then an anxiety neurosis may be said to have supervened. The patient is no longer in touch with the fact that he is quite simply scared. Instead, the anxiety symptoms themselves (especially the somatic concomitants) become a source of secondary anxiety, frequently experienced as a fear of a heart attack or of impending death. This may be chronic or episodic with panic attacks. The secondary anxiety snowballs and dwarfs the original concerns.

Management of these situations varies, but should always include a clear explanation to the patient of the nature of anxiety symptoms—especially of the somatic concomitants—and reassurance that he will not die of them. An explanation of secondary anxiety is useful in enabling a patient to simply register when he is having anxiety without getting further frightened by that very fact. Weekes's book has been very useful to many patients in teaching them cognitive strategies for dealing with the anxiety.[134] An important component of anxiety reaction is the sense of helplessness, of being out of control, of not understanding what is happening. An essential therapeutic tactic is to provide coping strategies that the patient can implement. Cognitive strategies and intellectual mastery allow the taking of some distance from the symptoms. The use of self-hypnosis or any of the wide variety of relaxation techniques as a self-control mechanism, ameliorates the anxiety both directly and by reducing the feeling of helplessness. The teaching of such techniques of self-control and anxiety management does not interfere with an exploration of the meaning of the anxiety symptoms. In fact, it may be necessary to reduce the anxiety to manageable levels before the patient is able to collaborate in an analytic exploration. Certainly, learning to use cognitive and relaxation strategies is preferable to reliance on tranquilizers or alcohol.

In view of the above emphasis on cognitive therapeutic processes, it may be useful to interpret preconscious derivatives of the active conflict situations even in patients who are not very psychologically minded; these patients will often be able to use intellectual insight in the service of mastery. For those patients who possess the requisite attributes described earlier, psychoanalytic psychotherapy is the treatment of choice.

For the others, especially if they have difficulty learning or applying relaxation techniques, EMG biofeedback combined with relaxation instructions on tape for home use, is a promising approach. If recurrent panic attacks are part of the picture, treatment with imipramine is helpful if combined with psychotherapy.

## CONVERSION REACTIONS[135-137]

The diagnosis of conversion reactions in the medical setting is fraught with danger. Two types of errors occur frequently. In the first type, the diagnosis is missed, and the patient is repetitively subjected to medical or surgical diagnostic and therapeutic procedures which not only carry a risk of their own (to say nothing of their expense), but delay or avoid appropriate psychiatric treatment. The second type is perhaps even more serious, since it entails falsely labeling as conversion symptoms, manifestations of an undiagnosed physical illness. The problem is confounded by the fact that organic disease and conversion reactions can and frequently do coexist, despite our fondness for either-or, reductionistic modes of thinking. Even when psychopathology can be established, this does not rule out the presence of organic pathology. In fact, life stress and emotional conflict increase one's vulnerability to physical illness.[138-141] By the process of secondary symbolization, psychodynamic meaning may accrue to symptoms of somatic origin. The initial lack of positive findings on physical and laboratory examination may be misleading, and sometimes a little "tincture of time" will clarify the diagnosis. Therefore, the psychiatric consultant should not be reluctant, when necessary, to defer a definitive diagnosis pending a period of observation.

Another diagnostic pitfall arises from the confounding of the notions of "hysteria" and "conversion." Patients with "hysterical personalities" will respond in a dramatic, histrionic, exhibitionistic, or pseudosexual manner when physically ill; and their "hysterical" behavior is *not* grounds for assuming that their pathology is not "real." Similarly, placebo reactors with bona fide organic disease may respond dramatically (at least temporarily) to placebo, and such a response cannot be used as a diagnostic test. Diagnostic caveats aside, conversion reactions *are* found in the general hospital, in association with neurotic conflict, adolescent identity crises, schizophrenia, and, importantly, depression. Pain is now the most common form of conversion symptom.

Rooms.[122] A variety of environmental manipulations such as transfer to a "normal" ward; replacing the patient's eyeglasses, hearing aid, dentures, cane, etc; alleviation of pain and sleeplessness; provision of personal belongings, pictures, clothing, calendars, newspapers, and a radio or television; and nursing care by a consistent familiar person who will repeatedly and clearly provide orienting and reassuring information; will usually facilitate psychological reintegration. Males undergoing homosexual panic are reassured by the presence of female caretakers. Haloperidol or phenothiazines may be necessary if the patient is violent, disruptive, or extremely paranoid. Therapy should be supportive and reality-oriented, avoiding interpretation of unconscious content. Explaining that he is merely "delirious" and not suffering from permanent mental illness is immensely reassuring to the patient and family.[143]

## DEVIANT ILLNESS BEHAVIOR[144-158]

The terms "disease," "illness," "illness behavior," and "sick role" convey important theoretical and practical distinctions, although they are not always precisely and consistently used. In simple terms, "disease" refers to objective physicochemical abnormalities at the cellular, tissue, and organ level of biological organization. "Illness" refers to the subjective organismic experience of not feeling well, usually attributed by the sufferer to the presence of disease. "Illness behavior" refers to aspects of behavior relevant to illness such as recognition or denial of symptoms; seeking or avoiding medical care; conformity or noncompliance with medical advice; etc. The "sick role" consists of behavioral expectations, rights, and obligations ascribed by the social system to the person who is ill.

Although disease and illness frequently coexist, each can be present without the other, as in hypochondriasis (illness without disease) and silent hypertension (disease without illness).[42]

Some important deviant illness behavior patterns consist of (1) rejection or avoidance of the sick role, even when this is harmful; or (2) adopting it readily and refusing to relinquish it. The first mentioned pattern is reflected in widespread nonadherence or noncompliance with medical regimens;[159-166] and delay in seeking medical care in the face of early symptoms of myocardial infarction, cancer, etc. This is related to the more general problem of altering life-styles to maximize health. Impressive improvements in morbidity and mortality from cardiovascular disease, cerebrovascular disease, cancer, and accidents could be accomplished with current medical knowledge by changes in life-style, and "health behaviors" involving physical exercise, diet, smoking, alcohol consumptions, wearing of automobile seat belts, breast self-examination, and adherence to chronic medication regimens (as in the treatment of hypertension).

Individual psychotherapeutic approaches have been notoriously ineffective in these areas except where depression is playing a major role. Group and family approaches have been more efficacious. Perhaps the most potent tools are public education and advertising techniques aimed at changing the value system and attitudes of whole populations. Comprehensive, prospective studies of multiple-risk factor intervention programs (e.g., MR. FIT) are currently in progress in the United

The principles of treatment planning are similar to those with depres
anxious patients. A psychodynamic assessment of the patient, his family, a
onset situation, is indicated. The therapeutic strategy may or may not includ
or lengthy insight-oriented therapy. The formation of conversion sym
probably shares common mechanisms with the hypnotic trance, so for patient
high trance capacities, hypnosis may be a powerful technique for implementir
of a variety of therapeutic strategies.[132, 133] The variety of therapies is as dive
the pleomorphic symptomatology, and ranges all the way from rude scare tac
classical psychoanalysis.

Mr. W. was a 36-year-old Jewish businessman hospitalized for "postcholecyst
syndrome." His father had died at age 40 when the patient was 13, of an abdominal c
He responded with strong affects during the psychiatric consultation when he su
"realized" that his own son was now the same age. The consultant, sensing that he wo
able to grasp and utilize an interpretation, told him that this was an "anniversary reac
and that his abdominal pain was at once a way of remembering and identifying with hi
father. To the consultant's pleasant surprise, the referring internist reported that the p
thereupon became free of pain for the first time in months, and remained so during a five
follow-up period.

Mrs. S., a 55-year-old married woman requested hypnotherapy for relief of intra
low back pain unrelieved by two laminectomies, physical therapy, and transcutaneous
stimulation. She also suffered from migraine headaches, depression, and a plethora of b
conversion reactions. A critical incident in therapy occurred during a home practice sessi
self-hypnosis. Without conscious intent or awareness, she produced a paralysis of her
hand. This led to a vivid emotional awareness that she really was unconsciously ab
produce somatic symptoms "against her will." From that point, the use of hypnosis
rapidly "faded," and she became engaged in meaningful therapeutic exploration o
unhappy marriage. She was concomitantly placed on a tricyclic antidepressant. Over the
two months there was a marked decrease in pain, and an almost total cessation o
headaches and other conversion symptoms.

Other patients respond to a therapeutic plan that provides reassurar
suggestion, allowance of a face-saving explanation for the symptoms to disapp
reduction of secondary gains, and encouragement of alternative sources
gratification.

## PSYCHOTIC REACTIONS

A psychotic reaction in a medically ill person should be presumed to b
delirium till proved otherwise. An exhaustive search for remediable physiolog
biochemical and pharmacologic etiologies must be carried out, and serial EE
obtained if possible.[142]

Delirioid psychotic reactions may occur in settings marked by sens
deprivation, sensory monotony, immobilization, disruption of the norn
sleep-wake cycle, pain, anxiety, and the absence of orienting environmental cu
Such conditions may obtain in Intensive Care Units and Surgical Recove

States; and Canada has recently launched a nationwide health promotion campaign called "Operation Lifestyle." On the individual level, preventative programs utilizing "health hazard appraisals," stress-testing, physical fitness evaluations, etc, are carried out in centers emphasizing health promotion and disease prevention. The rubric "holistic medicine" has been widely utilized to describe this movement. It has tended lately to become an ideological movement with an antimedical bias, embracing chiropractic, homeopathy, vegetarianism, shiatsu massage, and all manner of nonsense. This unfortunate development is fostered by the lukewarm response, if not outright resistance, of organized, orthodox medicine to health advocacy.[167-169]

Another nonmedical but thoroughly "respectable" thrust in this direction has been the development of "behavioral medicine" and "health psychology," primarily from the ranks of psychologists.[170-177] The use of behavior modification techniques, especially those based on operant conditioning, social-learning theory, and cognitive psychology, has great promise for the reduction of maladaptive "illness behavior," and the enhancement of adaptive "health behavior," as well as in the area of stress-management previously described.

The above discussion has emphasized the utilization of "educational" and nonmedical approaches.[108] The phenomena in question all share the feature of a refusal to adopt the "sick role." These individuals are reluctant to see their medical doctors, let alone a mental health professional, and are quite resistant to referrals for psychotherapy. Even for those individuals in therapy for other, "unrelated problems," it is not at all unusual for the therapist to ignore the health-related dimensions of the person's behavior, (e.g., cigarette smoking). This is unfortunate, for if the maladaptive defenses, such as denial, magical thinking, and rationalization, are dealt with; and the psychological meaning of overeating, nonadherence to medical regimes, and the like, are worked through, many individual patients will significantly modify their inappropriate behaviors (especially if the therapist is a good role-model, intentionally or otherwise). This, however, obviously does not represent a feasible strategy for effecting change across broad segments of the entire population.

A second major class of deviant illness behavior is represented by an inappropriate use of the sick role. One example of this is the problem of overutilization of health care resources by the "worried well," individuals who unconsciously translate their dis-ease in life into a feeling of being ill and attempt to adopt the sick role despite the absence of serious organic pathology.[178] Much of the morbidity found in studies of adjustment to bereavement, or as a sequel to accumulated life changes, consists of illness behavior of this type, and not necessarily the development of disease per se.

Another class of patients does indeed have chronic disease. Not all of the suffering and disability (i.e., not all of the illness) is actually due to the disease itself, however. For these patients, the sick role has become their primary role in life; they have embarked on an "illness career," and their identity has progressively constricted to that of a "patient" (sometimes referred to as a "professional patient"). These people have developed a pernicious "disuse atrophy" of their adaptive "well-behavior" and social roles, and have adopted illness as a way of life. These developments have been most intensely studied in the realm of chronic pain syndromes, and the subsequent discussion will review the analysis and management of patients with chronic pain as a paradigm of the eclectic approach to the therapy of the medically ill patient.

There are a sizeable number of patients with chronic benign pain for whom pain and suffering have become a way of life. They engage in a great deal of "pain behavior" and "illness behavior," with a progressive reduction in the amount of "well-behavior." Their very identity becomes that of a "pain patient," embarked on a "pain career."[179, 180] Similar concepts of the "pain-prone patient" and the "painful man" have been advanced by psychoanalytic writers.[181] Their interpersonal transactions are marked by the prominence of "pain games." We see here a confluence of psychoanalytic, behavioral, and transactional thinking around a common clinical phenomenon; supplementing but not supplanting the biological level of explanation. The treatment program is correspondingly multimodal. Such patients are most effectively treated as inpatients in a pain-center with a carefully designed therapeutic milieu.[182]

The behavioral view asserts that much of the pain behavior has become operant in nature because of the reinforcing contingencies provided by the social system (e.g., disability payments), the family ("T.L.C.," relief from responsibilities), and the hospital system (rest, narcotic analgesics, attention from professional staff). Consequently, a contingency-management, operant-conditioning approach is implemented by a staff carefully trained to extinguish illness behaviors progressively and reinforce adaptive, task-oriented, and healthy behaviors. Key members of the family have to be systematically trained to continue the program at home and interrupt the pathogenic family interactions.[183, 184]

Family and group therapy is also an integral part of the program oriented along transactional analysis principles to neutralize the "pain games" and learn healthier patterns of interacting. Atrophied social and vocational skills are redeveloped with the assistance of behavioral rehearsal techniques. At an individual level, the patient develops a treatment contract with the staff, and assumes an active, responsible role in his own treatment. Self-monitoring, self-management, and cognitive restructuring techniques are frequently included, as are biofeedback and hypnotic strategies.[185] As these active coping strategies are developed, reliance on analgesic medication is reduced, and the pharmacologic addiction is treated by gradual withdrawal. At the biological level, in addition to the above measures and traditional physiotherapy, transcutaneous nerve stimulation is often utilized. This procedure is frequently helpful, and probably acts by virtue of the effect of a strong afferent barrage on the postulated spinal "gate" leading to a blockade of nociceptive transmission. Tricyclic antidepressants are an important component of the treatment package. Chronic pain patients are almost always depressed, and their depression, in turn, magnifies and aggravates their suffering. In addition, the tricyclics probably act directly on pain-inhibiting serotonergic systems in the midbrain, perhaps accounting for their usefulness even in patients who are not markedly clinically depressed. Empirically, phenothiazenes have also been found to be helpful, either alone or in combination with tricyclics in many pain syndromes.[186]

The result of such a comprehensive intensive program is the functional rehabilitation of the patient. Surprisingly, even though the patients become more physically active and use less analgesic medication, they usually also experience a reduction in their subjective pain experience. Even when this reduction is of minor magnitude, however, the alteration of the maladaptive illness behavior is of major significance both in terms of the individual's quality of life and in terms of socioeconomic concerns.

## SUMMARY

The physician, faced with a medically ill patient, now has at his disposal an imposing array of treatment modalities, extensively reviewed in this volume. Formulation of a therapeutic strategy has been rendered more rational by the development of a comprehensive theory of the role of psychosocial factors in physical illness. By a careful analysis of the nature of the specific pathogenetic mechanisms in individual case, both psychophysiologic and somato-pyschic, a multimodal treatment package aimed at "target processes" can be devised. This approach differs from both a monolithic Procrustean application of a favored technique to all patients; and a "shotgun," purely empirical eclecticism.

Unconscious, intrapsychic conflict is seen as an important, but not exclusive, determinant of psychopathologic mechanisms; and insight-oriented therapy as only one aspect of a treatment approach. The use of an adaptational, coping model is heuristically more powerful in this context, and leads to a greater emphasis on cognitive and educational strategies for intervention.

Such a pluralistic, active, and flexible approach to treatment planning provides therapeutic leverage in many cases previously considered inaccessible to psychotherapy.

## References

1. Reiser MF: Changing theoretical concepts in psychosomatic medicine. In Arieti S (Ed.), American Handbook of Psychiatry, IV, 2nd ed. 1975, pp 477–500
2. Hill OW (Ed.): Modern Trends in Psychosomatic Medicine, 3. London, Butterworths, 1976
3. Leigh H, Reiser MF: Major trends in psychosomatic medicine. The psychiatrist's evolving role in medicine. Ann Intern Med 87:233–239, 1977
4. Lipowski ZJ, Lipsitt DR, Whybrow PC (Eds.): Psychosomatic Medicine: Current Trends and Clinical Applications. New York, Oxford University Press, 1977
5. Lipowski ZJ: Psychosomatic medicine in the seventies: an overview. Am J Psychiatry 134:233–244, 1977
6. Weiner H: The psychobiology of human disease: an overview. In Usdin G (Ed.), Psychiatric Medicine. New York, Brunner/Mazel, 1977, pp 3–72

7. Sachar EJ: The current status of psychosomatic medicine. In Strain JJ, Grossman S (Ed.), Psychological Care of the Medically Ill. New York, Appleton-Century-Crofts, 1975, p 54

8. Wittkower ED, Warnes H (Eds.): Psychosomatic Medicine: Its Clinical Applications. Hagerstown, Harper & Row, 1977

9. Lipowski ZJ: Consultation-liaison psychiatry: an overview. Am J Psychiatry 131:623–630, 1974

10. Usdin G (Ed.): Psychiatric Medicine. New York, Brunner/Mazel, 1977

11. Strain JJ, Grossman S: Psychological Care of the Medically Ill: A Primer in Liaison Psychiatry. New York, Appleton-Century-Crofts, 1975

12. Lipp MR: Respectful Treatment: The Human Side of Health Care. Hagerstown, Harper & Row, 1977

13. Pasnau RO (Ed.): Consultation-Liaison Psychiatry. New York, Grune & Stratton, 1975

14. Reading A, Wise TN (Eds.): The Medical Clinics of North America, 61. Symposium on Psychiatry in Internal Medicine. Philadelphia, WB Saunders, 1977

15. Lipowski ZJ: Psychosocial aspects of disease. Ann Intern Med 71:1197–1206, 1969

16. Lipowski ZJ (Ed.): Psychosocial Aspects of Physical Illness. Basel, S Karger, 1972

17. Lipowski ZJ: Psychiatry of somatic diseases: epidemiology, pathogenesis, classification. Compr Psychiatry 16:105–124, 1975

18. Lipowski ZJ: Physical illness, the patient and his environment: psychosocial foundations of medicine. In Arieti S, Reiser MF (Eds.), American Handbook of Psychiatry, 4, 2nd ed. New York, Basic Books, 1975, pp 3–42

19. Miller WB: Psychiatric consultation, I: a general systems approach. Psychiatry Med 4:135–145, 1973

20. Miller WB: Psychiatric consultation, II: conceptual and pragmatic issues of formulation. Psychiatry Med 4:251–271, 1973

21. Schwab JJ: Handbook of Psychiatric Consultation. New York, Appleton-Century-Crofts, 1968

22. Meyer E, Mendelson M: Psychiatric consultations with patients on medical and surgical wards: patterns and processes. Psychiatry 24:197–220, 1961

23. Strain JJ, Grossman S: Psychiatric assessment in the medical setting. In Psychological Care of the Medically Ill. New York, Appleton-Century-Crofts, 1975, p 11

24. Small IF, Foster LG, Small JG, et al: Teaching the art and skill of psychiatric consultation. Dis Nerv Syst 29:817–822, 1968

25. Mackinnon RA, Michels R: The Psychiatric Interview in Clinical Practice. Philadelphia, WB Saunders, 1971

26. Kimball CP: Techniques of interviewing, I: interviewing and the meaning of the symptom. Ann Intern Med 71:147, 1969

27. Franck JD: Faith that heals. Johns Hopkins Med J 137:127–131, 1975

28. Benson H, Epstein MD: Placebo effect: neglected asset in care of patients. JAMA 232:1225–1227, 1978

29. Luborsky L, Singer B, Luborsky L: Comparative studies of psychotherapies: is it true that "everyone has won and all must have prizes"? Arch Gen Psychiatry 32:995–1008, 1975

30. Ramsay RA, Wittkower ED, Warnes H: Treatment of psychosomatic disorders. In Wolman B (Ed.), The Therapist's Handbook: Treatment Methods of Mental Disorders. New York, Van Nostrand-Reinhold, 1976, pp 451–519

31. Keller R: Psychotherapy in psychosomatic disorders: a survey of controlled studies. Arch Gen Psychiatry 32:1021–1028, 1975

31a. Alexander F. Psychosomatic Medicine. New York, Norton, 1950

32. Dewald P: Psychotherapy: A Dynamic Approach. New York, Basic Books, 1964, pp 109–136

33. Karasu TB: Psychotherapies: an overview. Am J Psychiatry 134:851–863, 1977

34. Marty P, de M'uzan M: La "pensee operatoire." Rev Fr Psychanal 27, Suppl. B45, 1963

35. Nemiah JC, Sifneos PE: Affect and fantasy in patients with psychosomatic disorders. In Hill OW (Ed.), Modern Trends in Psychosomatic Medicine. London, Butterworths, 1970

36. Nemiah JC, Freyberger H, Sifneos PE:

Alexithymia: a view of the psychosomatic process. In Hill O (Ed.), Modern Trends in Psychosomatic Medicine, 3. London, Butterworths, 1976, pp 430–440

37. Schur M: Comments on the metapsychology of somatization, in The Psychoanalytic Study of the Child, Vol. 10. N.Y., International Universities Press, 1955, pp 110–164

37a. Sperling M: Psychotherapeutic techniques in psychosomatic medicine. In Bychowski G, Despert JL (Eds.), Specialized Techniques in Psychotherapy. New York, Basic Books, 1952, pp 279–301

38. Rosenbaum M: Personal communication

39. Schmale AH, Jr: Giving up as a final common pathway to changes in health. In Lipowski ZJ (Ed.), Psychosocial Aspects of Physical Illness. Basel, Karger, 1972, pp 20–40

40. Parkes CM: Bereavement. New York, International University Press, 1972

41. Balint M: The Doctor, His Patient and the Illness. London, Pitman, 1957

42. Cassell EJ: The Healer's Art: A New Approach to the Doctor-Patient Relationship. Philadelphia, JB Lippincott Co, 1976

43. Meissner WW: Family dynamics and psychosomatic processes. Family Process 5:142–161, 1966

44. Meissner WW: Family process and psychosomatic disease. Int J Psychiatry Med 5:411–430, 1974

45. Livsey CG: Physical illness and family dynamics. In Lipowski ZJ (Ed.), Psychosocial Aspects of Physical Illness. Basel, Karger, 1972, pp 237–251

46. Grolnick L: A family perspective of psychosomatic factors in illness: a review of the literature. Family Process 11: 457–486, 1972

47. Minuchin S, Baker L, Rosman BL, et al: A conceptual model of psychosomatic illness in children. Arch Gen Psychiatry 32: 1031–1038, 1975

48. Minuchin S, Baker L, Rosman BL, et al: A conceptual model of psychosomatic illness in children: family organization and family therapy. In Wittkower ED, Warnes H (Eds.), Psychosomatic Medicine: Its Clinical Applications. Hagerstown, Harper & Row, 1977, pp 116–128

49. Meyer JK (Ed.): Clinical Management of Sexual Disorders. Baltimore, Williams & Wilkins, 1976

50. Wagner NN: Sexual activity and the cardiac patient. In Green R (Ed.), Human Sexuality: A Health Practicioner's Text. Baltimore, Williams & Wilkins, 1975

51. Sifneos P: Short-Term Psychotherapy and Emotional Crisis. Cambridge, Harvard University Press, 1972

52. Malan DH: A Study of Brief Psychotherapy. New York, Plenum Press, 1976

53. Malan DH: The Frontier of Brief Psychotherapy. New York, Plenum Press, 1976

54. Mann J: Time-Limited Psychotherapy. Cambridge, Harvard University Press, 1973

55. Balint M, Ornstein PH, Balint E: Focal Psychotherapy: An Example of Applied Psychoanalysis. London, Tavistock Publications Ltd, 1972

56. Castelnuovo-Tedesco P: The Twenty-Minute Hour. Boston, Little, Brown, 1965

57. Davanloo H: Basic Principles and Techniques on Short-Term Dynamic Psychotherapy. New York, Spectrum Publishing Co, 1978

58. Fishman G, Nadelson T: Crisis intervention in psychosomatic medicine. In Wittkower ED, Warnes H (Eds.): Psychosomatic Medicine: Its Clinical Applications. Hagerstown, Harper & Row, 1977, pp 15–25

59. Stein EH, Murdaugh J, Macleod JA: Brief psychotherapy of psychiatric reactions to physical illness. Am J Psychiatry 125: 1040, 1969

60. Stunkard AJ: Presidential address—1974: from explanation to action in psychosomatic medicine: the case of obesity. Psychosom Med 37:195–236, 1975

61. Lazarus AA: Multimodal Behavior Therapy. New York, Springer, 1976

62. Shapiro D, Surwit RS: Operant conditioning: a new theoretical approach in psychosomatic medicine. Int J Psychiatry Med 5:377–387, 1974

63. Wilson GT: The behavior therapies. In Wittkower ED, Warnes H (Eds.), Psychosomatic Medicine: Its Clinical Appli-

cations. Hagerstown, Harper & Row, 1977, pp 138–145

64. Meichenbaum D: Cognitive Behavior Modification: An Integrative Approach. New York, Plenum Press, 1977

65. Suinn R: Behavior therapy for cardiac patients. Behavior Therapy 5:569–571, 1974

66. Richardson FC: Anxiety management training: a multimodal approach. In Lazarus AA (Ed.): Multimodal Behavior Therapy. New York, Springer, 1976, pp 103–115

67. Benson H, Greenwood MM, Klemchuk H: The relaxation response: psychophysiologic aspects and clinical applications. Int J Psychiatry Med 6:87–98, 1975

68. Benson H, Kotch JB, Crassweller KD: The relaxation response: a bridge between psychiatry and medicine. In Reading A, Wise TN (Eds.): The Medical Clinics of North America, 61. Symposium on Psychiatry in Internal Medicine. Philadelphia, WB Saunders, 1977, pp 929–938

69. Luthe W, Blumberger SR: Autogenic therapy. In Wittkower ED, Warnes H (Eds.), Psychosomatic Medicine: Its Clinical Applications. Hagerstown, Harper & Row, 1977, pp 146–165

70. Birk L (Ed.): Biofeedback: Behavioral Medicine. New York, Grune and Stratton, 1973

71. Hauri PP: Biofeedback and self-control of physiological functions: clinical applications. Int J Psychiatry Med 6:255–265, 1975

72. Shapiro D: Biofeedback. In Pasnau RO (Ed.), Consultation-Liaison Psychiatry. New York, Grune & Stratton, 1975, pp 87–101

73. Sargent JD: Biofeedback and biocybernetics. In Wittkower ED, Warnes H (Eds.), Psychosomatic Medicine: Its Clinical Applications. Hagerstown, Harper & Row, 1977, pp 166–171

74. Schwartz GE, Beatty J (Eds.): Biofeedback: Theory and Research. New York, Academic Press, 1977

75. Wickramasekera I (Ed.): Biofeedback, Behavior Therapy and Hypnosis: Potentiating the Verbal Control of Behavior for Clinicians. Chicago, Nelson-Hall, 1976

76. Schuster MM: Biofeedback treatment of gastrointestinal disorders. In Reading A, Wise TN (Eds.), The Medical Clinics of North America, 61. Symposium on Psychiatry in Internal Medicine. Philadelphia, WB Saunders, 1977, pp 907–912

77. Weiss T: Biofeedback training for cardiovascular dysfunctions. In Reading A, Wise TN (Eds.): The Medical Clinics of North America, 61. Symposium on Psychiatry in Internal Medicine. Philadelphia, WB Saunders, 1977, pp 913–928

78. Shader RI (Ed.): Manual of Psychiatric Therapeutics. Boston, Little, Brown, 1975

79. Solow C: Psychotropic drugs in somatic disorders. Int J Psychiatry Med 6: 267–282, 1975

80. Greenblatt DJ, Shader RI: Psychotropic drugs in the general hospital. In Shader RI (Ed.), Manual of Psychiatric Therapeutics, Practical Psychopharmacology and Psychiatry. Boston, Little, Brown & Co, 1975, p 1

81. Strain JJ: Psychopharmacological treatment of the medically ill. In Strain JJ, Grossman S (Eds.): Psychological Care of the Medically Ill. New York, Appleton-Century-Crofts, 1975, pp 108–122

82. Greenblatt DJ, Shader RI, Lofgren S: Rational psychopharmacology for patients with medical diseases. In Creger WP, Coggins CH, Hancock EW (Eds.): Annual Review of Medicine, 27. Chicago, Annual Reviews Inc, 1976, p 407

83. Mandell AJ: Pharmacotherapy. In Wittkower ED, Warnes H (Eds.), Psychosomatic Medicine: Its Clinical Applications. Hagerstown, Harper & Row, 1977, pp 172–179

84. Goldstein AP, Stein N: Prescriptive Psychotherapies. New York, Pergamon Press, 1976

85. Engel GL: A unified concept of health and disease. Perspect Biol Med 3:459–485, 1960

86. Engel GL: Psychological Development in Health and Disease. Philadelphia, WB Saunders, 1962

87. Engel GL: The need for a new medical model: a challenge for biomedicine. Science 196:129–136, 1977

88. Dubos R: Man, Medicine and Environment. New York, Praeger, 1968

89. Shagass C: The medical model in psychiatry. Compr Psychiatry 16:405–413, 1975

90. Kimball CP: Psychosomatic theories and their contributions to chronic illness. In Usdin G (Ed.), Psychiatric Medicine. New York, Brunner/Mazel, 1977, pp 259–333

91. Feinstein AR: Clinical Judgment. Baltimore, Williams & Wilkins, 1967

92. Susser M: Causal Thinking in the Health Sciences. New York, Oxford University Press, 1973

93. Peterson HW, Martin MJ: Organic disease presenting us a psychiatric syndrome. Postgrad Med 54:78–83, 1973

94. Strauss AL: Chronic Illness and the Quality of Life. St. Louis, CV Mosby, 1975

95. Sachar EJ: Evaluating depression in the medical patient. In Strain JJ, Grossman S (Eds.): Psychological Care of the Medically Ill. New York, Appleton-Century-Crofts, 1975, pp 64–75

96. Schwab JJ, et al: Diagnosing depression in medical inpatients. Ann Intern Med 67:695, 1967

97. Seligman ME: Fall into helplessness. In Wickramasekera I (Ed.), Biofeedback, Behavior Therapy and Hypnosis: Potentiating the Verbal Control of Behavior for Clinicians. Chicago, Nelson-Hall, 1976, pp 243–253

98. Bräutigam W, Rüppell A: Group psychotherapy. In Wittkower ED, Warnes H (Eds.), Psychosomatic Medicine: Its Clinical Applications. Hagerstown, Harper & Row, 1977, pp 94–106

99. Sclare AB: Group therapy for specific psychosomatic problems. In Wittkower ED, Warnes H (Eds.): Psychosomatic Medicine: Its Clinical Applications. Hagerstown, Harper & Row, 1977, pp 107–115

100. Rahe RH, Juffli CF, Suchor RJ, et al: Group therapy in the outpatient management of post-myocardial infarction patients. Psychiatry Med 4:77–88, 1973

101. Stein A: Group therapy with psychosomatically ill patients. In Kaplan HI, Sadock BJ (Eds.), Comprehensive Group Psychotherapy. Baltimore, Williams & Wilkins, 1971, pp 581–601

102. Milvy P (Ed.): Annals of the New York Academy of Sciences, 301. The Marathon: Physiological, Medical, Epidemiological and Psychological Studies. New York, The New York Academy of Sciences, 1977

103. Amsterdam EA, Wilmore JH, DeMaria AN (Eds.): Exercise in Cardiovascular Health and Disease. New York, Yorke Medical Books, 1977

104. Zohman LR, Phillips RE (Eds.): Progress in Cardiac Rehabilitation: Medical Aspects of Exercise Testing and Training. New York, Stratton Intercontinental Medical Book Corporation, 1973

105. Kavanagh T: Heart Attack? Counterattack! Toronto, Van Nostrand Reinhold, 1976

106. Kostrubala T: The Joy of Running. Philadelphia, J.P. Lippincott, 1976

107. Hackett TP, Cassem NH: The psychology of intensive care: problems and their management. In Usdin G (Ed.), Psychiatric Medicine. New York, Brunner/Mazel, 1977, pp 228–258

108. Mechanic D: Illness behavior, social adaptation and the management of illness: a comparison of educational and medical models. J Nerv Ment Dis 165:79–87, 1977

109. Beck AT: Cognitive Therapy and the Emotional Disorders. New York, International Universities Press, 1976

110. Mahoney MJ: Cognition and Behavior Modification. Cambridge, Ballinger, 1974

111. Sachar EJ: Psychiatric disturbances associated with endocrine disorders. In Reiser MF (Ed.): American Handbook of Psychiatry, 4: Organic Disorders and Psychosomatic Medicine (2nd ed.). New York, Basic Books, 1975, pp 299–313

112. Lesse S (Ed.): Masked Depression. New York, Jason Aronson, 1974

113. Warnes H: The problem of masked depressions in a clinical perspective. The Psychiatric J of the University of Ottawa, 2:37–43, 1977

114. Kielholz P (Ed.): Masked Depression. Bern-Stuttgart-Vienna, Hans Huber Publishers, 1973

115. Lesse S: Psychotherapy in combination with antidepressant drugs in the treatment of patients with masked depression. In Lesse S (Ed.): Masked Depression. New York, Jason Aronson, 1974, pp 253–272

116. Janis IL: Psychological Stress. New York, Wiley, 1958

117. Egbert LD, et al: Reduction of postoperative pain by encouragement and instruction of patients: a study of doctor-patient rapport. N Engl J Med 270:196–198, 1964

118. Visintainer MA, Wolfer JA: Psychological preparation of surgical pediatric patients: effect of children's and parent's stress responses and adjustment. Pediatrics 56: 187–202, 1975

119. Hackett TP, Weisman AD: Psychiatric management of operative syndromes. the therapeutic consultation and the effect of noninterpretive intervention. Psychosom Med 22:267–282, 1960

120. Weisman AD, Hackett TP: Psychosis after eye surgery: establishment of specific doctor-patient relationship in prevention and treatment of "black-patch" delirium. N Engl J Med 258:1284–1289, 1958

121. Abram H: Therapeutic consultation with the surgical patient. In Wittkower ED, Warnes H (Eds.), Psychosomatic Medicine: Its Clinical Applications. Hagerstown, Harper & Row, 1977, pp 42–48

122. Kornfeld DS: The hospital environment: its impact on the patient. In Lipowski ZJ (Ed.): Advances in Psychosomatic Medicine, 8. Psychosocial Aspects of Physical Illness. Basel, Karger, 1972, pp 252–270

123. Lipowski ZJ: Physical illness, the individual and the coping processes. Psychiatry Med 1:91–102, 1970

124. Verwoerdt A: Psychopathological responses to the stress of physical illness. In Lipowski ZJ (Ed.), Psychosocial Aspects of Physical Illness. Basel, Karger, 1972

125. Kiely WF: Coping with severe illness. In Lipowski ZJ (Ed.), Advances in Psychosomatic Medicine, 8. Psychosocial Aspects of Physical Illness. Basel, Karger, 1972, p 105

126. Yager J: Cognitive aspects of illness. In Pasnau RO (Ed.), Consultation-Liaison Psychiatry. New York, Grune & Stratton, 1975, pp 61–71

127. Lazarus RS: Psychological Stress and the Coping Process. New York, McGraw-Hill, 1966

128. Visotsky HM, Hamburg DA, Goss MA, et al: Coping behavior under extreme stress. Arch Gen Psychiatry 5:423–448, 1961

129. Coelho GV, Hamburg DA, Adams JE (Eds.): Coping and Adaptation. New York, Basic Books, 1974

130. Schachter S, Singer JE: Cognitive, social and physiological determinants of emotional state. Psychol Rev 69:379–399, 1962

131. Weiss JM: Influence of psychological variables on stress-induced pathology. In CIBA Foundation Symposium, 8 (New Series), Physiology, Emotion & Psychosomatic Illness. Amsterdam, Elsevier Excerpta Medical North-Holland, 1972, pp 253–265

132. Frankel FH: Hypnosis as a treatment method in psychosomatic medicine. Int J Psychiatry Med 6:75–85, 1975

133. Peterfy G: Hypnosis. In Wittkower ED, Warnes H (Eds.), Psychosomatic Medicine: Its Clinical Applications. Hagerstown, Harper & Row, 1977, pp 129–137

134. Weekes C: Hope and Help For Your Nerves. New York, Hawthorne Books, Inc, 1969

135. Ziegler F, Imboden JB, Meyer E: Contemporary conversion reactions. a clinical study. Am J Psychiatry 116:901–910, 1960

136. Ziegler F, Imboden JB: Contemporary conversion reactions, II. a conceptual model. Arch Gen Psychiatry 6:279, 1962

137. McKegney PF: The incidence and characteristics of patients with conversion reactions: a general hospital consultation service sample. Am J Psychiatry 124:542, 1967

138. Rahe RH: Subjects' recent life changes and their near-future illness susceptibility. In Lipowski ZJ (Ed.), Psychosocial Aspects of Physical Illness. Basel, Karger, 1972, pp 2–19

139. Rahe RH: Life stress and illness. In Pasnau RO (Ed.), Consultation-Liaison Psychiatry. New York, Grune & Stratton, 1975, pp 47–59

140. Hurst MW, et al: The relation of psychological stress to onset of medical illness. In Creger WP, Coggins CH, Hancock EW (Eds.), Annual Review of Medicine. Chicago, Annual Reviews Inc, 1976

141. Rabkin JG, Struening EL: Life events, stress and illness. Science 194:1013–1020, 1976

142. Lipowski ZJ: Delirium, clouding of consciousness and confusion. J Nerv Ment Dis 145:227–255, 1967

143. Folstein M, McHugh PR: Phenomenological approach to the treatment of "organic" psychiatric syndromes. In Wolman BB (Ed.), The Therapist's Handbook: Treatment Methods of Mental Disorders. New York, Van Nostrand Reinhold Company, 1976, pp 279–286

144. Reading A: Illness and disease. In Reading A, Wise TN (Eds.), Medical Clinics of North America, 61. Symposium on Psychiatry in Internal Medicine. Philadelphia, WB Saunders, 1977, pp 703–710

145. Mechanic D: The concept of illness behavior. J Chronic Dis 15:189–194, 1962

146. Mechanic D: Medical Sociology. New York, Free Press, 1968

147. Mechanic D: Stress, illness and illness behavior. J Human Stress 2:2–6, 1976

148. Kasl SV, Cobb S: Health behavior, illness behavior, and sick-role behavior, 1. health and illness behavior. Arch Environ Health 12:246–266, 1966

149. Kasl SV, Cobb S: Health behavior, illness behavior, and sick role behavior, 2. sick role behavior. Arch Environ Health 12:531–541, 1966

150. Bloom SW: The Doctor and His Patient. New York, Russell Sage Foundation, 1963

151. Zola IK: Problems of communication, diagnosis, and patient care: the interplay of patient, physician, and clinic organization. J Med Educ 38:829, 1963

152. Suchman EA: Stages of illness and medical care. J Health Soc Behav 6:114–128, 1965

153. Twaddle AC: The concepts of the sick role and illness behavior. In Lipowski ZJ (Ed.), Psychosocial Aspects of Physical Illness. Basel, Karger, 1972, pp 162–179

154. Sontag S: Illness as metaphor. The New York Review of Books, 26 Jan 1978, p 10

155. Sontag S: Images of illness. The New York Review of Books, 9 Feb 1978, p 26

156. Sontag S: Disease as a political metaphor. The New York Review of Books, 23 Feb 1978, p 29

157. Cobb S: Presidential address-1976: social support as a moderator of life stress. Psychosom Med 38:300–314, 1976

158. Moos RH: A social ecological perspective on medical disorders. In Wittkower ED, Warnes H (Eds.), Psychosomatic Medicine: Its Clinical Applications. Hagerstown, Harper & Row, 1977, pp 199–208

159. Blackwell B: Patient compliance. N Engl J Med 289:249–252, 1973

160. Gillum RF, Barsky AJ: Diagnosis and management of patient noncompliance. JAMA 228:1563–1567, 1974

161. Taglicozzo DM, Ima K: Knowledge of illness as a predictor of patient behavior. J Chronic Dis 22:765–775, 1970

162. Rosenstock IM: Patient's compliance with health regimens. JAMA 234:402, 1975

163. Sackett D, Haynes R (Eds.): Compliance With Therapeutic Regimens. Baltimore, Johns Hopkins University Press, 1976

164. Marston M: Compliance with medical regimens: a review of the literature. Nurs Res 19:312, 1970

165. Mitchell J: Compliance with medical regimens: an annotated bibliography. Health Education Monograph 2:78, 1974

166. Gentry WD: Noncompliance to medical regimens. In Williams RB, Gentry WD (Eds.), Behavioral Approaches to Medical Treatment. Cambridge, Ballinger Pub Co, 1977

167. Pelletier KR: Mind As Healer, Mind As Slayer: A Holistic Approach To Preventing Stress Disorders. New York, Delta, 1977

168. Medical Tribune: North Lies The Cradle of "Lifestyle Medicine," 22 Feb 1978

169. Kane RL (Ed.): The Behavioral Sciences and Preventive Medicine: Opportunities and Dilemmas, DHEW Pub No. (NIH)76-878. Washington, D.C., U.S. Gov't Printing Off., 1976

170. Schwartz GE, Weiss SM: What is behavioral medicine? Psychosom Med 39:377–381, 1977

171. Pomerleau OF, Bass F, Crown V: Role of behavior modification in preventive medicine. N Engl J Med 292:1277–1282, 1975

172. Pomerleau OF: Behavioral medicine: practical applications and future implications. (Paper presented at Annual Meeting of the Association for the Advancement of Behavior Therapy, New York), 1976

173. Katz RC, Zlutnick S (Eds.): Behavior Therapy and Health Care: Principles and Applications. New York, Pergamon Press, 1975

174. Williams RB, Jr, Gentry WD (Eds.): Be-

havioral Approaches to Medical Treatment. Cambridge, Ballinger, 1977

175. Weiss S (Ed.): Proceedings of the National Heart and Lung Institute Working Conferences on Health Behavior. DHEW Pub (NIH), Washington, D.C., U.S. Gov't Printing Off., 1975

176. Berni R, Fordyce WE: Behavior Modification and the Nursing Process. St. Louis, The CV Mosby Co, 1973

177. Suinn RM: Type A behavior patterns. In Williams RB, Gentry WD (Eds.), Behavioral Approaches to Medical Treatment. Cambridge, Ballinger Pub Co, 1977

178. Idzorek S: Functional classification of hypochondriasis with specific recommendations for treatment. South Med J 68: 1326–1332, 1975

179. Sternbach RA: Pain Patients: Traits and Treatment. New York, Academic Press, 1974

180. Weisenberg M (Ed.): Pain: Clinical and Experimental Perspectives. St. Louis, CV Mosby Co, 1975

181. Engel GL: Psychogenic pain and the pain-prone patient. Am J Med 26:899–918, 1959

182. Bonica JJ: Organization and function of a pain clinic. Adv Neurol 4:433–443, 1974

183. Fordyce WE: Treating pain by contingency management. In Bonica JJ (Ed.), Advances in Neurology, 4. International Symposium on Pain. New York, Raven Press, 1974, pp 583–594

184. Fordyce WE: Behavioral concepts in chronic pain and illness. In Davidson PO (Ed.), The Behavioral Management of Anxiety, Depression and Pain. New York, Brunner/Mazel, 1976, pp 147–188

185. Meichenbaum D, Turk D: The cognitive-behavioral management of anxiety, anger and pain. In Davidson PO (Ed.), The Behavioral Management of Anxiety, Depression and Pain. New York, Brunner/Mazel, 1976, pp 1–34

186. Merskey H: Psychologica aspects of pain relief: hypnotherapy, psychotropic drugs. In Swerdlow M (Ed.), Monographs in Anesthesiology, 1. Relief of Intractable Pain. London, Excerpta Medica, 1974

Morton F. Reiser

# 4

# Psychoanalysis in Patients with Psychosomatic Disorders

**INTRODUCTION**

Although much of modern psychosomatic *theory* is rooted in the abundant clinical observations and derivative theoretical contributions, of psychoanalytic pioneers like Alexander,[1] Deutsch,[2] Dunbar,[3] Garma,[4] Grinker,[5] Kubie,[6] Margolin,[7] Schur,[8, 9] and Sperling,[10, 11] as well as many others, the literature dealing specifically with psychoanalytic *treatment* of patients with psychosomatic disorders is relatively sparse. My examination of this important, controversial, but somewhat neglected, subject will be divided into four parts: first, a brief historical sketch and report on the "state of the art," second, a reconsideration—in the light of recent developments and possible modifications of psychosomatic theory—of the indications for (and rational expectations to have from) the psychoanalytic treatment of patients with psychosomatic disorders; third, a description of the technical issues as I understand them, of necessity emphasizing the anecdotal state of the art and the need for additional research in this area; and fourth, the conclusion, emphasizing the impressive potential of the psychoanalytic method for contributing to basic theoretical research, as well as to treatment in psychosomatic medicine.

This chapter will confine itself to issues centering on treatment of patients with the "classical" psychosomatic disorders—i.e., those in which psychogenetic forces are considered to have played important contributing roles in proximal etiology and pathogenesis. The best studied of these include mainly peptic duodenal ulcer, essential hypertension, thyrotoxicosis, neurodermatitis, ulcerative colitis, rheumatoid arthritis, and bronchial asthma. Limiting the scope of the discussion to

---

This chapter represents a somewhat modified version of the Fourth Annual Melitta Sperling Lecture of the Psychoanalytic Association of New York, February 27, 1978.

these illnesses will serve to keep the paper within manageable limits and to concentrate attention on central and important theoretical issues about which there is considerable research and clinical psychoanalytic data, such as specificity.* At the same time, it should be pointed out that interest in this small group of diseases represents only a limited sector of the now more broadly defined field of consultation-liaison psychiatry. Consequently, many of the points to be discussed cannot be taken as immediately or directly applicable to that broader context.

## STATE OF THE ART

When interest in psychosomatic medicine was reaching its ascendancy following the Second World War, psychoanalytic treatment of patients with psychosomatic disorders was undertaken with enthusiasm by many analysts, but after awhile, enthusiasm began to wane somewhat and the idea of psychoanalytic treatment of psychosomatic disorders developed something of a bad press, much of it outside the literature. Some patients developed serious, occasionally even fatal, exacerbations of illness during the course of the analytic work, and understandably analysts who had or heard of such experiences began to shy away. Lindemann was one of the first to point out that the active and aggressive uncovering of unresolved, repressed psychological conflicts could lead to psychotic states and/or serious exacerbations of ulcerative colitis, and he was, I think, convinced that classical psychoanalytic procedure was contraindicated in patients with that disease.[12, 13] Others, like Alexander, were not convinced of the inevitability of such untoward reactions, and continued actively to use analytic techniques with such patients during periods of relative clinical quiescence and remission.[1] Sperling and her followers went even further, and reported very dramatic clinical improvements following vigorous analytic work during active stages of the disease, using techniques of confrontive attack on the defenses and the gratifying use of symptoms, giving the patient symbolic interpretations of the meaning of symptoms and their relationship to the transference. She writes describing the treatment of a 7½ year old girl:

> In the ward she began immediately to tell me how unhappy she was and beg to be allowed to go home. When I said that "little Barbara" (as we spoke of her unconscious impulses) was responsible for her plight because she was so angry that in her attempt to "get even" with everybody she did not care what happened to "big Barbara," the child screamed, "Stop it! Stop it!" She writhed and called for the bedpan. While sitting on the bedpan, straining to defecate, I continued to talk of her rage and destructiveness, adding that she now included me in her anger because I was telling her these things.

*In general, decisions regarding appropriateness and/or feasibility of undertaking psychoanalysis with other classes of physically ill patients rests upon the usual indications and contraindications for psychoanalysis, though special attention should be given to issues of pain and other physical discomforts, severity of illness, life expectancy, degree of incapacitation, etc.

I now reassured her that I could and would help her if she wanted me to, and if she herself would fight "little Barbara." She became calm and we parted with my promise to get her some concessions in the matter of food and other liberties in the ward. When next I saw her she was much quieter and an arrangement was made, with her approval, that she be taken in a wheelchair to the clinic to see me regularly twice a week.[14]

Many of her students, including L. Deutsch, G. Fraiman, and C.P. Wilson have continued the use of this active approach with apparently favorable results.[14 a,b,c,] Knapp, Mushatt, and Nemetz, who have carried out detailed longitudinal covariance studies combining tape recordings of analytic hours with physiologic measurements in patients with bronchial asthma, report in detail one especially dramatic instance of a patient who died suddenly and unexpectedly on the way to his first ("reunion") hour following a summer interruption of the analysis:

In both of these last sessions (August 6 and 8) he also had one other, highly specific group of associations. These concerned a television program he had seen recently, about an artist who killed his wife. The man was seeing a psychiatrist, who took him to the police. There the crime was confirmed by an analysis of the murderer's paintings. Unlike a number of surrealistic and violent creations which were brought before an expert, the painting by this man was of a beautiful woman. "The fellow that painted this picture could certainly kill" was the final verdict. And this remark, which was ushered in by a brief spell of wheezing devoid of manifest emotion, was virtually the patient's final association as he departed.

During the ensuing month, according to his wife, he was unusually well. He stopped taking ACTH on August 8, 1962. A week later he and his immediate family left to visit his brother in the South. He was so optimistic that he brought only a two-day supply of medication along—for him, an almost unheard of step. Actually he remained symptom-free, without the aid of steroid or other medication for three weeks, until September 1, 1962, toward the end of his return trip home. He had had a happy visit, but had spoken of dreading the return to his job and to analysis. He mentioned the fantasy of moving to Texas, though only to say that step was impossible, because he needed his doctors too much. Once he had arrived at home, his asthma continued to mount. On September 6 he had a severe exacerbation, treated with ACTH, to which, as usual, he appeared to respond. He was still taking it on September 10, the day he was scheduled to resume work and analysis. He left home in apparent health, but while driving to work, suddenly stopped his car at the side of the road and slumped over the wheel. Two workmen saw this and approached the car. They reported that he was smiling. They opened the door. He was dead.

Was death in some way a welcome solution? We remember the alleged smile as he died. In the past he had had fantasies of dying on the way to his sessions, a sort of hari kari on the doorstep of the analyst. They forecast what we interpret to have been his grim escape—namely, to make a final assault on himself and join the beautiful mother in death.[15]

But this was an exception and not the rule in their experience; Knapp and his coworkers still continue undaunted in their combined psychoanalytic and physiologic studies of patients with bronchial asthma.

The main questions to emerge ultimately from these conflicting experiences focused upon the capacity (or tolerance) of such patients for "working through" in traditionally conducted analysis of the transference neurosis. If they were not capable of doing so, could classical techniques be modified, as in the schizophrenias and severe borderline conditions, so as to render psychoanalytic work with them feasible and productive?

Attempts to research these questions inevitably encounter the myriad and well-known difficulties of obtaining reliable and objective observations and evaluations of psychoanalytic process. In the case of psychosomatic disorders, these difficulties are compounded by the fact that investigators confront complicated diseases with unknown multiple-factor etiology, and clinical courses characterized by sometimes frequent, but irregularly occurring, remissions and exacerbations. Consequently, despite the provocation provided by anecdotal accounts of dramatic experiences and conflicting reports of results, the amount of objectively based data that is available to answer these questions is necessarily limited. In the face of these problems it may be worthwhile to review, even very briefly, some of the theoretical implications that emerge from recent neurobiologic and psychophysiologic research, in the hope that they might furnish clues to formulation of new questions, or reformulations of old questions, that would point to rational ways out of the present therapeutic dilemmas.

## THEORETICAL CONSIDERATIONS—THEIR IMPLICATIONS REGARDING INDICATIONS FOR PSYCHOANALYSIS IN PATIENTS WITH PSYCHOSOMATIC DISORDERS

Early theories in psychosomatic medicine initially developed as multiple factor linear theories which assigned psychological-psychosocial factors one place among several factors in etiology and pathogenesis. Alexander's theory, prototypical of many, included formulations of specific psychological configurations of conflict and psychological defenses; specific precipitating social situations; and specific constitutional psysiologic anlagen, and considered all of them to be "necessary but not sufficient" causes of psychosomatic illnesses.[1] Such models implied that psychotherapy would constitute an essential component of effective treatment since the etiologic model embodied linear cause and effect sequences, with psychological conflict as one of the links in the causal chain.

It is beyond the scope of this chapter to review the newer neurobiologic and psychophysiologic data and their implications for psychosomatic theory. I have discussed these issues in a previous paper.[16] Of importance for the present discussion is the fact that these data so powerfully implicate central nervous mechanisms, particularly those connected with the psychoneuroendocrine system, as key functions linking events in the psychosocial realm with events in the physiological realm. It has now become abundantly clear that states of health and illness are best understood in terms of three parameters: the biological, the psychological, and the social; and that the brain occupies a central position between the psychosocial and the physiological realms.

These new data from neurobiological sciences indicate that a biopsychosocial systems model (which assigns little or no importance to linear causal sequences) is probably more appropriate than the older linear models. By implication, curative effects from psychotherapy might well be considered as less immediately and directly expectable than they were considered to be from the earlier models. While the newer models still would logically assign a highly significant and meaningful place to psychological (including psychoanalytic) techniques in management, they would not in my understanding necessarily justify mandatory indication for psychotherapeutic intervention as the earlier theories did. If this should be so, then there are important implications to be drawn regarding indications for psychoanalysis in patients with these conditions. Formerly it was considered by many that the presence of one of the major psychosomatic diseases *in and of itself* justified psychoanalytic treatment if it was not psychologically contraindicated. The implicit expectation was that successful analysis should (or could) lead to cure, or at least to very major improvement in the status of the disease. Such a position no longer seems fully supportable to me; rather it would seem more correct to say that psychoanalysis should be undertaken in such patients for psychological indications *in their own right*. The expectation would then be that: if in the individual patient, psychological factors were found to be interacting with social and biological ones in such a way as to be sustaining, exacerbating, or otherwise aggravating the disease process, one could then anticipate that successful analysis might well yield an incidental dividend in the form of substantial improvement in medical status. Put another way, I do not feel that it is any longer justified *in the absence of clear psychological and psychosocial indications* to undertake psychoanalysis just because the patient has one of the classical psychosomatic diseases such as duodenal peptic ulcer or bronchial asthma. Another corollary would follow: if it should turn out that the medical disorder is currently being sustained by physiologic mechanisms that are currently functionally independent of psychological and psychosocial forces, it seems possible that psychoanalysis, even when undertaken for valid psychological indications and carried through to a satisfactory termination, might have little or no effect upon the medical condition. This could be so even though psychological conflict had been embedded in early epigenetic developmental sequences and had in fact played an important etiologic role, e.g., in programming the capacity for the particular disease in the individual. The original preverbal pathogenic conflict and associated physiologic mechanisms could be *currently* archaic and beyond the therapeutic reach of psychological methods.* In such cases, failure to influence the medical disease would not necessarily reflect upon the psychological efficacy or success of the psychoanalytic treatment per se.

The new data also have important implications for the place of psychoanalytic method in research. They serve to refocus serious attention upon the phenomenon of consciousness and the fact that it consists of a broad continuum of states, ranging from vigilance and alertness at one end to deep sleep at the other. In ego-psychological terms, this spread might be referred to as a continuum of

---

*Similar reservations must also pertain to limitations of biofeedback techniques in long-established medical disorders such as essential hypertension.

differing ego states. Regardless of semantic considerations, it seems clear from the empirical data that functional changes in states of the central nervous system may manifest themselves in the psychological realm as altered states of consciousness and cognitive function; and simultaneously in the physiological realm as altered patterns of autonomic integrative and homeostatic mechanisms, and altered patterns of neuroendocrine secretion. These are the very mechanisms and patterns that regulate visceral function, and so can exert profound effects upon the individual's state of health. Elsewhere I have proposed the hypothesis that a particular kind of alteration in the state of the central nervous system may in fact provide the necessary psychologic and physiologic substrate or condition that would be permissive of, or facilitate, precipitation or major worsening of psychosomatic disorders.[16] Speculative as this idea may be, it is nonetheless reasonable to expect that: psychosocial stresses, emotional experiences, and/or psychotherapeutic techniques that are capable of inducing changes in psychological state, and presumably in the underlying functional organization of the central nervous system, would accordingly hold the capacity to modify integrative and regulatory mechanisms so as to induce either relaxation and cessation of pathogenetic output to the viscera, or its reverse if the effects are such as to induce physiologic arousal and stimulation. From a clinical point of view, such a conceptual view may help to explain some of the contradictory and conflicting impressions and opinions of the effects of psychoanalysis upon patients with psychosomatic disorders that were referred to earlier. The altered brain states implicated above are of a type that could be expected to occur when ego defenses have failed and hypothalamic anterior pituitary adrenocorticotrophic hormone systems have been activated.[17] Circulating andrenocorticotrophins and catecholamines affect not only higher cognitive functions[18, 19, 20] but also enzyme systems regulating biosynthesis and breakdown of critical neurotransmitter biogenic amines in the central nervous system, as well as in the rest of the body.[21, 22] The important implications to emphasize are: (1) that serious breakdown of ego defenses (and coping mechanisms) may set the stage for activation of pathogenic autonomic and neuroendocrine outflow to visceral systems; and conversely, (2) that resolution of conflict, and/or institution of more effective defenses, may set palliative mechanisms into motion—or at least permit them to operate. Psychoanalytic process, in providing unique and unparalleled opportunities for longitudinal observations of and influence upon the very psychological phenomena that are associated with altered states of the central nervous system, should indeed constitute a powerful therapeutic and research tool.

## TECHNICAL ISSUES**

In psychoanalytic treatment, the management of the transference neurosis, as suspected earlier, may well turn out to be the critical factor. After all, it embodies the capacity for disrupting, reinforcing, or instituting new ego defenses, and for

---

**It is assumed throughout the discussion that follows that patients with active medical disease will concurrently be under continuing medical observation and care.

reactivating or resolving core conflicts. As in the case of other conditions such as severe borderline and schizophrenic states, modifications in technique that would be proposed by conservative analysts would emphasize careful, perhaps even gentle, analysis of ego functions with particular attention to analysis of defenses so as to insure that the patient will always be in possession of a repertoire of effective defenses and coping devices that can be supported by the analytic relationship, especially the therapeutic alliance. Further, in managing the transference neurosis, the intensity of frustration that may safely be allowed to develop would be seen as limited, perhaps to a considerable degree, when compared to the classical symptom neuroses and neurotic character disorders. This leads to extremely important theoretical questions that should be amenable to research. For example, if the required modifications in technique are so extensive as to preclude thorough (i.e., as complete as possible) analysis of the transference neurosis, would this accordingly limit the changes that could be expected in the physiologic realm, e.g., would the treatment then fall short of influencing the central nervous system so as to modify pathogenic outflow mechanisms? It may well be the two-edged sword of the transference neurosis—with its potential for "storm" and associated aggravation of the medical condition on the one hand, or its potential for amelioration of pathogenic central nervous system outflow on the other hand—that accounts for discrepancies between the experiences of clinicians like Sperling and Lindemann.

I believe that some technical questions and issues can be reconsidered in the light of new data and theoretical perspectives. Schur considered that patients with active pathological somatization reactions undergo ego regression in two important ways: (1) alterations in the ego's capacity to perceive and evaluate dangers, including regression to extensive use of thought processes organized according to the primary process; and (2) use of unneutralized energy in resomatized reactions to (mis-) perceived danger signals.[8, 9] Clinical observations of psychosomatic patients indicate that the alterations in ego state are not total and homogeneous; rather, they are observed to be uneven, partial, and limited to selected spheres, or limited periods, of regressed function. In most respects, and for much of the time, patients with psychosomatic disorders may display highly mature and adaptive ego functions; e.g., memory, intelligence, *general* reality-testing, synthetic, executive functions, etc. Defensive ego functions also may be unevenly disrupted although regression to more primitive defenses is generally seen with altered ego states. This is particularly apparent in the ego's eventually unsuccessful attempts to master the external and internal pressures of the stressful situations that precede the onset of the clinical disorder. Giovacchini and Muslin offer important observations on ego function that are relevant to this point.[23, 24] The neuroendocrine consequences of failure of defensive function of the ego have been discussed above. All of this would lend support to arguments that emphasize the importance of reinforcing existing, or supplying effective new, ego defenses.

Engel has emphasized the possible role of object loss and the reactive affects of "helplessness and hopelessness" as central issues in the ego reactions associated with serious medical illness.[25] Schmale, working with Engel, emphasized the role of separation—real, symbolic, or threatened.[26] They emphasize the importance of paying close attention to object relations and to the variety of major "conservative" affects which may be involved when they are disrupted—this in contrast to previous theories that had emphasized anxiety and activation ("fight-flight") states. This calls attention to the clinical importance of attending to and dealing technically with overt and covert manifestations of depression in treatment of patients with psychosomatic illness.

The psychological issues just discussed are of a general nonspecific nature. They do not address the question of why individual patients develop one psychosomatic disease rather than another. This requires further brief digression into theory. As noted earlier, Alexander et al evolved a theory that postulated specific unresolved core conflicts and specific ego defensive configurations against specific affects that were thought to be associated with concomitant disease-specific physiological patterns of arousal.[1] This theory includes a constitutional (perhaps genetic) predisposition in its conceptual scheme and is a (linear) multiple-factor theory which proposes specific necessary, but not sufficient, causes in both psychological and physiological spheres.

Mirsky discovered the physiological (genetically determined) condition necessary, but not sufficient, for the development of duodenal ulcer (that is, the hypersecretion of pepsinogen into the blood), and postulated that this inborn trait, through its influence on the mother-infant relationship, played a central role in personality development and in determining the types of ego defenses that would develop and the types of social conflict situations that would later be pathogenic for the individual in adult life.[27] This, then, was an epigenetic, developmental, and circular system rather than a linear one, embodying somato-psycho-somatic sequences rather than psychosomatic ones.

Grinker,[5] Deutsch,[2] and Schur[8, 9] also recognized the incompleteness of the psychological explanations alone, and saw choice of organ system as dependent mainly upon genetic factors and/or early conditioning like psychophysiological fixations of infantile patterns of function. In other words, they believed specificity to be determined by genetic factors or by early psychophysiological life experiences which may have occurred at crucial developmental stages. Primitive and global affect states characteristic of infantile patterns of arousal were postulated to occur when defenses fail in the adult rather than patterns of specific physiological concomitants of affects, as they are ordinarily encountered in the adult. Note the compatability of these psychoanalytic epigenetic developmental models with the modern biopsychosocial systems model described above.

In a different vein, Sperling[10, 11, 14] and Garma[4] evoked purely psychological mechanisms as determining factors in choice of disease. They conceptualized the physiological changes of disease as symbolic expressions of the ego's attempts to master intrapsychic conflict. Deutsch also was impressed with the possible role of symbolic function and conversion mechanisms, and did not rule them out; but not seeming to feel satisfied with them as sole explanatory concepts, let them ride as additions to the more complex formulations described above.[2] Engel and Schmale also consider that conversion may be important; perhaps indirectly, by inducing nonspecific trophic changes in psychologically hypercathected organs, leading to lowered resistance in these organs.[28] Accordingly, they feel that the final disease state should be regarded as a complication of the conversion rather than as having primary symbolic meaning.

I have pointed out previously that after a disease has manifested itself clinically and the diagnosis has been established, the patient may then elaborate fantasies about the disease and the lesion, assign symbolic meanings to them, and then incorporate the fantasies, symbolic meanings, and other psychological reactions to the illness into his/her body image and ongoing psychological life.[16] Such symbolic elaborations are regularly encountered in the associations of patients with psychosomatic diseases. Most of them probably represent psychological reactions to disease and can be thought of as somato-psycho-somato-psychic phenomena—i.e., as reactive to the illness without having played a role in proximal etiology and pathogenesis. This is an issue that can be answered only by prospective research. As will be noted below, they might still constitute matters of central importance in psychoanalytic therapeutic process, even if they did not antedate the illness and contribute to its original development.

Returning now, in the context of specificity, to therapeutic issues: it may be that symbolism and conversion can be importantly involved in treatment—but in a second-order role, if one takes the perspective that *levels* of function and integration are of primary importance. Knapp has recently pointed out that, in analytic treatment, one may deliberately direct efforts at *relatively* superficial layers of the patients' psychic economy without exerting effects on deeper layers.[29]

It seems to me that it would be analytic work at the deeper levels that might be expected to influence visceral functions. This would imply that it should be possible explicitly to set the set therapeutic goals accordingly, and that limiting therapeutic ambition in respect to the medical disorder, i.e., short of expecting "cure," may not necessarily mean conducting an analysis that is seriously flawed, incomplete, or superficial. This is what I had in mind when I mentioned earlier that successful analysis undertaken for psychological indications might leave the basic medical disorder unaltered. In other words, if it is not feasible safely to "reach into" or "activate" preverbal, pregenital levels of psychological integration (the corresponding physiological level of integration would be the hypothesized special nervous system states referred to above), neurotic layers of the patients' personality still might be dealt with analytically—not merely supportively—without affecting the "psychosomatic disorder." All the same, it is conceivable that in particularly and specially skilled hands, (e.g., Sperling et al) these primitive levels could be penetrated or entered in ways that would permit the more mature observing ego to "understand" and to use symbolic translations of the meanings of psychobiological behavior so as to facilitate healthier, integrated psychological and physiological function. (I realize that this argument runs counter to the logic of my earlier discussion—such is the "state of the art.") I think that Deutsch[2] probably "believed" this to be possible, as perhaps do Knapp and his coworkers, Mushatt and Nemetz.[15]

The "particular ways and skills" referred to above as permitting such to occur might very well include a number of personal capacities in the analyst: (1) to establish and maintain an appropriately supportive therapeutic alliance that can weather stormy alterations in ego state; (2) to permit such states to develop and be sustained for limited phases of the analytic work; and (3) to translate primitive body fantasy meanings that emerge during such states into meanings that are understandable to the patient in the mode of secondary process thought. In current psychobiologic perspective, this would imply to me that it would be necessary to utilize CNS circuits subserving mature cognitive functions at the very same times when CNS circuits subserving more primitive infantile patterns of limbic-brain stem hypothalamic—anterior pituitary mechanisms and outflow pathways are active and malleable! This may sound fanciful—indeed it does to me. Enough speculation! Only research—empirical methods and data—will uncover the actual facts. Perhaps among the most important phenomena to study would be the work of analysts with the "special" capacities described above. It is well known that analysts of similar theoretical persuasion nonetheless differ considerably in their individual technical styles and practices.[30]

To summarize the therapeutic technical implications as I am able to understand them at present:

1.  A decision to undertake psychoanalysis with a psychosomatic patient should rest upon the usual psychological-psychosocial indications and contraindications.

2.  Psychoanalytic process with psychosomatic patients can be thought of in terms of levels. Analysis of neurotic layers of the personality—with particular attention to maintenance of adequate ego defenses, nurturance of supportive aspects of the therapeutic alliance, and avoidance of intense frustration in the transference neurosis—can probably take place without direct or fundamental influence on basic pathophysiologic processes involved in the medical illness.

3.  Work at "deeper" levels seems possible, but clearly carries risks of serious psychotic developments and/or exacerbations of the medical process. Conversely, there is some evidence that, carried out with just the proper combination of skills, it may have quite salutary effects. At the moment this possibility embodies challenging and important research questions, but is not to be generally recommended.

## RESEARCH IMPLICATIONS

It should not be necessary to belabor the obvious. I have tried to identify a variety of research questions throughout this chapter. Dahl,[31] Sampson et al,[32] Horowitz et al,[33] Gill et al,[34] Luborsky and Spence,[35] and many others, are systematizing psychoanalytic observations methods. Weiner[36] has recently reviewed the myriad of physiologic mechanisms and systems that may be involved in developing and sustaining psychosomatic disorders. The time is ripe for careful and responsible application of psychoanalytic process in psychosomatic research. Longitudinal, detailed psychoanalytic observations of (even subtle) alterations in levels of consciousness, ego states, and cognitive processes, could now well be combined with simultaneous physiologic measures reflecting relevant functions of body systems. It may be true that "nature guards her secrets jealously"—but perhaps some times more than others. This may be one of the "better" times for research.

# References

1. Alexander F, French TM, Pollack GH: Psychosomatic Specificity. Chicago, University of Chicago Press, 1968
2. Deutsch F: The Psychosomatic Concept in Psychoanalysis. New York, International University Press, 1953, pp 158–161
3. Dunbar HF: Psychosomatic Diagnosis. New York, Hoeber, 1943
4. Garma A: Peptic Ulcer and Psychoanalysis. Baltimore, Williams & Wilkins, 1958
5. Grinker R, Sr: Psychosomatic Research. New York, Norton, 1953.
6. Kubie LS: Instincts and homeostasis. Psychosom Med 10:15–30, 1948
7. Margolin SG: Genetic and dynamic psychophysiological determinants of pathophysiological processes. In Deutsch F (Ed.), The Psychosomatic Concept in Psychoanalysis. New York, International University Press, 1953, pp 3–36
8. Schur M: The ego in anxiety. In Loewenstein RM (Ed.), Drives, Affects, Behavior, 1. New York, International Universities Press, 1953, pp 67–103
9. Schur M: Comments on the metapsychology of somatization. In Eisser RS, Freud A, Hartmann H, Kris E (eds.): The Psychoanalytic Study of the Child, 10. New York, International Universities Press, 1955, pp. 110–164.
10. Sperling M: The role of the mother in psychosomatic disorders in children. Psychosom Med 11:377–385, 1949
11. Sperling M: A psychoanalytic study of bronchial asthma in children. In Schineer HI (Ed.), The Asthmatic Child. New York, Hoeber, 1963, pp 138–165
12. Lindemann E: Modifications in the course of

ulcerative colitis in relationship to changes in life situations and reaction patterns. In Wolff H (Ed.): life stress and bodily disease. Res Publ Assoc Res Nerv Ment Dis 29:706, 1950
13. Lindemann E: Psychiatric problems in conservative treatment of ulcerative colitis. Arch Neurol Psychiatry 53:322, 1945
14. Sperling M: Psychoanalytic study of ulcerative colitis in children. Psychoanal Q 15:302–329, 1946
14a. Wilson CP: Theoretical and clinical considerations in the early phase of analysis of patients suffering from severe psychosomatic symptoms. Bull Phil Psychoanal Assoc 20:1, 1970
14b. Wilson CP: On the limits of effectiveness of psychoanalysis: early ego and somatic disturbances. Panel report. J Am Psychoanal Assoc 19(3):552–564, 1971
14c. Wilson CP: The psychoanalytic treatment of hospitalized anorexia nervosa patients. Unpublished manuscript.
15. Knapp PH, Mushatt C, Nemetz SJ: Asthma melancholia and death, I. psychoanalytic considerations. Psychosom Med 28:114–133, 1966
16. Reiser MF: Changing theoretical concepts in psychosomatic medicine. In Reiser MF (Ed.), American Handbook of Psychiatry, IV. New York, Basic Books, 1975, pp 477–500
17. Sachar EJ, Mason J, Kolmer HS, et al: Psychoendocrine aspects of acute schizophrenic reactions. Psychosom Med 25: 510–537, 1963
18. Pollin W, Goldin S: The physiological and psychological effects of intravenously ad-

ministered epinephrine and its metabolism in normal and schizophrenic men, II. J Psychiatr Res 1:50–67, 1961

19. Levitt EE, Persky H, Brody JP, et al: The effect of hydrocortisone infusion in hypnotically induced anxiety. Psychosom Med 25:158–161, 1963

20. Callaway E, Thompson SV: Sympathetic activity and perception. Psychosom Med 15:433–455, 1953

21. Maas JW: Adrenocortical steroid hormones, electrolytes, and the disposition of the catecholamines with particular reference to depressive states. J Psychiatr Res 9:227–241, 1972

22. Henry JP, Stevens PM, Axelrod J, et al: Effect of psychosocial stimulation on the enzymes involved in the biosynthesis and metabolism of noradrenaline and adrenaline. Psychosom Med 33:227–237, 1971

23. Giovacchini PL: The ego and the psychosomatic state. Psychosom Med 21:218–227, 1959

24. Giovacchini PL, Muslin H: Ego equilibrium and cancer of the breast. Psychosom Med 27:524–532

25. Engel GL: A psychological setting of somatic disease: the "giving up—given up" Complex. Proc R Soc Med 60:553–555, 1967

26. Schmale AH, Jr: A relationship of separation and depression to disease. Psychosom Med 20:259–277, 1958

27. Mirsky IA: Physiologic, psychologic, and social determinants in etiology of duodenal ulcer. Am J Dig Dis 3:285–314, 1958

28. Engel GL, Schmale AH, Jr.: Psychoanalytic theory of somatic disorder: conversion, specificity, and the disease onset situation. J Am Psychoanal Assoc 15:344–365, 1967

29. Knapp PH: Unpublished manuscript. emotion and learning—psychoanalytic cross currents in psychosomatic medicine. Presented at Annual Meeting, American Psychiatric Association, Toronto, Ontario, May 1977.

30. Glover E: The Technique of Psychoanalysis, Part II, Questionnaire. New York, International Universities Press, 1938, pp 259–350

31. Dahl H: A Quantitative Study of a Psychoanalysis, 1. Psychoanalysis and Contemporary Science. New York, The MacMillan Co, 1972.

32. Sampson H, Weiss J, Mlodnosky L, et al: Defense analysis and the emergence of warded-off mental contents: an empirical study. Arch Gen Psychiatry 26:524–532, 1972

33. Horowitz M, Sampson H, Siegelman EY, et al: On the identification of warded-off mental contents. J Abnorm Psychol 84:545–558, 1975

34. Gill MM, et al: Studies in audio-recorded psychoanalysis, I. general considerations. J Am Psychoanal Assoc 16:230–244, 1968

35. Luborsky L, Spence DP: Quantitative research on psychoanalytic psychotherapy. In Bergin AE, Garfield S (Eds.), Handbook of Psychotherapy and Behavior Change: An Empirical Analysis. New York, Wiley, 1971

36. Weiner H: Psychobiology and Human Disease. New York, Elsevier North-Holland, Inc, 1977

Toksoz B. Karasu

# 5
# Psychotherapy with the Somatically Ill Patient*

The most significant development in the field of psychotherapy with psychosomatic patients came from application of psychoanalytic principles to the study of the so-called "holy seven"—bronchial asthma, dermatitis, hypertension, thyrotoxicosis, peptic ulcer, rheumatoid arthritis, and ulcerative colitis. Dunbar attempted to correlate particular personality dimensions with their respective diseases,[1] while Alexander demonstrated the existence of specific intrapsychic conflicts in different psychosomatic disorders.[2]

These principles still form the core of the working hypothesis of practitioners engaged in the treatment of patients with psychosomatic disorders. Later work of Wolff,[3] Rahe,[4] and others addresses itself to environmental friction in the life of these patients, opening an era of stress-oriented, short-term psychotherapy, application of which extends beyond the traditional psychosomatic disorders to include psychophysiological reaction as well as such problems as myocardial infarction (MI), headaches, anorexia nervosa, etc.

The current application of psychoanalytic concepts to the treatment of psychosomatic disorder is reflected in the works of Sperling,[5] Jessner,[6] and Castelnuovo-Tedesco.[7] The psychodynamic thesis of Sperling, based on her work with children with ulcerative colitis and bronchial asthma, is that every case of psychosomatic disorder has its origin in the dependency of the mother-child relationship; that is, no matter how independent and self-sufficient a patient's life may appear to be, we find on closer inspection that the patient lives in an emotional symbiosis with one object in his environment. This does not have to be the actual mother but someone who, in the patient's unconscious, serves the dynamic function of a mother figure. The psychosomatic patient cannot consciously tolerate his

*This paper was read at the Fourth Congress of the International College of Psychosomatic Medicine and appeared in the Congress Proceedings as "Psychotherapy in Psychosomatic Disorders."

pregenital impulses. He denies them completely and converts them into somatic symptoms, thus gratifying them. Castelnuovo-Tedesco emphasizes the role of fantasized or real alterations in important object relations of the patient in the exacerbation of his symptoms.[8]

Research findings have not confirmed some success that has been reported by individual therapists. In any case, the application of analytic approaches to the treatment of psychosomatic disorders has not gained wide application and practice. There are very few therapists still continuing to treat these patients with traditional psychoanalytic technique. There is no doubt that the general opinion of the public and the referring physicians also has been less than favorable in the treatment of psychosomatic patients with psychotherapy.[9]

Not much help has come from our own profession. Sperling stressed the uneconomic aspect of therapy with these patients.[5] Sifneos suggested that dynamic psychotherapy is contraindicated in the majority of the patients with psychosomatic disorders.[10] These assertions certainly have not encouraged psychosomatotherapists in continuation of their difficult work.

Most psychiatrists in the field have confined their work with these patients to consultation-liaison services, using brief intervention approaches. A difficulty has been the lack of theory and working hypothesis about which one can be relatively sure. This, I believe, is the main source of countertransference in the therapist working with these patients (as discussed in the writings of Fain and Marty[11] and Wolff.[9]

Nevertheless, a modest amount of work has continued to develop. Lazarus & Hagens have attempted to decrease postoperative delirium in cardiotomy patients with brief psychotherapy;[12] Layne & Yudofsky claim similarly favorable results with even simple interviews.[13] Surman et al have replicated the former study mentioned above, but not the latter.[14] These brief psychotherapies utilized greatly supportive, as well as educational, techniques in treatment of the patients by clearing up possible misconceptions about forthcoming procedures and teaching them simple autohypnotic techniques, etc.

The focus of this paper is on the specifics of long-term individual psychotherapy with patients who have a medical illness which may have some psychological components on either initiation or maintenance or in the etiology of the disease.

One can argue that all medical diseases may have some form and degree of psychological component. Researchers have not been able to confirm the earlier assertions that there are specific factors in the psychological make-up of those patients susceptible to certain somatic diseases, although some controversies are still quite alive in regard to others, such as the dependency struggle of ulcer patients and the hard-driven personalities of patients with MI disorders. Most of the contributors have focused their attention on the patients' personality organization; their defense mechanisms, such as denial of conflict and resistance to therapy, etc. Reckless and Fauntleroy have interpreted such denial as an archaic defense against anarchy, and stressed the inability of these patients to express neurotic feelings, especially aggression.[15] Meanwhile, O'Connor has stressed the psychosomatic patient's need to use his physical symptoms to ward off psychological insight.[16] Wolff thinks that somatic disorders often develop because emotional conflicts and individual impulses are not allowed a direct expression. There is a general agreement that most somatically disturbed patients are usually unaware of stress[17] and will deny the psychological contributions to his illness, either because they regard emotional problems as signs of weakness or as synonomous with malingering.[18] Others focused on character problems of patients with psychosomatic disorders, elucidating lack of libidinal affect on their object relationships, impoverished use of language, operational thinking, inability to regress, and lack of neurotic behavior.[19] Sifneos discusses these patients' impoverished fantasy of life, emotional constriction, and inability and restriction of self-examination (which he terms "alexithymic").[20] McDougall interprets the "psychological hardiness" of these patients as a need to refuse one's dependency, disappointment, anger, despair, etc.[21] Castelnuovo-Tedesco speaks of the ulcerative colitis patient's aloofness, detachment, and contentious demands.[8] Reckless and Fauntleroy describe this posture of psychosomatic patients in treatment as "a negative attitudinal set."[15]

Unfortunately, these hypotheses have not been translated into the language of practice which may be useful in therapy.

Treatment of psychosomatic disorders in a hospital setting utilizes a great deal of physical and psychological rest and removal of the patient from the life situation. The role of the psychiatrist in such cases is usually limited to identifying the conflict and stress in the life of the patients, areas which most patients may not volunteer to discuss. In general, the support and availability of the therapist are all that is needed and tolerated by the patient and his family and physicians. Unfortunately, patients are usually discharged to the same situation following treatment of the acute phase; these medical illnesses are usually chronic, and stresses in the life of an individual are everlasting. Of course, one can hardly recommend an early retirement to these individuals, nor should one help to promote the fantasy of a nonstressful existence. Nevertheless, the therapist may temper the indulgence in the stress, as these patients seem prone to do, if a relationship with the patient can be established. Most patients, however, tend to drop out at an earlier stage of the treatment.

The psychodynamic working theory for somatic patients is based on certain assumptions: (1) unconscious impulses are manifesting themselves in pathology of the organs; (2) the affective experiencing is somewhat inhibited or repressed and/or somatically manifested; and (3) developmental stages of the individual are somewhat arrested and have never reached the symbolic-verbal-expressive stage, operating at a more primitive organ representation. Regardless of the validity of these theoretical formulations, such generalizations are not only of little practical use but they may actually interfere with the clinician's careful evaluation of the patient as they provide ready-made explanations. Such categorical approaches may only help to comfort the therapist. The psychotherapist in the treatment of psychosomatic illness should get away from a generalized formula that may be applicable to all diseases. Rather, he should explore with the patient the role of the symptoms in his life, whatever conscious and unconscious meanings they may have taken on, and whether there are stresses that initiate, or conflicts that maintain, the patient's disease. Individual patterns of somatization, coping and defense, instinctual patterns, and character organization would require careful individual attention prior to determining the patient's suitability for psychotherapy. The criteria used to assess whether the neurotic patient and his character disorders are suitable for psychotherapy—insightfulness, the ability to relate, psychological mindedness, motivation, etc.—are quite applicable to medically ill patients. Relative lack of desirable qualities for psychotherapy, more rule than exception among somatically ill patients, should not deter the therapist from attempting to treat the patient by modifying his approach. Practitioners modify their approaches all the time to accommodate psychotics, less intelligent patients, severe borderlines, etc.

At the end of the initial evaluation, the patient and therapist may have a sense that the patient's medical illness is either reactive to the external stresses or is the result of his failing coping mechanism with or without primary or secondary gains associated with illness. Then one may formulate a treatment approach that may be acceptable to the patient. Such negotiation is quite an important aspect of working with somatic patients. On the other hand, if the therapist does not find external stresses or failure of coping mechanism but identifies certain characterological structures of the patient as perhaps either causing or participating in the initiation or maintaining of the illness, he may only attempt to do psychotherapy by recognizing that such an assumption is only an inferential one. At this time, psychotherapy may be offered to the patient. Whether the therapy is geared toward the maturation of the individual or resolution of psychodynamic conflicts, it must be understood that the therapist can only state that the patient's illness may be secondarily helped by such a process. It is important that the patient agree to such a working relationship at the beginning, otherwise the question of "what has all this got to do with my illness" will become a major obstacle in therapy, and the patient will sooner or later drop out of the treatment.

It is well known that these patients are difficult to keep in treatment. This might be partly due to factors relating to a patient—defensiveness or characterological aspects discussed earlier—and partly due to our inability to present convincing evidence that we might be of some help to them. Certainly, most training programs do not provide experience in the treatment of psychosomatic diseases. That, compounded with insecurities related to limited knowledge in the field itself, creates an unfavorable condition from the beginning. These uncertainties are easily conveyed to the patient in the earlier stages of treatment, which results in the disruption during those times, as is the case with typical psychotherapeutic situations. Mushatt's[19] findings from ulcerative colitis patients confirms that they could not tolerate the therapists' silences.[22] Therapists should be most encouraging, and actively try to engage the patient to speak. Sifneos noted that psychosomatic patients had little to talk about.[10] Most of these patients will respond by saying nothing to the question "what are you thinking?" They usually are thinking about trivial matters in their lives and are embarrassed to mention them unless the therapist insists and also reassures them that such realities are important to talk about. Most disconcerting about these patients is that material necessary for psychotherapy may not be so easily forthcoming. One can talk about such triviality as a defensive posture of the patient and an avoidance of a therapeutic situation. Nevertheless, such an approach proves to be rather useless and further alienating.

The countertransference of the therapist to these patients manifests itself in annoyance, boredom, or belittling statements of an aggressive nature, either in the guise of attacking defenses or interpreting the affective distance, further reducing the potential for therapeutic alliance. As the traditional therapeutic frame of reference is inoperative, the therapist tends to become defensive. Fantasies of impotence, rejection, and self-doubt and defeat will emerge. Such painful experience on the part of the therapist is not conducive to a sense of confidence in the patient. The vicious cycle will continue with a sense that the patient is neither motivated nor suitable for psychotherapy. Fain and Marty point out a countertransferential lack of interest in the patient's character which constitutes a chronic narcissistic blow to the therapist's interpretive powers—the patient appears impervious to his special skills.[11] In truth, the patient may have come to explore the possibilities at least, but the working hypothesis of the therapist may not be suitable for him.

## CONCLUSION

Therapists treating psychosomatic patients must be able to create a climate of therapeutic acceptance, warmth, understanding, and empathy, as well as provide all the other nonspecific elements for a supportive environment. Specific techniques for the treatment of the psychosomatically ill have to be flexible enough to include a consideration of the broad dimensions of psychosomatic theories, such as the psychogenesis of the illness, the psychological contribution or psychological predisposition to the disease, psychodynamic configuration, and character structures which may be specific to any particular somatic disorder. In some instances, none of these elements may be represented. In others, one or more of these possibilities may exist. Therefore, an individualized approach to each patient including assessment of the specific psychological factors involved is an important prerequisite to successful initiation or formulation of therapy.

On intake, a thorough psychological history should be taken. The therapist must be familiar with the disease in question, as well as its medical treatment.

Initally, the patient should not be seen more than once or twice a week because such intensive involvement generates excessive anxiety and exacerbation of symptoms. The therapist, without competing with the internist in "physicianhood," should be able to discuss the questions of the patient with regard to his illness. This will help to increase the confidence of the patient in that he may not have had all his questions handled by his internist. The patient's misconceptions and misunderstandings about the illness may have to be corrected, and his undue anxieties, fears, and concerns dealt with. Topics for early discussion may include the vulnerability and mortality of the patient, his/her fear of dying, issues of separation, etc. At one level, medical illness and its medical treatment is discussed and at the other, psychological parameters of the illness are explored. Interpretation of maladaptive defenses in psychosomatic patients at an early stage of the treatment, as Sperling pointed out, may aggravate the patient's somatic condition.[5] It is common, too, that the patient's psychological condition may deteriorate simultaneously, though feared precipitation of psychotic breakdown is rather unlikely.

In terms of technique, the therapist has to engage the patient initially in issues such as trivial daily affairs, business, etc. (operational subjects). In the case of adolescents, he might be interested in talking football, rock music, etc., in order to establish common grounds.

At the beginning, the therapist must address himself to the patient's understanding of the psychiatrist referral itself. There are fears and concerns about it as well as expectations. Most patients do show up for the first interview to pass the test of sanity, not necessarily to be helped by a psychiatrist. It is important to discuss this phenomenon at an early session; it has an educational value for the patient, as well as helping to create positive relations with the therapist.

The therapist should recognize that he is not treating medical illness, whether it is MI or ulcers, but is concerned about identifying psychosocial contributors in the patient's life to his illness, helping patients to recognize their responses to the medical illness if they are not adaptive and working to modify them. His job is to identify secondary gains associated with the illness in order to prevent maintenance of the symptoms and to anticipate and prevent psychological conflicts which might promote somatic disorders.

I suggest that the therapist should establish an authentic object relationship with the patient which serves to support him in dealing with affect and experience in the therapeutic context, flexible enough to utilize all potential therapeutic elements suitable to his patient and to formulate an approach that satisfies both therapist and patient as acceptable and workable.

## References

1. Dunbar F: Emotions and Bodily Changes. New York, Columbia University Press, 1938
2. Alexander F: Psychosomatic Medicine: Its Principles and Applications. New York, Norton, 1950
3. Wolff H: Stress and Disease. Springfield, Charles C. Thomas, 1953
4. Rahe R: Subjects' recent life changes and their near-future illness susceptibility. In Lipowski Z (Ed.), Advances in Psychosomatic Medicine, 8: Psychosocial Aspects of Physical Illness. Basel, Karger, 1972, pp 2–19
5. Sperling M: Psychotherapeutic techniques in psychosomatic medicine. In Bychowski G, Despert JL (Eds.), Specialized Techniques in Psychotherapy. New York, Basic Books, 1952, pp 279–301
6. Jessner L: Psychoanalysis of an eight-year-old boy with asthma. In Schneer HI (Ed.): The Asthmatic Child: Psychosomatic Approach to Problems and Treatment. New York, Harper and Row, 1963, pp 118–137

7. Castelnuovo-Tedesco P: Psychiatric observations on attacks of gout in a patient with ulcerative colitis. Psychosom Med 28:781–788, 1966

8. Castelnuovo-Tedesco P: Ulcerative colitis in an adolescent boy subjected to a homosexual assault. Psychosom Med 24:148–155, 1962

9. Wolff HH: The psychotherapeutic alproach. In Hopkins P, Wolf HH (Eds.), Principles of Treatment of Psychosomatic Disorders. London, Pergamon Press, 1965, pp 83–94

10. Sifneos P: Is dynamic psychotherapy contraindicated for a large number of patients with psychosomatic diseases? Psychother Psychosom 21:133–136, 1972–3

11. Fain M, Marty P: A propos du narcissisme et de sa genese. Rev Fr Psychanal 29: 561–572, 1965

12. Lazarus H, Hagens J: Prevention of psychosis following open-heart surgery. Am J Psychiatry 124:1190–1195, 1968

13. Layne O, Yudofsky S: Postoperative psychosis in cardiotomy patients: the role of organic and psychiatric factors. N Engl J Med 284:518–520, 1971

14. Surman O, Hackett T, Silverberg E, Behrendt D: Usefulness of psychiatric intervention in patients undergoing cardiac surgery. Arch Gen Psychiatry 30:830–835, 1974

15. Reckless J, Fauntleroy A: Groups, spouses, and hospitalization as a trial of treatment in psychosomatic illness. Psychosomatics 13:353–357, 1972

16. O'Connor J: A comprehensive approach to the treatment of ulcerative colitis: In Hill OW (Ed.): Modern Trends in Psychosomatic Medicine, Vol. 2. New York, Appleton-Century-Crofts, 1970, pp 172–187

17. McDougall J: The psychosoma and psychoanalytic process. Int Rev Psychoanal 1:437–459, 1974

18. Raft D, Tucker L, Toomey T, Spencer R: Use of conjoint interview with patients who somatize. Psychosomatics 15:164–165, 1974

19. Marty P, M'Uzan M, David C: L'Investigation Psychosomatique. Paris, Presses University de France, 1963

20. Sifneos P: The prevalence of "alexithymic" characteristics in psychosomatic patients. Psychother Psychosom 22:255–262, 1973

21. McDougal J: The psychosoma and psychoanalytic process. Int'l Rev Psychoanal 1:437–459, 1974

22. Mushatt C: Psychological aspects of non-specific ulcerative colitis. In Whittkower ED, Cleghorn RA (Eds.), Recent Development in Psychosomatic Medicine. Philadelphia, Lippincott, 1954, pp 345–363

Wilbert E. Fordyce

# 6

# Behavioral Methods in Medical Practice

## INTRODUCTION

The emergence of behavioral methods as a therapeutic tool in the past two decades has had enormous influence on concepts and methods in human service settings. The driving force behind these methods is the idea that behavior has clinical significance in its own right and is not to be seen solely as an extension or reflection of "underlying processes." Traditional perspectives, particularly those embodied under the term "psychodynamic concepts," have tended to view behavior virtually exclusively as the product of forces within the organism (e.g., intrapsychic forces, intrapsychic dynamics, personality traits, defense mechanisms, motivations, drives, need states). In order to understand why people behave the way they do, it was held that one needed to understand those underlying factors. And, if one were to help a person who comes asking for help, it was essential to modify those underlying factors in order to permit their troublesome behavior to change.

The basic point of departure for behavioral methods, as contrasted with traditional psychiatric views, including but not restricted to psychoanalytic concepts, is that behavior—what a person says or does—has clinical significance in its own right. Significant and enduring changes in what a person does or says may result in highly beneficial therapeutic effects for that person, whether or not one can demonstrate that there have been concomitant changes in some inferred underlying state of the organism. Behavior is not to be properly understood as solely the automatic extension or manifestation of underlying forces within the organism. Behavior is subject to influence by a variety or forces. Some of those forces may be understood in terms of states within the person (e.g., tissue needs, sets of expectancies, perceptions or discriminations of stimuli). Yet even in those instances, changes in behavior may be brought about by changing events outside the person. There are other forces which may effectively influence behavior and which reside in the stimulus environment and not within the person. Changes in that stimulus environment may also result in behavior change. A measure of impact of behavioral methods on health care is illustrated in Figure 6-1, which reports the number of articles in Index Medicus under the heading of behavioral therapy or behavioral methods.

Behavioral approaches have not been uniform or tightly homogeneous. They have ranged widely. One extreme has been the long outmoded and discarded tenets of early Watsonian Behaviorism, which sought to deny the existence of "mind" and to reduce all behavior to muscle movements and glandular secretions alleged to be virtually totally controlled by environmental factors. Anchor points at the other end of the spectrum are the more recently emerging and increasingly important methods based, in part, on the idea that much behavior, and learning or behavior change, is cognitively mediated. These cognitive processes are seen as a proper and empirically useful medium to which therapeutic attention should be directed and through which change may be brought about.

The emphasis in this chapter will be on setting forth a sampling of applications of behavioral methods to a range of medically related problems. The broad field of behavioral methods has burgeoned so enormously in the past decade, it is quite impossible to review and illustrate the full spectrum of possible applications in the space available. Some choices will be made and those will be set forth below. The examples chosen have been selected to illustrate a range of medical targets for which these methods may be used and to describe briefly how to apply behavioral technology. That technology is, for the most part, not complex; but, it is impractical to attempt to set forth a near full array of tactical details in the confines of one chapter. Readers should consult other references such as cited below for more complete descriptions of behavioral technology.

In view of the many controversies which have arisen about behavioral methods, to say nothing of the numerous misconceptions as to what the methods and their underlying conceptual bases really are, it is necessary to direct some attention first to background and contextual matters.

There is a methodological perspective or emphasis which often, though not exclusively, characterizes behavioral approaches. Behavioral methods often are "characterized by an adherence to some form of operationism, microscopic determinism, logical positivism, and pragmatism (p. 15)."[1] To make the point another way, from the behavioral perspective, there is not only a focus on the actions or behavior of people, but also an emphasis on operationalizing the procedures to be used in helping people to bring about desired changes and in assessing the effectiveness of those efforts in terms of the ensuing behavior displayed by the person. If a therapeutic endeavor does not result in some discernible and measurable change in behavior or action, both its validity and its utility are to be questioned.

As Lazarus states so eloquently, "Of course, nearly everyone, apart from ESP enthusiasts, will agree that the only way we can know anything about another

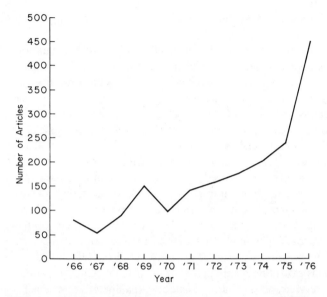

**Fig. 1.**   Behavior therapy references in Index Medicus.
(Adapted from Budd. )

person is through his or her *behavior* (verbal and nonverbal responses) . . ."[2] We
are quite unable to assess, for example, therapeutic benefits, unless we can
demonstrate (measure and count) changes in patient behavior. Without such
changes, we have accomplished nothing. The key question then becomes that of
identifying methods which will help people who come asking for help to bring about
those changes. Behavioral methods represent an increasingly important and
effective way of achieving those ends.

One of the major implications of a behavioral perspective concerns the use of
the concept of motivation. Traditional perspectives tend to characterize motivation
as something a person *has:* he/she is (or is not) motivated; i.e., he/she has (or
doesn't have) motivation. It is seen as an attribute of the person, as something which
somehow resides within the organism, and the behavior displayed is seen as an
extension of it. The occasion for some observer to identify a problem with
motivation is nearly always that the person is doing too little or too much of
something. Patients, for example, are identified as having a problem of motivation
if they fail to behave in the prescribed or therapeutically desired ways. They may do
too little of therapeutic effort or too much of some behavior incompatible with such
effort. Identification of the motivational problem stems from what they *do,* their
behavior.

A behavioral perspective on "motivational problems" addresses the question
of what behaviors are occurring and explores the contingencies or environmental
consequences which appear to relate to the incidence of those behaviors. The
remedy to motivational problems for the behaviorally oriented approach lies in

analyzing behavior-consequence relationships and seeking to modify those relationships.

There have been many challenges and criticisms of behavioral methods. Like the methods themselves, these criticisms have been too wide-ranging for all to be dealt with here, nor would it be essential to do so for the objectives of this chapter. There are three often raised issues which merit attention, however briefly. The first is conceptual. Naive critics of behavioral methods often continue to insist that those methods somehow deny that there is "mind" or "feeling states" or "conscious processes." As Franks and Wilson state, ". . . is a corpse which is intermittently exhumed by behavioral critics who seem to delight in its logical inadequacies (p. 15)."[1] There should be no need to belabor the point. As is self-evident in the previous reference to attention to cognitive processes, modern behavioral methods do not deny or ignore mental or affective processes. In the individual case of a therapeutic approach, those processes may or may not play central roles in the treatment process, depending on a variety of circumstances.

A second issue is an ethical one. Critics of behavioral methods often assert that those methods constitute manipulation of the patient. All professional interventions in human service settings are potentially manipulative whether they be, for example, surgery, prayer, medication, or psychotherapy. They are manipulative to the extent that they seek to produce effects without the informed consent of the recipient of the efforts, the patient. The issue is easily enough disposed of simply by noting that behavioral methods are not hampered in the least by fully informed consent and discussion regarding every step of the treatment plan, all to be done beforehand, as well as during the process. There are no empirical contraindications to informed consent and all of the obvious ethical and legal reasons for it. This is no less and no more true for behavioral methods than for any other treatment approach. Failure to adhere to that principle is a flaw in therapist and not in the methods.

The final issue is philosophical. Behavioral methods are sometimes characterized as "dehumanizing." That is a more complex issue; one which cannot be fully explored in a limited space. Two brief points will be made, however. The first is that behavioral methods are based, to a significant degree, on the empirical observation, verified countless times, that behavior is sensitive to consequences. It follows that one method for helping people to change their behavior is to help them to modify the consequences to the behavior and its alternatives. To argue somehow that such an enterprise is "dehumanizing" seems to be based on the premise that humans are not humans. The facts are that behavior is sensitive to consequences. To argue that that is "dehumanizing" is to argue from an incorrect view of the human organism. The essence of that argument usually appears to be that the person would prefer that behavior were not sensitive to consequences. That is logically a perfectly acceptable proposal, but is not unlike arguing that one would prefer the law of gravity did not exist. The second part of this "dehumanizing" issue usually concerns the claim that behavioral methods are "insensitive." The implication appears to be that behavioral methods are applied in an insensitive way. That certainly could be true, particularly if the therapist proceeded in some kind of heavy-handed fashion which proceeded with little attention to the ongoing feedback from the patient as to what effects treatment approaches are having. Indeed, one will encounter on occasion professionals who received the bulk of their training in learning and behavior concepts in laboratory settings and who naively assume the relatively simple laboratory setting is comparable to the complex interactional setting of the clinic or hospital. They may give behavioral methods a bad name. It is the writer's impression that they rarely do more damage than to discourage patients from persisting in their efforts to get help because patients tend simply to drop out of these naively conceived or naively executed therapeutic regimens.

These introductory remarks can be concluded by one additional point. It is axiomatic in behavior change that a behavior which is reduced or eliminated must and inevitably will be replaced with some other behavior. What that "other" behavior is ought not to be left to chance. Here we are concerned with helping people to reduce sick behaviors, to be replaced with more effective "well" behaviors. Sick behaviors and well behaviors tend to encounter different contingencies or consequences in the environment. It follows that the reduction of one does not automatically lead to its replacement by an increase in the other. For example, the reduction of visible and audible displays of pain, including particularly much guarding in physical movement, does not automatically and inevitably lead to a corresponding increase in activity level: a widening and accelerating of physical movement. The therapeutic regimen must concern itself with helping the patient to develop effective alternatives to the sick behavior and not leave that matter to chance. Often the reduction of sick behavior will be followed by corresponding increments in well behavior, but not always and not inevitably. This point certainly is central to developing treatment strategies with behavioral methods, though it would appear to be no less important for any other kind of conceptual or tactical approach in the helping professions.

## TYPES OF BEHAVIORAL APPROACHES

Any attempt to subclassify behavioral methods is fraught with complications. The methods are diverse and often overlapping. In addition, it is a rapidly growing field, making it difficult to keep up with new approaches. Somewhat arbitrarily, five families of methods will be identified and the rationale for the divisions will be stated briefly. These families of methods seem not to have anywhere near equivalent relevance, at least in the present state of the art, to management of chronic illness and related medical problems. The broad classes of approaches might be characterized as follows.

### Operant Conditioning or Contingency Management

Operant conditioning refers to the programming of environmental stimuli or consequences or contingencies as a way of helping people to bring about behavior change. It is a potentially powerful therapeutic tool. It has probably the best developed experimental and theoretical underpinning of any of the behavioral methods. Operant methods are perhaps also the behavioral approach most frequently misused by naive therapists. The misuse problem is sometimes that the methods have been applied to the wrong problem and sometimes that the right problem has been tackled with sloppy, superficial, or naive procedures.

Operant methods will be the central focus of this chapter for several reasons. The two main reasons are that they have much relevance to the problems encountered in management of chronic illness and that they lend themselves particularly well to use in chronic illness settings.

The central thrust of operant methods is that the problem is analyzed into rather precisely defined behavioral components and then the cues leading to, or the contingencies or consequences following, these behaviors (those to be decreased and those to be increased) are examined and rearranged in a fashion designed to promote the desired behavior changes.

Operant methods are not based on the assumption that behavior is changed only by changes in consequences or that appropriate changes in consequences have unlimited capability for producing behavior change. The methods are based on extensive clinical and experimental evidence that systematic management of stimuli and contingencies can indeed produce striking changes in behavior.

### Cognitive Behavior Modification

The basic distinguishing feature of cognitive approaches is that there is studied use of inner language and thought processes as one of the treatment tools. These methods are a form of self-control. The person may use, for example, either overt or covert speech as a way of cueing himself to stop or alter some behavior. For example, a person beset with intense desires to engage in a particular unwanted behavior (e.g., smoking) might develop a set of covert word signals designed to inhibit or interrupt the undesired behavior. To continue with the smoking example, a person might, when beginning the act of reaching for a cigarette, immediately begin to recite a set of reasons for not smoking, or he might fix mental attention on an alternative behavior, e.g., a visual image of a peaceful scene.

Behavior change methods utilizing cognitive components do so basically because of the evidence indicating that learning or behavior change is not simply a mechanical relationship between behaviors, on the one hand, and environmental stimuli or cues signalling the impending availability of a reinforcing consequence, on the other. There are thoughts and there is private speech and both exert influence on behavior. How much and in what ways varies enormously according to a variety of factors. Clearly, to rely solely on the behavior-change capability of such approaches is often insufficient. To deny the utility of these methods is to ignore potentially useful tools.

### Modeling

We often change our behavior in response to our observations of how others behave. The effects of modeled behavior can be very considerable. The current focus of attention on the influence of television on child behavior is one obvious illustration of the relevance of modeling.

Modeling can be a potent force in helping people to change behavior. There appear, however, to be limited ways in which modeling can be systematically applied as a studied treatment tool in reference to the kinds of settings making up the focus of this book. In the context of chronic illness, probably the major uses of modeling are: (1) to demonstrate and instruct in regard to complex motor actions (e.g., standing pivot transfers in physical therapy); and (2) to use patients who have previously undergone some procedure and who now come back to demonstrate to patients just entering the procedure that the future is brighter than the patient might now recognize. Illustrations of this approach are to be found in arranging for postmastectomy patients to visit patients about to undergo the procedure or bilateral below-knee amputees demonstrating their mobility to patients convalescing from such a procedure. Though an important behavior change process, because of the seemingly narrow range of applications to consultative psychiatry, it will receive no further attention here.

### Systematic Densitization: Including Flooding, Implosion Therapy, and More or Less Classical Wolpian/Lazarus Desensitization Methods

A central theme which runs through these methods is that there is some kind of symptom behavior, usually fear, anxiety, or muscle tension, which is associated with one or more stimulus situation in the environment. The thrust of treatment is to "de-fuse" the connection between that stimulus situation and the adverse symptom behavior so that, when encountering the stimulus, the patient will no longer emit the adverse symptom behavior. Those methods are more often used in relation to phobias and the like. They seem not often to have important utility in medical management problems. Accordingly, they will receive limited consideration here. That is not to diminish their importance, overall. Readers interested in exploring their use can consult many references, some of which are listed below.

### Biofeedback

Biofeedback is a special instance of treatment based on learning technology. As it is dealt with elsewhere in this book, it will receive no further consideration here.

### APPLICATIONS OF BEHAVIORAL METHODS IN CONSULTATIVE PSYCHIATRY

A review of the literature in relation to this chapter must have two objectives. One is to direct readers to the broad subject of behavioral methods: what they are and how they are used. The second is the more focal question of how behavioral methods have been applied to the specific context of medical problems. These will be treated separately.

Table 6-1 has given one indication of the burgeoning number of publications which have been concerned with behavioral methods. In the interests of brevity, there will be presented only a sampling of sources from which one can gain an understanding of the history, the methods, and their applications.

Lalonde[3] and Pomerleau et al[4] discuss and illustrate why behavioral methods are of such potential importance to health care.

Each year, beginning with 1973, there has been an *Annual Review of Behavior Therapy: Theory and Practice*. The introductory section to Volume 2 (pp. 1–40) provides an excellent review of theoretical and ethical issues and discussion of common misconceptions regarding the use of behavioral methods.[1]

Another excellent review of the field, with in-depth discussion and illustration of a number of areas of application is found in Leitenberg.[5]

The most comprehensive treatment of cognitive behavior modification is the recent book by Meichenbaum.[6]

The methods of systematic desensitization, or reciprocal inhibition, are set forth in detail, as well as a review and illustrations of many applications in Wolpe and Lazarus.[7]

There are numerous texts which set forth the basic procedures for operant conditioning, or contingency management, as applied to human service settings, only a few of which will be listed. Patterson presents the essentials in easily handled programmed text format.[8] Berni and Fordyce present the rudiments in stepwise fashion, with study questions and case examples based on medical settings.[9] Another programmed text approach, using a cartoon format, is found in Brethower.[10] Another excellent text is Becker.[11]

Applications of behavioral methods to medically related problems are illustrated or reviewed in several places. In addition to the *Annual Review*,[1] an excellent review of the subject is found in Katz and Zlutnick.[12]

Fordyce describes conceptual issues, underlying behavioral principles and methods, and gives detailed accounts of the use of behavioral methods in the evaluation and treatment of chronic pain.[13] Leitenberg also reports a number of medically relevant applications.[5]

We have now briefly defined a set of methods, but there remains the formidable task of relating those methods to a range of consultation problems. Behavioral methods are no respector of the classificatory schema encountered in medical practice (e.g., either specialty jurisdictions—cardiology, orthopedics, chest surgery, etc.—or body system classifications—gastrointestinal, cardiovascular, nervous system, etc.). We shall move in a different direction in trying to bring some order to the subject. The four-part classification used is somewhat arbitrary. It classifies applications into different groups of operational problems. The classifications are not mutually exclusive, nor do they correspond either to body systems or to specific behavioral methods. Each refers to a different aspect of patient behavior and/or the relationship of that behavior to the health care delivery system.

Examples selected to illustrate applications to the problem groupings will be chosen in part to demonstrate use of different behavioral methods. It should be evident, however, that the confines of a single chapter will not permit detailed presentation of the full range of essential elements to behavioral technology. The examples chosen, and the methods used, will be described specifically, but more detailed texts should be consulted to explore more fully the use of these methods.

It should be emphasized again that the examples chosen were applied with full knowledge, consent, and participation of the patients involved.

Finally, certain operation rules of thumb should be kept in mind in applying behavioral methods. These can be stated briefly.

1. Change behavior, not feelings or attitudes.
2. Clarify precisely what behavior(s) is to be increased or decreased.
3. It is easier to increase or accelerate a behavior than to decrease or decelerate it. Therefore, if possible, when seeking to decrease a behavior, proceed by working to increase a desirable behavior which is an effective alternative incompatible with the undesired behavior.
4. Always be sure that the person has an alternative behavior to move to. That is, one must not only move *from* a behavior, but also *to* a behavior.
5. Never ask a person to do something he/she cannot do. If the desired response is not in the repertoire, it must be learned before its rate can increase.
6. Positive reinforcement for performance nearly always works better than punishment for nonperformance. The major exception is in the early phases of reducing the frequency of a very high-strength, high-frequency behavior (e.g., heavy smoking, incessant scratching).
7. For a reinforcer to be effective, it must be contingent.
8. Any behavior change process using contingent reinforcement should move in the direction of diminishing reinforcement per unit of performance and, ultimately, toward termination of the special reinforcement arrangements set up to initiate behavior change.
9. High strength or preferred activities are usually the most direct and most readily available reinforcers. When programmed as contingent upon increasing amounts of the behavior to be increased, they can be very effective. This is the Premack Principle.[14]

Before proceeding with this aspect of task analysis, it is timely to portray a sampling of the range of problems which have been addressed by behavioral methods. In every kind of example cited, there will have been at least one such effort made within the past decade, usually within the past five years. Those are reported in Table 6-1.

The four subgroupings formed are identified as follows:

1. Problems of patient performance or compliance. This group of examples refers to programs designed to change the rate at which patients perform in some aspect of self-care or adherence to a prescribed regimen. The essence of this grouping is that one simply seeks to increase the rate of effectiveness of some

**Table 6-1**
Medical Problem Targets of Behavioral Methods—A Partial Listing

|                      | Reference Number                     |
| -------------------- | ------------------------------------ |
| Anorexia             | 25, 26, 27, 16, 28, and 29           |
| Asthma               | 30, 31, 32, 33, 21, 22, and 34       |
| Bowel Retention      | 35                                   |
| Dermatology          | 40                                   |
| Eczema               | 41, and 42                           |
| Neurodermatitis      | 17                                   |
| Dysmenorrhea         | 43                                   |
| Encopresis           | 44, 45, and 46                       |
| Enuresis             | 47 and 48                            |
| Epilepsy             | 20, 49, and 50                       |
| Exercise             | 9, and 13                            |
| Gagging              | 51                                   |
| Headaches            | 52, 53, and 54                       |
| Heart Problems       | 19, 55, 56, 57, 23, and 58           |
| Insomnia             | 59                                   |
| Medication Addiction | 60 and 13                            |
| Obesity              | 15, 16, and 61                       |
| Pain                 | 13, and 60                           |
| Pressure Sores       | 62                                   |
| Raynauds             | 63                                   |
| Tics                 | 64, 24, 65, and 66                   |
| Torticollis          | 67 and 68                            |
| Ulcers               | 69                                   |
| Vomiting             | 36, 37, 38, and 39                   |

well behavior. Examples in this group probably best illustrate a behavioral perspective on the concept of motivation.

2.  Reduction of unwise behavior. A brief sampling of methods which have been used to attempt to reduce smoking, overeating (obesity), and excessive drinking will be presented. The difficulty of producing significant and lasting behavior change in those problems cannot be overstated. Behavioral methods will offer no panaceas. They have been shown to produce more results than the alternatives extant—but there is a long way to go before sure methods, useful with a wide range of people, will be at hand.

3.  Changing illness behavior (symptoms) supported by environmental contingencies. This grouping will focus on chronic pain, where it is often the case that the pain problem arose for one set of reasons (nociception), but gradually has evolved to a problem now maintained by the consequences to pain and well behaviors.

4.  Direct reduction of somatic symptoms. The possible range of examples here is too vast for consideration in a single chapter. The scope of applications which might be considered is implied by the list presented in Table 6-1. The examples

chosen for illustration were selected both to indicate the range of possibilities and to illustrate a variety of behavioral approaches which might be used.

## Problems of Patient Performance or Compliance

As noted before, here we are dealing with problems of "motivation," not of skill deficits or of inability to inhibit some response. In each case cited, the desired or target behavior was in the patient's repertoire. The problem was that he was not expressing that behavior at the needed rate.

SELF-CARE IN A DIABETIC REGIMEN

Patient was a 45-year-old male schoolteacher diagnosed as diabetic three years previously and requiring 40 units of NPH insulin daily. He had three prior admissions, two for hypoglycemia and one for "diabetic coma." He had relied on his wife, a licensed practical nurse, to care for his condition. He had not mastered testing his urine and adjusting insulin intake accordingly and had repeatedly failed to maintain an appropriate diet. Both he and his wife had received (several times) the appropriate information as to what self-care procedures should be followed but, as is usually the case, information alone is a low-power way of changing behavior.

The behavior change problem could be reduced to that of helping him to (1) each six hours, collect and test urine samples, chart their color and the reaction in terms of sugar; and (2) prepare the insulin syringe, draw the appropriate amount of insulin, and inject same subcutaneously.

The strategy used was to arrange that certain consequences or reinforcers would become contingent upon units of performance of these self-care tasks. Selection of reinforcers was made by mutual discussion with the patient. The patient expressed that he felt cigarettes would be an effective incentive. Though it is a bit tangential, it should be noted that the patient also desired to reduce his smoking rate from his usual one-and-a-half to two packages per day. Therefore, these two diverse missions, increasing self-care and decreasing smoking, were blended together. (That is not usually a wise procedure, but in this case it was done and it worked.)

A point or token system was used. There were six behaviors to be performed: collect urine, test, and chart; prepare syringe, draw insulin, and inject. Each was to be done four times daily: 24 tasks. Initially, each two tasks performed at the designated times earned one cigarette. His wife participated by monitoring the cigarette supply and delivering the earned number immediately following performance. The initial reinforcement schedule was set by the patient and represented his effort to reduce smoking, as well. Each week the reinforcement schedule was cut, i.e., the second week each three points earned a cigarette and the third week each four points earned a cigarette. By that time the self-care behavior was well established, the formal reinforcement pattern was discontinued, and the patient voluntarily joined a diabetic group and a no-smoking group.

Results are shown in Figure 6-2.

One should note in this example that a high-strength behavior, smoking, was used as the reinforcer and was made contingent upon performance of the desired, but low-strength, self-care behaviors; all with the patient's full approval. It isn't always that easy.

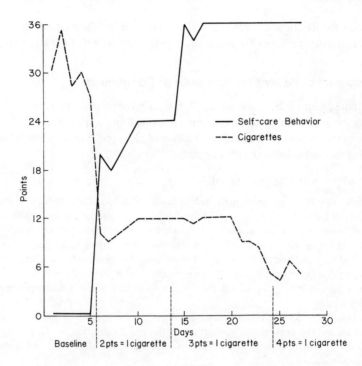

**Fig. 2.** Diabetic self-care behaviors. (Project completed by S. K. Shah, M.D. and the author.)

## PARTICIPATION IN EXERCISE: REST OR "TIME-OUT
## FROM WORK" AS A REINFORCER

Patient was a 67-year-old woman with multiple and diffuse somatic complaints, including low back pain and a history of psychiatric treatment for depression. The problem was to get her to do her prescribed walking in Physical Therapy.

Initially, a baseline (i.e., current performance level) was obtained by asking her to walk to tolerance: ". . . until pain, weakness, or fatigue cause you to want to stop. . . " Amount walked was measured as number of 200-foot laps completed without pausing. After discussion, patient agreed that rest was likely to be an effective incentive or reinforcer. Her initial performance level was three laps. Thereafter, for sessions 1–9, each lap increment yielded three minutes of rest. That is, quotas were set equaling one more lap each session. Meeting the quota led to the rest period or time out from work. For sessions 10–22, each lap increment yielded two minutes of rest. Thereafter, no fixed reinforcement plan was used. The walking session simply ended when she had met the assigned ceiling of laps, in her case 20, or 4,000 feet.

The quota method or using rest or time-out as a reinforcer is often questioned by noting the patient could also rest if she simply refused to perform. That is true, but the additional reinforcers of therapist attention and approval are also extant and, if kept contingent upon performance, usually suffice. Moreover, absolute refusal to

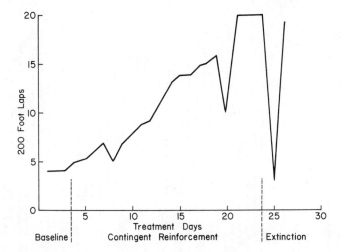

**Fig. 3.** Rest as a reinforcer to increase walking. (Project completed by Marjorie Keely, M.D. and the author.)

participate is grounds for ending treatment for the justification for continuing would appear in most cases to have fled. At any rate, in the practical case, the quota system has been used with dozens of patients for more than a decade and rarely has failed. But its effective use assumes an initial tolerance level or baseline has been established by observation, the rate of increment of quotas is set prudently (the most common rate is one unit or repetition per session) and the whole plan is explained and discussed with the patient before proceeding. Results are shown in Figure 6-3.

MAINTAINING ADEQUATE FLUID INTAKE:
USE OF SOCIAL REINFORCEMENT

Patient was a 33-year-old female with partial paraparesis, secondary to an accident. She had a history of pylonephritis, multiple urinary tract infections, and multiple suicide gestures. The problem was to help her to establish an effective daily fluid intake level (4000cc) to maintain bladder and kidney function. She found it difficult to do this despite ample instruction and reminders from ward staff and her physician.

The initial behavioral management approach used by her physician was the simplest and, in this case, proved sufficient. Physician and nurse attention in problems of this sort usually tend to be illness-contingent, i.e., special attention (lectures, pep talks, urging, etc.) tend to occur when there is nonperformance. Praise for adequate performance tends to be delayed until the next day when urinary output measures indicate adequate intake. Her physician, working with the team, reversed this. Staff worked hard to be prompt with praise and general social responsiveness on each occasion the patient was observed to request fluids, reach for them, or take them. Staff attention was withdrawn from nonperformance. In short, staff attention as regards the fluid intake issue and, to the extent practicable, in relation to other interactions with the patient, as well, became performance contingent.

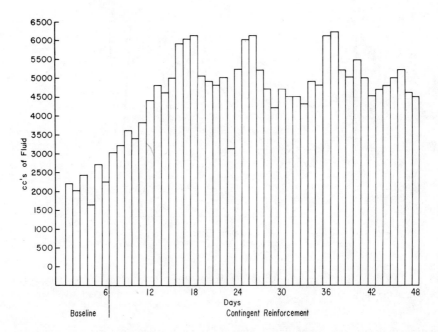

**Fig. 4.**   Attention as a reinforcer to increase fluid intake. (Project completed by Joel DeLisa, M.D. and the author.)

Figure 6-4 shows the results.

The impact and importance of the health care professional's attention on patient performance in the context of management of chronic illness can hardly be overstated. Social responsiveness is often overlooked as a way of helping patients to accomplish self-care or treatment performance tasks with which they are encountering difficulty. Sometimes staff responsiveness is misused, as when it becomes illness-contingent. The pattern then becomes a variant of the cliche, "The squeaking wheel gets the grease." To let staff attention or social responsiveness become performance-contingent does not mean the patient is ignored. One does not withdraw social attention by, for example, stalking out of the room when nonperformance is observed. One instead simply becomes neutral or nonresponsive in style: no coaxing, no casual conversation, no reassurance, no changing of the subject. Concomitantly, units of performance are followed as promptly as possible with attentiveness, praise, etc. In such a regimen, the total of patient/staff interaction should not diminish. The change is that it is programmed.

A useful variation of attention as a reinforcer is to prepare performance graphs such as that shown in Figure 6-4. When posted at the bedside, they can become powerful reinforcers for they tend to elicit from all who see special response for performance.

This section on compliance or encouraging patient performance illustrates several different methods. Point systems, leading to whatever reinforcers the patient helps you to identify as promising, have great flexibility. Similarly, the use of rest or "time-out from the low strength task" and of attention or staff responsiveness, can be applied to almost any performance task or nonperformance problem.

### Reduction of Unwise Behavior

The title of this section is arbitrary and may read as semantic moralizing. Operationally, the central theme is concern with helping a person to change well-established or extremely high-strength behaviors; behaviors which are being maintained by potent reinforcers. Moreover, because, in most instances, the behaviors have been occurring for many months and years, they almost certainly will have become associated with many environmental cues which now elicit them. For example, in the case of a long-standing smoking habit, many cues, when encountered, are followed immediately by the beginning of the chain or sequence of behaviors which culminate in lighting a cigarette. Rare is the inveterate smoker who does not reach for a cigarette the instant "The End" flashes on a movie screen, or the fork is returned to the table following the last bite of dessert, or the waitress brings the coffee or a cocktail, or the car has reached the street en route to work. In the presence of those cues promising the "benefits" of a cigarette, the desire for a cigarette is virtually irresistible.

A psychiatrist in the consultation role is not likely often to be confronted with these kinds of problems, not because they are infrequent but because it is unlikely anyone expects much can be done about such difficult problems within the confines of a consultation role. Some attention will be given to them, however, in order to illustrate some of the general strategies which have been tried—and which sometimes succeed. It would be an error to lose sight of the difficulty of these problems.

As in all behavior change projects, it is important first to pinpoint the behavior to be changed. In the case of smoking, that is easy. In the case of obesity and associated overeating, pinpointing is not always selfevident. It is essential first to identify the precise contours of the problem or the eating behavior patterns. For example, some overeaters do so only by snacking between meals; others overeat at virtually every meal; still others over-eat only by excessive intake of sweets during, for example, evening hours. Without pinpointing the problem, one would not know where to focus the change effort. In the case of eating, it is also well to keep in mind that the objective is not to eliminate eating, but rather to produce changes in the amount and type of eating. Without that precision of aim, there is minimal chance of enduring success.

Two alternative approaches to eliminating smoking will be described briefly. If one of these is to be used, the choice should be based on consultation with the patient.

The first tactical step in any approach to eliminating smoking, once there has been concurrence of patient and therapist as to the method to be used, is to reduce the environmental hazards to the program. As much as possible, the cigarette supply should be controlled. If the plan includes quitting "cold turkey," cigarettes are to be removed from the household (or hospital room). Matches and cigarette lighters are to be given away, and ash trays are to be stored. If the plan is to quit by stepwise decreases, the spouse or a confederate should be given control of the supply. Whatever the plan, if a spouse or other member of the household is continuing to smoke heavily, the plan is probably doomed to failure and serious consideration should be given to refusing even to attempt to work with the patient under such conditions.

## PLAN I: AVERSIVE CONDITIONING

Initiation of the smoking sequence may, if paired systematically with an aversive stimulus, become so aversive as to obliterate the desire for a smoke. Small, portable, low voltage shock devices can be purchased for a few dollars. The shock may be delivered to a fingertip. A series of trials, usually of many dozens, should be set up in which the patient goes through the smoking sequence (reaching for a cigarette, lighting a match, putting cigarette in the mouth, inhaling, etc.). At variable points in the sequence he administers himself a shock. These sessions should be distributed over several days and should occur at different times of day and, if possible, at different locations, corresponding as much as possible to the kinds of places in which the patient typically smokes. The arrangement is that the person can smoke as much as is desired, so long as each cigarette is accompanied by $x$ number of shocks. Assuming the program rapidly leads to cessation of smoking, there should be periodic follow through sessions spanning several weeks in which additional shock sessions occur. Those can occur with diminishing frequency, if smoking remains at zero level.

It should be obvious that few subjects will agree to this approach and, of course, it should not be attempted unless there is convincing agreement to go all the way with it. For those who do go this route, however, there is considerable probability of at least short-term success, e.g., no smoking for several weeks or months. And, if smoking is resumed, the aversive conditioning regimen can also be resumed. Those resumption regiments usually need be very brief, e.g., a dozen shocks spread across three days.

## PLAN II: REDUCTION CONTRACTING

Patient negotiates contracts with self or with therapist which specify a rate of reduction. That rate should be prudent and not naively optimistic. For example, once the daily rate is known, reduce it by one per day or one every other day. There should be clear agreement that failure to adhere to a given day's contract does not constitute total failure and justification/rationalization either for abandoning the whole enterprise or for returning to the starting point. Instead, the next day's contract becomes the same as the day of failure. Of course, any person could use that arrangement as a way of maintaining a fixed level of smoking, simply by failing each day; but the social pressures from the therapist and family members usually can overcome that kind of difficulty.

The next step is to attack the conditioned relationships between environmental cues and the smoking behavior chain. One of the simplest ways to do that is to negotiate an agreement with the patient that all smoking will occur only when standing before a toilet bowl. That choice has several advantages. Particularly, there is a low probability that that environmental stimulus has been conditioned to smoking. Secondly, your patient is never far from a bathroom and so knows smoking is always available when the demand for it is high.

A variation of this plan is to focus on the time interval between cigarattes rather than negotiating a daily quota. For example, suppose the person smokes three cigarettes each hour, and further suppose each cigarette lasts approximately 12 minutes; the average time gap to the next cigarette is then approximately eight minutes. The initial contract, once the baseline of daily consumption and average time between cigarettes has been identified by several days of observation, might then be that 10 minutes of waiting earns a cigarette. The waiting interval could then be increased by some preset rate, e.g., one minute per day. Carried to its logical conclusion, this plan ultimately leads to 24 hours of waiting between cigarettes.

CONTROL OF OVEREATING

Approaches to two different kinds of overeating problems will be described to illustrate a range of methods which have been used. There are several possible variations to each.

*Reduction of snack or focally undesired eating.* The problem here, the contour of the poor eating habit, is that the person does all right except for a circumscribed deviant or undesired pattern (e.g., evening snacking or "candy orgies"). The circumscribed character to the problem will have become evident by having your patient keep an eating diary for 3–4 days in which is recorded the time, place, amount, and kind of eating, with the units of eating shown as mouthfuls or bites.

In the arbitrarily selected example, it shall be assumed the person tends to snack in the evening while sitting before television and that it is popcorn or candy which is consumed. A contract is negotiated in which access to television becomes contingent upon remaining within a quota of mouthfuls of snack food. If the baseline averaged 30 mouthfuls, for example, when 25 mouthfuls have been reached, off goes the TV; thence on to 20, etc., across several days. Alternatively, if absence of TV proves not to be an effective deterrant, the *place* of snacking can be manipulated. For example, it might be contracted that all snacking occur from a small TV table or tray. That tray can then easily be moved. Initially, it is before the TV; then it is moved to the back of the room; then into the next room; etc.

*Reduction of generalized overeating.* Calorie counting is rarely sufficient for the person with a well-established and persisting problem of overeating. Moreover, calories are not behavior. Eating is behavior. What needs to be changed is eating.

Calories are but a reflection, and only an indirect one, of eating behavior. Weight is also not a behavior. Like calories, weight records are only reflections of eating behavior, and loose ones at that. In addition, weight can be seen as a consequence or outcome of eating behavior; but a consequence which can be known only many hours after the eating behavior has occurred. That delay is often fatally long, and so reliance on checking weight often proves not to be by itself an effective deterrent to well established eating problem behavior.

One of the simplest methods is first to establish, via diary recording, the daily consumption of mouthfuls. In the case of fluids, ignore low calorie fluids, but record each swallow of high calorie fluids (beer, soft drinks, sugared coffee) as a mouthful. Concomitantly, daily weight checks are made under standard conditions: same scale, same time of day, same garb (or lack of it). Weights are graphed, as are mouthfuls. Next, a rate of weight loss is agreed upon. This is an important issue. It should be remembered that the ultimate objective is to establish effective eating habits, not to lose weight. An eating regimen which results in rapid weight loss is ultimately risky and, during the course of such a regimen, there cannot, by definition, be rehearsal of long-term effective eating behavior. Assuming the patient is many pounds overweight, a prudent weekly weight loss rate might range from 1.5 to 2.5 pounds per week. Accordingly, after the baseline, on the weight and mouthful graph, a sloping line is drawn to reflect a projected weight loss rate of 2.0 pounds per week. Each morning the person weighs and plots that weight. If the amount recorded falls below the weight loss slope line, he is on course and may continue with the same number of mouthfuls recorded the preceding day. If the weight is on or above the weight loss slope line, that day's mouthful quota cannot exceed 10 fewer than what was recorded the preceding day. The next day, if the weight again falls on or above the line, the daily quota of mouthfuls must be cut by an additional 10. That continues until the weight again falls below the line. When that is achieved, mouthfuls remain at the lower level until three consecutive days of weight below the slope line is recorded, at which point the daily mouthful quota can be raised by 10 mouthfuls each day until weight again falls on or above the line. This method has great flexibility as to what is eaten. The person quickly learns that expending only a few mouthfuls on high calorie foods still results in a weight increase and that the need for prudence in food selection is not diminished by the plan. The plan also has the advantage of helping the person to find how much eating behavior constitutes a near maintenance level of intake so that when the target weight is reached, there is little need to make significant additional changes in eating behavior.

The approach just described necessarily relies heavily on patient adherence to the regimen. Programmed use of spouse as a treatment confederate can help in that regard.

More impact to this approach can be added by assigned differential mouthful count values to different kinds of food (e.g., three points for a mouthful of dessert, one for a cooked vegetable).

The work of Stuart and Davis[15] and Stunkard and Mahoney[16] on this subject should be consulted for more details and alternative approaches.

TREATMENT OF ANOREXIA

In a sense, anorexia nervosa is the obverse of obesity. In both cases, the central problem is that the person has a well-established but destructive or harmful eating habit. Both problems, obesity and anorexia nervosa, have proven responsive to behavioral interventions. But in the case of anorexia, the problems tend to be more circumscribed and focal. The problem occurs primarily among females, particularly in adolescence. The problem seems usually to have its origins in an excessive, phobic-like fear of obesity for which the person undertakes extreme protective efforts. That is, obesity must be avoided at all costs, and gradually there evolves a pattern of excessively restricted eating. An excellent review of the problem and of treatment methods for it can be found in Stunkard and Mahoney.[16]

There are two basic approaches which have been used: systematic desensitization and contingency contracting (or operant conditioning). They may be used separately or concomitantly. Systematic desensitization is aimed at removing the "fat phobia" so that the person is no longer concerned about obesity to the point of having to restrict dietary intake. The essentials of the approach begin by identifying the cues or body sensations which signal impending obesity (i.e., what is it that seems to tell the person, "I am (feeling) (looking) fat."). Usually, the key sensations are found to be in the eating act itself. A few mouthfuls of food, for example, are found to lead to a sensation of extreme fullness in the stomach; a bloated, extended feeling unrealistically related to the amount consumed. Alternatively, after eating, visual inspection in the bathroom mirror may lead the person to perceive himself as perceptibly fatter. In either case, or in relation to whatever other body sensation or visual cue triggers fear or concern about obesity, the standard systematic desensitization methods may be employed. A hierarchy of steps leading to the extreme of sensation intensity is then constructed in consultation with the patient. Where the key is found to relate to the amount eaten, the hierarchy may be nothing more than increasing numbers of mouthfuls consumed. The patient is then trained in achieving deep relaxation, and the steps of the hierarchy are then presented via imagery and are successively paired with relaxation until they no longer elicit the "fat fear." The imagery phase should then be followed by in vivo rehearsal. Hunger is induced. A relaxation state is produced. Then, successive increments of mouthfuls are consumed.

The contingency management approach arranges that high-strength behaviors become accessible, contingent upon increasing amounts of eating behavior. Baseline periods of eating observation are made using, for example, mouthful counting to permit precise recording of amounts eaten. In addition, daily weight checks are made, and prescribed rates of weight increment are specified (e.g., a weight graph with an upward sloping line at a pitch equaling one kilogram per week). Patient high-strength behaviors are observed to identify probable effective reinforcers. In the case of most anorexia nervosa cases, this proves usually to be a simple matter, as nearly all of them are observed to be active, restless people. One reason that is so often observed is that they probably associate activity with losing weight and avoiding obesity. It then becomes a simple matter to arrange that activities become contingent upon mouthfuls consumed. This might proceed at two levels. The most immediate is use of a wrist counter to tally mouthfuls. Selected morning activities become contingent upon $x$ breakfast mouthfuls; afternoon activities on $y$ lunch mouthfuls; evening activities on $z$ dinner mouthfuls. The required mouthful quotas can then be gradually increased. Additional activities, particularly those most intensely desired, might then be programmed to become contingent upon the daily weight check recording falling on or above the weight slope line.

It is rarely necessary in this kind of approach to be concerned about calorie counting. If they didn't know it already, and they nearly always do with exquisite precision, patients soon learn what kinds of mouthfuls help to get the weight graph record on or above the slope line, without the burden of counting calories.

## CONTROL OF SCRATCHING BEHAVIOR
## IN TACTILE DERMATITIS

Incessant or too frequent scratching which produces visible tissue damage is usually a more easily reduced or eliminated behavior than smoking or overeating. That tends to be the case for two reasons: the behavior likely has not been established as long as overeating or smoking, and therefore, has fewer cues which have been strong enough to elicit the behavior; and the adverse consequences to the behavior are more immediate and apparent.

Ratliff and Stein report treating such a problem using electric shock.[17] The shock was terminated after the scratching stopped and the person said, "don't scratch." They augmented their therapy with relaxation training, a step more likely to be important in patient's reporting marked tension associated with inhibiting scratching.

Aversive conditioning methods should, of course, never be used without full consent of the person. In addition, tactically, that approach is usually not indicated except early in the treatment of an extremely high-strength behavior which must be reduced. There are instances in which something like incessant scratching or engaging in some socially adverse behavior such as putting one's fingers to one's mouth, or nose-picking, or toying with or tugging at one's hair, occurs with great frequency and often without the person's awareness. An example patterned after a number of case studies aimed at reducing those kinds of high-strength, high-frequency behaviors will be used to illustrate. In doing so, the example will also illustrate use of a more innocuous and logistically available aversive stimulus.

We shall assume the problem is a case of tactile dermatitis, though it just as well could be toying with one's hair, etc. The first step, once agreement has been reached to proceed with the behavior change process, is to help the person to restore awareness of when the behavior is occurring. A diary form can be provided on which is tallied each instance of the behavior, noted as to time of day and place of occurrence. A sampling of 2–3 sessions in which a confederate also observes and records for 30–60 minutes and in which they then compare tallies, is usually enough to restore awareness. If not, more observation and immediate signaling by the confederate should be used. It is rarely necessary to reach a point of absolute agreement as to rate of occurrence, only to narrow the discrepancy to modest levels. Thereafter, the patient simply wears a fairly heavy rubberband around one wrist at all times. When he begins to scratch, a firm snap of the rubberband is substituted. If there is incomplete performance, additional periods with the confederate may suffice; periods during which the confederate both helps to identify scratching and insures the rubberband is suitably snapped.

It is usually helpful in the kinds of problems just described to help the person to find a more suitable way to use his hands for a few moments (e.g., interlace them and hold in the lap for 10 seconds, place each hand on the thighs and hold for 10 seconds, etc.).

Even scratching which occurs during one's sleep tends to be influenced by this approach.

### Changing Illness Behavior (Symptoms) Supported by Environmental Contingencies

There are many ways in which a person may communicate to his environment that some form of distress is being experienced. When such signals are transmitted, the environment often either sanctions and supports the protective actions of the person or takes action itself designed somehow to make the person feel more comfortable. Perhaps the most common examples are to be found in pain behaviors; behaviors a person communicates by word, action, or sound, to those around him, that there is pain and it is necessary to take protective action (lie down, take medications, walk slowly, terminate effort at the chore underway). While pain behavior is the more common example, analogous phenomena are not uncommon in chronic care facilities such as psychiatric institutions. In those settings, the display of disturbed or bizarre behavior often has the effect of reauthenticating the need for institutionalization or, in other terms, sanctioning the continued separation from life responsibilities outside the ward or outside the institution. Sometimes they occur because of the social consequences to which they lead (e.g., nurse attention, authentication of need to remain in the hospital).

A pain problem nearly always begins with some body trauma and associated noxious stimulus arising from the site of body damage. That noxious stimulus leads to suffering, which in turn is communicated to the environment in the form of pain behaviors. If the cause of the pain is appropriately diagnosed and treated, the problem diminishes and the pain behaviors cease to occur. If the problem is not effectively treated or if pain behaviors lead to highly reinforcing consequences in the environment, however, there is always the risk that those pain behaviors will come under control of environmental contingencies or reinforcers. It is beyond the scope of this chapter to explore why and how that occurs. A more detailed account of this subject, including methods for evaluating and treating such problems can be found in Fordyce.[13] For the purposes here, we shall assume we are faced with a pain problem which has existed for many months, one for which the physical findings are simply unable to account for the pain behaviors or, at the least, their magnitude *and* close inspection appear to demonstrate that there are pain-behavior-contingent environmental consequences which appear likely to be effective reinforcers for that person. The prototype of this kind of problem is "chronic benign pain," by which is meant that physical findings, currently active, cannot be found sufficient to account for displayed pain behaviors. Tumors impinging on nerve endings, arthritis in an inflammatory phase, causalgias, or sympathetic dystrophies, are examples not falling under the rubric of chronic benign pain.

Identification of what has come to be termed "operant pain"[13] proceeds essentially first by establishing by medical evaluation that physical findings do not account for the persistence of the pain behaviors. Secondly, by interview and direct patient observation, essentially two sets of questions are explored: one is, to paraphrase, "What 'good' things happen when pain behaviors occur?." Examples would be pain contingent medications, pain contingent rest, and special attention. The second set of questions concerns, again to paraphrase, "What bad things (other than 'pain') don't happen when pain behaviors occur?." This corresponds approximately to the concept of secondary gain. That is, when the person displays pain behaviors and takes protective action to limit activities, not only does such protective action apparently ease "pain," but it also effectively avoids other activities which, if engaged in, tend to be aversive. Examples are such things as staying home from a job when a recent promotion has raised one to a level one can no longer handle, avoidance of intercourse when that is an aversive activity, avoiding a social obligation when one feels uncomfortable at such affairs, or simply avoiding responsibility when one is diffusely inadequate.

The consultation psychiatrist often will be asked to evaluate a pain patient to assess whether there is "psychogenic pain." Operationally, asking about that term means one wishes to know whether the pain behaviors are controlled virtually exclusively by nociception from physical findings or whether they are controlled in significant degree—or altogether—by environmental contingencies. That is, "When I hurt do good things happen?" or, "When I hurt do bad things not happen?" These are another way of saying it hurts more to be well than to be limited by a pain problem.

To the existing experience and skills of psychiatric evaluation, only the following suggestions will be added regarding the evaluation process:

1.  The Minnesota Multiphasic Personality Inventory (MMPI) is a useful tool to help identify people who demonstrate a readiness to be sensitive to or to readily display somatic complaints, and who are seemingly not as worried about their somatic complaints as one might expect.[13]
2.  A few days of diary recording, in which is indicated when and how much the person is sitting, standing or walking, or reclining, and when, what kind, and

how much medications are taken, can be very helpful. There are often marked discrepancies between what people say and what they do. Diaries help to clarify and solidify the data.

3.  The spouse should be interviewed as well as the patient in order to get his perspective and data report.

It should be emphasized that the alternative to "respondent pain" (pain behaviors controlled essentially by nociception) is not necessarily some form of mental illness, personality disturbance, or motivational problem. For example, the absence of diagnosis of hysterical personality, conversion reaction, or hypochondriasis, etc., does not rule out presence of operant pain. Many pain patients' pain behaviors have come under control of conditioning effects simply because they received poor or disadvantageous treatment, i.e., the problem is iatrogenic. Yet others, nominally highly functional, have been subjected to extended and very militant overprotection by excessively worried spouses or parents.

When one is satisfied that there is much operant pain in the picture, there are a number of treatment tactics likely to be useful, depending upon the particular configuration of the pain problem and associated pain behaviors. Particularly, management of medications, of rest/exercise, and of family or hospital staff attention or social responsiveness should be considered.

MEDICATIONS

In all cases of chronic benign pain, pain medications should be given orally only. If narcotics are to be used, one should shift to Methadone because it is slow-acting and avoids the "soar-crash" effect of fast-acting narcotics.[18] Medications should be given only on a time contingent basis. Observe the typical time intervals before the patient requests medications. Prescribe accordingly so that the medications arrive slightly sooner (e.g., if the interval is about five hours, place the patient on a four-hour regimen), unless there is a shift to Methadone. In that case, every six hours will nearly always suffice. In either instance, the 24-hour totals should approximate what you have observed your patient as needing during 2–3 days of observation preceding instigation of the medication management regimen.

By delivering the medications in a color and test masking vehicle (e.g., cherry syrup) one can then also gradually fade the active ingredients, e.g., at the rate of 10 percent each 10 days. The order to the pharmacist should be to provide the prescribed active ingredients in the prescribed number of daily doses such that the total volume of the active ingredients plus the masking vehicle equals 10cc, and the 24-hour totals are specified.

Each step of this procedure should be explained to the patient fully before beginning, omitting only the detail as to the rate the active ingredients will be reduced. When the cocktail reaches zero active ingredients, tell the patient.

Most chronic pain patients are also depressed. A tricyclic antidepressant can be added to the ingredients making up the cocktail mix. For more details, see Fordyce and Halpern (pp. 18 and 157–167).[13]

REST/EXERCISE

Chronic pain patients who display either guarded motion or a more generalized reduction in exercise and activity level often can be helped considerably by rather simple alterations in existing rest/exercise patterns. Most pain patients, when they engage in physical activity likely to be productive of pain, do so in a "work-to-tolerance" mode. They are active until pain begins, until it accelerates significantly, or until it is intolerable, and then they rest. Rest and termination of the activity is pain contingent (i.e., if there was no pain or increase in it, they would continue with the activity. The working-to-tolerance mode is often prescribed by physicians. Or, it may be simply that family members admonish the patient to stop when pain begins or increases. A perhaps even more important reason for patients using that pattern is that the patient interprets the pain signal as an indication that, were he to continue with activity, pain would worsen and there would be a risk of further tissue damage, thereby worsening the pain problem. That is the "warning function" interpretation of pain. It is one we have all learned, particularly pain patients. But in cases of chronic benign pain, after a few weeks following onset, all indications are that continued activity would not result in additional tissue damage; perhaps a temporary increase in pain, but not additional body damage. In short, "pain" no longer has the "warning function" meaning in many cases of chronic pain—but the patient and the family do not understand that.

In those chronic pain patients where overall activity level has been lowered by much reclining or sitting instead of moving around, or where specific kinds of activities or body motions are avoided because of anticipated pain, there is much that can be done on a consultative basis to help reduce the problem. The objectives are to increase activity; to restore lost function.

Physicians suitably trained in exercise selection and prescription should define what exercises or body motions are not tissue destructive and the ceilings of each exercise which should not be exceeded. Given this set of prescribed activities, and nearly always walking and stair climbing should be included unless specifically contraindicated, a handful of working-to-tolerance sessions are set up. The patient is instructed to do as many, for example, pelvic tilts, or deep knee bends, or laps walked on a measured course (without pausing to rest) ". . . until pain, weakness or fatigue cause you to want to stop. You decide when to stop. We need to know how much you can now do so that we can design a treatment program to help." The number of repetitions of each procedure is recorded each time. This yields a baseline or starting point. Next, one shifts to working-to-quota. Quotas are set such that rest or the end of the exercise becomes contingent upon accomplishing a specified amount, rather than according to how one feels. Quotas are to be met but not exceeded. Initial quotas should be clearly lower than baseline values (e.g., slightly below average of the baseline values). Quotas then are set to increase at a preset rate (e.g., one repetition per session or one repetition each two sessions). The rate of increment is a judgment based on estimates of probable patient tolerance. When in doubt, increment slowly, but do it at a preset rate and not according to how the patient feels. This arrangement has the effect of helping the patient out of the trap of setting activity level according to whether any pain is experienced.

Continued recording of performance and transfer to graphs can add an important source of reinforcement as the patient displays to family and staff the increases in performance.

ATTENTION

Attention or social responsiveness becomes important for many chronic pain patients' management programs in two ways. First, in the hospital or treatment setting, it is often the case that health care professionals tend to let their attention become illness or pain contingent. If a nurse, for example, sees a patient suffering, that nurse may be particularly ready to provide reassurance and emotional support. If, on the contrary, there is no display of distress, that busy nurse may see no need for input and may proceed about her business. She then will have let her attention become illness contingent and will have, to some extent, withheld it from activity or well behavior. In the case of chronic illness with a history of extensive contacts with health care professionals, the staff attention factor can become a potent force. Often it is misused to the disadvantage of patient and all others involved.

Attention as a treatment tool in behavioral management of chronic benign pain can be outlined briefly:

1.  On rounds and in patient contacts, ask not how the patient feels. To do that is to attach professional responsiveness to pain behaviors. Ask what the patient has done (e.g., how many laps did you walk? how many situps?). That both attaches attention to the desired well behaviors of increased activity and also adds additional sanction to the value and safety of increases in activity, thereby reassuring the patient that it is safe to continue with more exercise.
2.  Do not ignore patients, nor information they provide you regarding pain. That would be both unethical and imprudent. Maintain eye contact and a socially neutral manner while the patient tells you about pain developments (this is now in the treatment phase, not in evaluation). If there is new information suggesting some complicating change in the picture, act accordingly. Assuming one is simply hearing a renewal of previously well rehearsed pain behaviors, however, wait until the patient is finished, shrug as if not worried about what you've heard, and say something like ". . . okay, but how many laps did you do yesterday afternoon?"
3.  Be sure that therapists working with the patient are appropriately attentive and responsive when the patient does perform to meet quotas. Praise, recording of performance, and assistance in preparing graphs are all helpful.

Again, it is entirely appropriate and desirable to indicate to the patient at the outset of such a regimen that staff attention is considered an important aspect of treatment. Moreover, how others respond to one's indications of pain can have significant effect. Therefore, professional responsiveness will tend to be withdrawn from signals of pain—non-responsiveness, not ignoring expressions of pain—and will, so far as possible, be attached to exercise and activity.

The second dimension to the attention issue concerns family members. Spouses in particular often have come to be militantly attentive in response to pain behaviors to the point of vigorously chastizing the patient to take it easy, to be protective of oneself. Sometimes spouse responsiveness is a potent force helping to maintain pain behaviors, sometimes not. Care should be exercised in studying this problem with each patient and spouse. The kinds of spouse reactions which may positively reinforce pain behaviors are sometimes quite subtle and obscure. Sometimes all that is needed from the spouse for reinforcement to occur is an indication by eye contact that the pain behavior was seen or heard. In effect, the patient has reauthenticated that the pain problem still exists and the spouse has acknowledged the same. Whatever the pattern, it often proves helpful and sometimes crucial to help that spouse to change those responses. Procedures for helping them to accomplish this can also be outlined briefly:

1. Be sure the spouse can identify what verbal or nonverbal behaviors signal there is "pain."
2. Help the spouse to identify precisely what responses in fact occur by the spouse when pain behaviors are observed.
3. Work out alternatives which move in the direction of withdrawing attention, social responsiveness, or support to pain behaviors while, concomitantly, being sure that there is militant responsiveness and attention toward each increment of activity and movement toward well behavior.

In closing this section, it should be emphasized that these methods assume that there will have been a thorough and competent medical evaluation preceding the behavioral intervention. Success of the methods also will depend in large measure on how precisely they are applied. If the effort is to occur on an outpatient basis, the changes for success, while not eliminated, are diminished considerably if the patient lives in an environment which continues richly to reinforce pain behaviors and/or to discourage activity and well behavior. Finally, in the space available, there has been only a sampling of the tactical steps one might use to help restore function to the chronic pain patient.

## Direct Reduction of Somatic Symptoms

As shown previously in Table 6-1, the range of symptoms found in medical settings which have undergone treatment by some form of behavioral methods is enormous. With few exceptions, the behavioral approaches used have proceeded along one or a combination of these lines:

1. The "medical" or physiological defect illness problem leads to occurrence of behavior which is disadvantageous to the patient and which, as an operant, may be influenced by contingency management approaches. An example of this would be a postmyocardial infarction patient who so fears a recurrence he

excessively guards movement and interprets proprioceptive and other cues elicited by movement as precursors of cardiac pain. In such an example, the behavior of overguarding, overprotecting, restricting activity, originates from an illness but, as an operant, may be changed by systematic conditioning procedures. It is not the original symptom which is changed, but a spin-off from it.

2.  The "medical" symptom is likely to occur under certain stimulus conditions or in certain physiological states (e.g., tension) and may be prevented or reduced in frequency by interrupting the chains of stimulus events which otherwise culminate in the symptom, or by modifying those physiological states. Examples of the former are found in the work done to interrupt chains of behavior leading to seizures. Examples of the latter are found in training asthmatics to achieve mastery over relaxation so that they become more effective in inhibiting or reducing the intensity of asthmatic attacks.

3.  The "medical" symptom itself, while generally identified as a "medical problem," can be understood as well as an occurrence of an operant which has come under control of contingent reinforcement and whose rate may be reduced by operant conditioning methods. Some cases of so-called projectile vomiting, encopresis, enuresis, gagging, bowel retention, and, in at least one study, premature ventricular contractions, illustrate.

Examples of each class of problem will be presented to illustrate the possibilities.

Rapp and Thomas treated, by use of systematic desensitization procedures, a post-myocardial infarction patient who was overprotecting himself.[19] They identified first the activities which, when attempted, resulted in "angina episodes." They then trained the patient in relaxation techniques, in the Wolpian mode, and reconditioned him to experience a response incompatible with the angina pains, i.e., relaxation. This was first done in imagery and then transferred to in vivo rehearsal, as in driving a car.

The work previously described on chronic benign pain also illustrates this kind of problem. Nearly all chronic pain patients will have sustained body damage either at the onset of their pain problems or as a result of surgeries. As noted above, it is often not pain, per se, but guarding behaviors which get them into trouble.

The work of Zlutnick, Mayville, and Moffat regarding seizure control illustrates analyzing behavior chains leading to occurrence of a symptom and then, by interrupting the chain and leading the person to an incompatible response, reducing symptom occurrence.[20] The one essential requirement for this approach to hold promise is that there are behaviors which reliably precede seizures. They report work with 19 such patients. All of their patients had formal diagnoses of epilepsy and had seizure rates of at least one per day. Their basic procedure was first to observe the patient in order to identify behaviors which systematically preceded seizures. Next, they devised ways of interrupting those behaviors so that they could not be completed. They used punishment procedures by forcibly interrupting the behaviors. For example, one youngster would, as the first link in the behavior chain leading to a seizure, stare with fixed gaze at a flat surface (wall or table top). When that behavior was observed during treatment sessions, the punishment procedure was applied. That procedure consisted of the therapist shouting "No!"; seizing the youngster by the shoulders and giving one vigorous shake. If the chain proceeded on its way and a seizure occurred, there were no contingencies applied to the seizure, nor was there any special attention given to it. The treatment phase was a six-hour observation period for three five-day weeks. The rate of minor seizures dropped from approximately twelve per day to near zero. Treatment effects carried over into other environments and persisted through the six-month follow-up.

Lukeman reviews treatment of a series of asthmatics by combinations of relaxation, systematic desensitization, counterconditioning, etc., with the treatment methods applied at the initiating or precipitant stage of attacks.[21] Additional work has been done with biofeedback, but that will be left for another chapter.

Neisworth and Moore report a case study in which a seven-year-old asthmatic male was able to reduce frequency of asthmatic attacks simply by receiving monetary reinforcement for reduction in the rate of attacks.[22]

A wide range of "medical" symptoms have been directly attacked by behavioral methods.

Weiss and Engel report treating eight patients with premature ventricular contractions (PVC). The procedure they use is described:

. . . the patient lay in a hospital bed in a sound-deadened room. At the foot of the bed was a vertical display of three differently colored light bulbs, an intercom, and a meter.

The three lights provided the patient with feedback information about his cardiac function. The top light (green) and the bottom light (red) were cue lights. The middle light (yellow) was the reinforcer; it was on when the patient was producing the correct heart rate response. Our system enabled us to feed back this information to the patient on a beat-to-beat basis.

When the fast (green) cue light was on, a relative increase in heart rate would turn on the reinforcer light. When the slow (red) cue light was on, a relative decrease in heart rate would turn on the reinforcer light.

The meter accumulated time. Whenever the patient was performing correctly, the meter arm moved, and when he performed incorrectly, it stopped.[23]

Further details as to number of trials, duration of treatment, etc., will not be related here. The important point is to note that they were able to demonstrate significant reduction in PVC's in several of their patients.

Thomas, Abrams, and Johnson describe treatment of tics and associated involuntary vocalizations and body movements in a case of Gilles de la Tourette's Syndrome.[24] Careful and extensive observation of the patient in a variety of settings indicated considerable variability in the rate of symptom occurrence in different stimulus settings in a way suggesting tension/anxiety was one element in the picture. Accordingly, treatment consisted essentially of two elements. First, relaxation training was carried out and a systematic desensitization program followed. The hierarchy, in this case, consisted of an ordering of stimulus situations from lesser to greater probability of evoking high-symptom rates. When that task had been completed, a second element was added, self-monitoring of symptom occurrence. The act of monitoring and recording symptom occurrence served both to assist the patient better to identify the target behaviors in order to promote inhibition and to provide reinforcing feedback as to changes in symptom rate under the impact of treatment. Eventually, symptom rate diminished from a starting baseline of approximately 4.5 per minute to virtually zero.

## PROMISING FUTURE DEVELOPMENTS

Perhaps the most important impact on medical practice of behavioral concepts and methods has been to help people to look at patient problems from more than simply a disease model perspective. Particularly in relation to chronic illness, the behavioral implications of patient problems become ever more evident.

One of the areas of application, not considered in this chapter, mainly because it is still in such a state of infancy, concerns the use of precision teaching methods for the modification of performance capabilities in the brain-injured. It is well understood that the single most common functional impairment associated with cortical defect is a reduction in learning rate or efficiency. Yet the methods by which therapy seeks to restore and retrain a function draw heavily on imprecise and not well designed (from a learning technology viewpoint) reteaching approaches. Bioengineering and behavioral engineering have begun to produce increasingly sophisticated electronic and mechanical equipment which make possible the use of precision signals and feedback systems for fine mesh units of patient performance. This support equipment and technology make it increasingly possible to apply precision teaching approaches to perceptual, motor, language/speech, and body postural behaviors which are often impaired by brain injury. Social behavior problems resulting from the disinhibitory effects of brain stem contusion, for example are also now becoming more accessible to intensive therapeutic intervention by precision teaching methods. The methods are still in their early development stages and the tactical steps in developing therapy programs require much more experimentation and experience, but it seems likely in the next few years that there will be significant gains by use of these methods in the restoration of function, including complex social behaviors, in people with cortical defects.

## CONCLUSION

It is evident that the surface has hardly been scratched in regard to the use of behavioral concepts and methods, including but not restricted to biofeedback, in the evaluation and management of chronic illness, as well as in preventive medicine. A host of major strategy and administrative questions are raised by the emergence of behavioral methods.

One of the most difficult problems to contend with is that most of health care is based implicitly on a mind-body dualism, i.e., the problem is physical or it is mental. Jurisdictional lines are drawn on that basis (e.g., medicine versus psychiatry), and third party payment policies often delimit one to the advantage of the other. One need only consider, however, the work done with biofeedback regarding migraine headaches or the work with operant methods regarding chronic pain, to recognize that what we knew all along was not valid, indeed is not valid—namely, that mind-body dualism is a philosophical and empirical fallacy. Alas, this belief persists and limits patients' opportunity for treatment. Any number of chronic low back pain, or postwhiplash patients, have been denied treatment, when there was an abundance of evidence to indicate, had they undergone an operant approach, their pain likely would have been relieved and health care utilization costs would have been markedly reduced. Treatment was denied because the frame of reference for classifying their pain was either "body" (e.g., physical findings) or "mind" (e.g., psychological or conversion reaction), which are often held to be *the* alternatives to pain related to physical findings and which are then often identified as indicative of some mental disturbance.

Examination of illness from both a disease and behavioral, or learning model, perspective, makes evident that each has its place and neither is exclusive of the other. Illness must be viewed from both perspectives and treatment strategies must take both into account.

A related issue, which likely will become more visible in the coming years, concerns the concept of Behavioral Medicine. Conceptually, that is somewhat the subject of this chapter. There is the question of whether it is better strategy to attempt to equip health care purveyors with the rudiments and experience in the use of behavioral science or behavioral medicine modules. Those are not mutually exclusive alternatives. Although, after several years of clinical practice in the use of behavioral methods in medical settings and in teaching their use to medical students, residents, etc., this writer is now persuaded that the range of interests, skills, and personal priorities, is too broad to expect that one can simply add behavioral science components to medical education and get the job done. Health care delivery units will need to add to their resources adequately trained and experienced behavioral scientists. That task, in turn, is not accomplished by reliance on traditionally trained psychiatrists who sometimes characterize themselves as behavioral scientists, but who, as that term is used here, appear to be not at all equipped in the application of behavioral methods for a range of health care problems. Nor is it accomplished by adding a handful of credit hours to a psychiatric training program which has significant other priorities, as well. An increasing number of psychiatrists, as well as psychologists, are becoming knowledgeable about, and skilled at, behavioral analysis of patient and illness problems and at applying behavioral methods to their remediation. They are not getting there by a smattering of training.

In short, it is this author's view that health care, in order to be effective, must have behavioral science as one of its central themes. The importance of that point increases as we are faced more and more with chronic illness and disability instead of acute, recent onset, short-term illness problems. The importance of the point also increases as it is more fully recognized that, as the Lalonde monograph points out so clearly, many of the chronic illness problems are themselves products of persisting patient behaviors which are destructive of health.[3] To cope with these issues the system will need people who are extensively trained and experienced in use of these methods, else patient care and illness incidence and prevalence will suffer from sins of omission and commission.

## References

1. Franks CM, Wilson TG (Eds.): Annual Review of Behavior Therapy: Theory and Practice. 2. New York, Brunner/Mazel, 1974
2. Lazarus AA: Has behavior therapy outlived its usefulness? American Psychologist 32:552–557, 1977
3. Lalonde M: A New Perspective on the Health of Canadians: A Working Document. Ottawa, Ministry of National Health and Welfare, 1974
4. Pomerleau O, Bass F, Crown V: Role of behavior modification in preventive medicine. N Engl J Med 292:1277–1282, 1975
5. Leitenberg H (Ed.): Handbook of Behavior Modification and Behavior Therapy. Englewood Cliffs, New Jersey, Prentice-Hall, Inc, 1976
6. Meichenbaum D: Cognitive Behavior Modification: An Integrative Approach. New York and London, Plenum Press, p. 305, 1977
7. Wolpe J, Lazarus A: Behavior Therapy Techniques: A Guide to the Treatment of Neuroses. London, Pergamon Press, 1966
8. Patterson G: Families: Applications of Social Learning to Family Life. Champaign, Illinois, Research Press, 1971
9. Berni R, Fordyce W: Behavior Modification and the Nursing Process. St. Louis, Missouri, CV Mosby Company, 1973
10. Brethower DM: A Total Performance System. Kalamazoo, Michigan, Behavior Delia, Inc., 1972
11. Becker W: Parents are Teachers: A Child Management Program. Champaign, Illinois, Research Press, 1970
12. Katz R, Zlutnick S (Eds.): Behavior Therapy and Health Care: Principles and Applications. Elmsford, New York, Pergamon Press Inc, 1975
13. Fordyce W: Behavioral Methods for Chronic Pain and Illness. St. Louis, Missouri, CV Mosby Company, 1976
14. Premack D: Toward empirical behavior laws, I. positive reinforcement. Psychol Rev 66:219–233, 1959
15. Stuart R, Davis B: Slim Chance in a Fat World: Behavior Control of Obesity. Champaign, Illinois, Research Press, 1972
16. Stunkard A, Mahoney J: Behavioral treatment of the eating disorders. In Leitenberg (Ed.), Handbook of Behavior Modification and Behavior Therapy. Englewood Cliffs, New Jersey, Prentice-Hall, Inc, 1976, pp. 45–73
17. Ratliff R, Stein N: Treatment of neurodermatitis by behavior therapy: a case study. Behav Res Ther 6:397–399, 1968
18. Halpern L: Analgesics and other drugs for relief of pain. Postgrad Med 53:91–100, 1973
19. Rapp M, Thomas M: Alleviation of angina pectoris following systematic desensitization. Can Psychiatr Assoc J 20:96, 1975
20. Zlutnick S, Mayville W, Moffat S: Behavioral Control of Seizure Disorders: The Interruption of Chained Behavior. London, Pergamon Press Inc, 1975, pp. 317–336
21. Lukeman D: Conditioning methods of treating childhood asthma. J Child Psychol Psychiatry 16:165–168, 1975
22. Neisworth J, Moore F: Operant conditioning of asthmatic responding with the parent as therapist. Behav Ther 3:95–99, 1972
23. Weiss T, Engel B: Operant conditioning of heart rate in patients with premature ven-

tricular contractions. Psychosom Med 33: 301–321, 1971

24. Thomas E, Abrams K, Johnson J: Self-Monitoring and reciprocal inhibition in the modification of multiple tics of Gilles de la Tourette's Syndrome. J Behav Ther Exp Psychiatry 2:159–171, 1971

25. Garfinkel P, Kline S, Stancer H: Treatment of anorexia nervosa using operant conditioning techniques. J Nerv Ment Dis 6:428–433, 1973

26. Leibman R, Minuchin S, Baker L: An integrated treatment program for anorexia nervosa. Am J Psychiatry, 131:432–436, 1974

27. Schaefer K, Schawartz D: Behavior therapy with anorexia nervosa. Z Klin Psychologie Psychother 22:267–284, 1974

28. Mann R: The behavior-therapeutic use of contingency contracting to control an adult behavior problem: weight control. J Appl Behav Analysis 00:99–109, 1972

29. Mahoney M, Moura N, Wade T: Relative efficacy of self-reward, self-punishment, and self-monitoring techniques for weight loss. J Consult Clin Psychol 40:404–407, 1973

30. Alexander A, Miklich D, Hershkof H: The immediate effects of systematic relaxation training on peak expiratory flow rates in asthmatic children. Psychosom Med 34: 388–394, 1972

31. Creer T: The use of time-out from positive reinforcement procedure with asthmatic children. J Psychosom Res 14:117–120, 1970

32. Cooper A: A case of bronchial asthma treated by behavior therapy. Behav Res Ther 1:351–356, 1964

33. Davis M, Saunders D, Creer T: Relaxation training facilitated by biofeedback apparatus as supplemental treatment in bronchial asthma. J Psychosom Res 17:121–128, 1973

34. Reckless J: A behavioral treatment of bronchial asthma in modified group therapy. Psychosomatics 12:168–173, 1971

35. Tomlinson J: Treatment of bowel retention by operant procedures: a case study. J Behav Ther Exp Psychiatry 1:83–85, 1970

36. Hubel K: Voluntary control of gastrointestinal function: operant conditioning and biofeedback. Gastroenterology, 66:1985–2090, 1974

37. Lang P, Melamed B: Case report: avoidance conditioning therapy of an infant with chronic ruminative vomiting. J Abnorm Psychol 1-8, 1969

38. Kohlenberg R: The punishment of persistent vomiting: a case study. J Appl Behav Anal 3:241–245, 1970

39. Wolf M, Birnbrauer J, Williams T, Lawler J: A note on apparent extinction of the vomiting behavior of a retarded child. In Ullmann L, Krasner L (eds.): Case Studies in Behavior Modification. Holt, Rinehart and Winston, Inc., 1965.

40. Bar L, Kuypers B: Behavior therapy in dermatological practice. Br J Dermatol 88:591–598, 1973

41. Miller R, Coger R, Dymond A: Biofeedback skin conductance conditioning in dyshidrotic eczema. Arch Dermatol 109:737–738, 1974

42. Waxman D: Behavior therapy of psoriasis, a hypno-analytic and counter-conditioning technique. Postgrad Med J 49:591–595, 1973

43. Tasto D, Chesney M: Muscle relaxation treatment for primary dysmenorrhea. Behav Ther 5:668–672, 1974

44. Ayllon T, Simon S, Wildman R: Instructions and reinforcement in elimination of encopresis: a case study. J Behav Ther Exper Psychiatry 6:235–238, 1975

45. Bach R, Moylan J: Parents administer behavior therapy for inappropriate urination and encopresis: a case study. J Behav Ther Exper Psychiatry 6:239–241, 1975

46. Wright L: Handling the encopretic child. Professional Psychology 4:137–144, 1973

47. Foxx R, Azrin N: Dry pants: a rapid method of toilet training children. Behav Res Ther 2:435–442, 1973

48. Atthowe J, Jr; Controlling nocturnal enuresis in severely disabled chronic patients. Behav Ther 3:232–239, 1972

49. Parrino J: Reduction of seizures by desensitization. J Behav Ther Exper Psychiatry, 2:215–218, 1971

50. Forster F: conditioning in sensory evoked seizures. Conditional Reflex, Vol. 1, No. 4, Philadelphia, J.B. Lippincott Company, 1966

51. Epstein Hersen M: Behavioral control of hysterical gagging. J Clin Psychol 30:99–100, 1974

52. Warner G, Lance J: Relaxation therapy in migraine and chronic tension headaches. Med J Aust 1:298–301, 1975

53. Sargent J, Walters D, Green E: Psychosomatic self-regulation of migraine headaches. Semin Psychiatry 5:415–428, 1973

54. Koppman J, McDonald R, Kunzel M: Voluntary regulation of temporal artery diameter by migraine patients. Headache 14:133–138, 1974

55. Suinn R, Brock L, Edie C: Behavior therapy for type A patients. Am J Cardiol 36:269, 1975

56. Blanchard E, Haynes M: Biofeedback treatment of a case of Raynaud's Disease. J Behav Ther Exper Psychiatry 6:230–234, 1975

57. Scott R, Blanchard E, Edmunson E, Young L: A shaping procedure for heart rate control in chronic tachycardia. Percept Mot Skills 37:327–338, 1973

58. Lang P, Gratchel R, Troyer W, Twentyman C: Differential effects of heart rate modification training on college students, older males, and patients with ischemic heart disease. Psychosom Med 37:429–446, 1975

59. Nicassio P, Bootzin R: A comparison of progressive relaxation and autogenic training as treatment for insomnia. J Abnorm Psychol 83:253–260, 1974

60. Fordyce W: Operant conditioning in the treatment of chronic pain. Arch Phys Med Rehab 54:399–408, 1973

61. Hall S, Hall R, Borden B, Hanson R: Follow-Up strategies in the behavioral treatment of overweight. Behav Res Ther 13:167–172, 1975

62. Malament I, Dunn M, Davis R: Pressure sores: an operant conditioning approach to prevention. Arch Phys Med Rehab 56:161–165, 1975

63. Blanchard E, Young LD: Clinical applications of biofeedback training. Arch Gen Psychiatry 30:573–589, 1974

64. Rafi A: Learning theory and the treatment of tics. J Psychosom Res 6:71–76, 1962

65. Hersen M, Eisler R: Behavioral approaches to study and treatment of psychogenic tics. Genet Psychol Monogr 87:289–312, 1973

66. Haidar A, Clancy J: Case report of successful treatment of reflex trigeminal nerve blepharospasm by behavior modification. Am J Opthamol 75:148–149, 1973

67. Cleeland C: Behavioral techniques in the modification of spasmodic torticollis. Neurology 23:1241–1247, 1973

68. Brierley H: The treatment of hysterical spasmodic torticollis by behavior therapy. Behav Res Ther 5:139–142, 1967

69. Welgan P: Learned control of gastric secretions in ulcer patients. Psychosom Med 36:411–419, 1974

Richard I. Shader
Daniel R. Weinberger
David J. Greenblatt

# 7

# Psychopharmacological Approaches to the Medically Ill Patient

## INTRODUCTION

Psychotropic drugs have become the most frequently prescribed class of pharmacological agents in the world. Many patients who receive these medications for symptomatic relief also suffer from concomitant medical illness. When symptoms of emotional distress appear in patients with serious medical diseases, physicians often resort to therapy with psychotropic drugs because they may offer relatively rapid symptomatic benefit and are usually simple to administer. Surveys of drug usage in hospitals and medical clinics reveal high percentages of patients receiving this form of therapy.[1-4] In some recent surveys, physicians have treated over 50 percent of their hospitalized medical patients with antianxiety or hypnotic drugs.[5, 6] In another such study, over 65 percent of patients visiting an ambulatory general medical clinic had a history of psychotropic drug use.[2] The Boston Collaborative Drug Surveillance Program showed that the frequency of psychotropic drug treatment in the long-term management of certain chronic diseases such as cardiac disease, hypertension, and gastrointestinal disorders, ranged from 27 to 32 percent.[1]

Further analysis of drug dispensing patterns indicates that the vast majority of psychotropic drug prescriptions come from nonpsychiatric physicians. Internists, surgeons, and family practitioners write more than 70 percent of all such prescriptions.[7] Thus, physicians commonly encounter patients, physiologically compromised by medical disease and already undergoing medical therapy, who may require additional pharmacologic intervention for treatment of emotional disturbances associated with, or perhaps caused by, their primary medical problems or treatment.

Polypharmacy, or use of multiple drugs concurrently, has generated considerable concern due to the possibility of adverse drug reactions caused by drug interaction. Psychotropic agents, because of their common use in medical patients, have the potential for participating in many such interactions. Furthermore, many psychopharmacological agents in themselves possess multisystem effects which can alter metabolic or physiological processes already compromised by disease. Accordingly, the physician called upon to administer a drug for emotional symptoms in a medical patient faces many potential problems. He must first assess whether such treatment offers the symptomatic benefit sought in the medical setting. This requires an understanding of certain relationships between emotional symptoms and medical illness, relationships which are often misleading. For example, just as digitalis-induced tachyarrhythmias must be differentiated from those requiring a digitalis glycoside, depression associated with methyldopa therapy or myxedema must be approached with treatment other than tricyclic anti-depressants. Next, untoward pharmacological effects that may complicate a medical condition require consideration. If a post-myocardial-infarction patient in the coronary unit becomes psychotic, a drug such as chlorpromazine with pronounced alpha-adrenergic blocking properties could drastically diminish coronary perfusion pressure.

In addition to such physiological considerations, an understanding of possible drug interactions also governs the rational use of these drugs. Psychopharmacological agents may alter, for example, absorption, protein-binding, and/or metabolism of medical drugs and vice versa. The barbiturate-anticoagulant interaction is a familiar example. In essence, the physician faced with emotional symptomatology in a medical patient must decide whether psychotropic drugs are indicated, whether they will affect the medical illness and/or its treatment, and, conversely, whether the illness and/or its treatment will alter the effects of the psychotropic drug.

This chapter will review this subject in three sections: first, the major psychotropic agents will be discussed, with particular attention to factors having implications for medical patients; second, indications for their use with such patients will be reviewed; and, finally the current issues relevant to psychotropic drug use in selected medical conditions will be considered.

## PSYCHOTROPIC DRUGS

Psychotropic drugs are a vast, heterogeneous group of pharmacological agents, which can be rationally used for medical patients only when their diverse effects and interactions are appreciated. A massive literature has been devoted to describing these properties; only those aspects with particular importance to the medical patient will be considered here.

## Sedative-Hypnotics: General Considerations

Included in this group are the hypnotic, or so-called soporific drugs and the sedative agents or antianxiety tranquilizers. Table 7-1 lists the commonly available agents and certain of their pharmacological properties. These drugs have many similar effects: they all induce dose-dependent central nervous system (CNS) depression, having antianxiety effects at low dosage, hypnotic effects at higher dosage, and causing coma in extreme doses; in general they are lipophilic chemicals, favoring rapid oral absorption but poor dialyzeability; they are biotransformed in almost all cases by hepatic enzyme systems; and their CNS effects are exaggerated in the presence of other depressant influences (i.e., opiates, ethanol, hypoxia, uremia, etc.). Anticonvulsant effects can be demonstrated for all the drugs in this group. In addition, habituation, abuse, and physiological addiction may occur with repeated use. Another property of many sedative-hypnotics, and of particular significance for medical patients, is their extensive, although reversible, binding to serum proteins. Under normal physiological circumstances, the majority of circulating drug is in an inactive, protein-bound form.

## Hypnotic Agents

Several different hypnotic agents are commonly administered to treat insomnia. They all seem to be equally efficacious during short-term treatment when given in adequate dosage; the frequency of morning hangover, psychomotor impairment, and electroencephalographic (EEG) abnormalities reported with these agents does not differ significantly from one to another.[8] To choose rationally among them, the clinician must consider their relative liabilities and subtle pharmacokinetic differences.

BARBITURATES

All derivatives of barbituric acid can depress respiration and effect a significant reduction in REM sleep time.[9] In some studies, REM duration was decreased from the usual 25 percent of total sleep time to as little as 10 percent.[10] REM rebound, an occasionally nightmarish experience, often follows the termination of barbiturate therapy and can actually cause subsequent insomnia.[11] Patients may then innocently continue the drug to avoid these withdrawal phenomena, initiating a repetitive cycle which contributes to the familiar problems of barbiturate dependence. Moreover, barbiturates are potent inducers of the hepatic enzyme system responsible for the biotransformation of many otherwise unrelated pharmacological agents. By stimulating this enzyme system, other drugs may undergo accelerated biotransformation, rendering them less effective clinically.[12-14] Microsomal enzyme induction augments the removal of coumarin anticoagulants,[15] phenothiazines,[16, 17] tricyclic antidepressants,[18, 19] antipyrine,[20] tolbutamide,[21, 22] digitoxin,[23] rifampin,[24] doxycycline,[25] vitamin D,[26] corticosteroids,[27]

**Table 7-1**
Some Sedative-Hypnotic Drugs

| Drug Group | Duration of Action | Significant Active Metabolites | REM Sleep Depression | Hepatic Microsomal Enzyme Induction | Significant Protein-Binding Interactions |
|---|---|---|---|---|---|
| *Barbiturates* | | | | | |
| Amobarbital | I-L | No | Yes | Yes | No |
| Butabarbital | L | No | Yes | Yes | No |
| Phenobarbital | L | No | Yes | Yes | No |
| *Chloral Derivatives* | | | | | |
| Chloral Hydrate | S | Yes | Probably Yes | No | Yes |
| *Piperidinediones* | | | | | |
| Glutethimide | I | — | Yes | Yes | ? |
| *Propanediols* | | | | | |
| Meprobamate | S-I | No | ? | No | No |
| *Benzodiazepines* | | | | | |
| Chlordiazepoxide | I-L | Yes | Probably Yes* | No | No |
| Chlorazepate | L | Yes | Probably Yes* | No | No |
| Diazepam | L | Yes | Probably Yes* | No | No |
| Flurazepam | L | Yes | Probably Yes* | No | No |
| Lorazepam | I | No | Probably Yes* | No | No |
| Oxazepam | S | No | Probably Yes* | No | No |
| Prazepam | L | Yes | Probably Yes* | No | No |

S=T½<10 hours
I=10 hours<T½<24 hours
L=T½>24 hours
*=with more than brief administration

phenylbutazone,[28] meprobamate,[29] phenytoin,[30-34] and possibly methyl-dopa.[35] Despite this imposing list of potential interactants, however, clinically important effects have been implicated in only a few areas. Many studies have confirmed the antagonism between barbiturates and coumarin anti-coagulants.[36-47] One case report implied that enzyme-induced hypermetabolism of vitamin D could cause osteomalacia.[26] Steroid-dependent asthmatics may deteriorate when treated with phenobarbital.[48] Several investigators have reported that barbiturates significantly lower antidepressant drug plasma levels.[18, 19, 49] Although the clinical importance of this particular interaction is unclear from these reports, other evidence supports a significant correlation between blood levels and therapeutic response to tricyclic antidepressants.[50-53] With geriatric patients, a population requiring special considerations whenever any psychotropic drug is administered, barbiturate-induced confusion, paradoxical excitement, or delirium occurs to the extent that some authors advise against their use with such patients.[54-56] It is also important to remember that barbiturates are absolutely contraindicated in patients with acute intermittent porphyria.

GLUTETHIMIDE

Glutethimide, a piperidinedione derivative, is another potent respiratory and REM sleep depressant[57] which also stimulates hepatic microsomal enzymes.[58] Abuse and serious overdose are well-known hazards; it offers no advantages over safer hypnotics.

CHLORAL DERIVATIVES

Chloral derivatives, including chloral hydrate, chloral betaine, and trichloroethyl phosphate (triclofos) are relatively safe, effective hypnotics with few potential hazards for medical patients. The suspected gastric irritant effect of chloral hydrate may render it a less desirable choice for patients with gastritis and peptic ulcer disease. Trichloroacetic acid, a metabolic by-product, binds tightly to serum albumin and may potentiate the clinical effects of other protein-bound drugs by displacing them from their albumin-binding sites. This has been reported with coumarin anticoagulants,[59, 60] and may also occur with phenytoin[61] and tolbutamide.[62] Chloral derivatives do not seem to cause clinically significant hepatic enzyme induction, although they do undergo biotransformation in the liver. Anecdotal reports suggest that chloral hydrate, like other sedative-hypnotics, may exacerbate confusion and nocturnal delirium in geriatric patients.[63]

ANTIHISTAMINES

Clinical lore indicates that antihistamines provide a "gentle and safe" pharmacological treatment for insomnia, especially in elderly patients. Familiar antihistamines, such as the ethanolamine derivative, diphenhydramine, the phenothiazine, promethazine, and hydroxyzine, do induce mild sedation, but lack direct and consistent hypnotic properties in adults.[64] Furthermore, there is no objective evidence to support claims that these agents are safer than other hypnotics.

In fact, elderly patients are particularly sensitive to the strong anticholinergic side effects of these drugs; cases of toxic delirium have been reported even with therapeutic doses.[65] Antihistamines are also metabolized in the liver, but their effects on inducible enzyme systems have not been established.

BENZODIAZEPINES

Flurazepam appears at the present time to be the pharmacological treatment of choice for most cases of insomnia for which drug treatment is chosen. In short-term controlled studies using a 30 mg dose, its effectiveness has been equal or superior to other hypnotic drugs,[66] and its potential hazards are considerably less. Pertinent benzodiazepine pharmacology will be discussed later, but in comparison to the other drugs mentioned, benzodiazepines depress REM sleep minimally, and cause no clinically important enzyme induction or interferenre with albumin binding sites. Other available hypnotics used for the treatment of insomnia offer no advantages over the drugs already mentioned and have greater liabilities.

## Antianxiety Agents

For years, there has been widespread controversy surrounding the pharmacological treatment of anxiety. Although some studies have not demonstrated the superiority of one group of antianxiety drugs over another or placebo, the majority of the evidence consistently gives a therapeutic advantage to the benzodiazepine derivatives.[67] Using barbiturates or antihistamines to treat anxiety in the medical patient involves many of the considerations given above. In addition, adverse CNS effects (e.g., sedation or ataxia) are more likely to occur with chronic daily use, as opposed to intermittent bedtime dosage. For the barbiturates in particular, their nonspecific action and addiction potential argue against their use despite possible savings in the health care dollar.

PROPANEDIOLS

Since its introduction in 1955, meprobamate, a propranediol, has failed to live up to its promoted reputation as a safer and more effective antianxiety agent than barbiturates. Controlled studies have generally revealed the opposite; namely that the clinical pharmacology of meprobamate does not offer significant advantages. The superiority of meprobamate over placebo in treating anxiety is minimal,[68, 69] and approximately equivalent to various barbiturates. Microsomal enzyme induction does occur in animals,[70] but a clinically significant effect has not been established in man.[71] Meprobamate abuse and addiction occur frequently. There is still insufficient controlled data to support claims that tybamate, a more expensive propranediol, has greater clinical efficacy with less addiction potential.[72]

BENZODIAZEPINES

Seven benzodiazepine derivatives are currently available in the United States for clinical use (see Table 7-1). They have many similar properties. As antianxiety agents, they are equally efficacious when used in appropriate dosages. They do not cause significant microsomal enzyme induction and their potential for abuse and addiction is small.[73, 74] In the absence of other sources of CNS depression, lethal overdose rarely, if ever, occurs.[75-77] Despite these similarities, the various benzodiazepines have important pharmacological differences.

Pharmacokinetic studies reveal that both diazepam and chlordiazepoxide are long-acting drugs which undergo slow biotransformation in the liver and yield active metabolites having even longer half-lives than the parent compounds.[67] In the elderly and in those with liver disease, the first hepatic degradation step—demethylation—may be impaired or slowed, thereby further prolonging the half-life of the drug. The clinical significance of these observations is twofold: first, because of their long half-lives, diazepam and chlordiazepoxide are most rationally given in a once-daily, and not more than twice-daily, regimen; and second, certain drug effects such as sedation or CNS depression may intensify during the first few weeks of treatment, despite constant dosage, as the active compounds accumulate. Likewise, therapeutic effects, which have been inapparent for several days, may subsequently appear as accumulating active compounds reach a therapeutic level. These effects may then persist after drug therapy is discontinued. In patients with already impaired CNS function, the potential for unwanted accumulation effects is greatest. Some investigators have suggested that the paradoxical excitement and hostility occasionally manifest by patients receiving these drugs is related to the presence of active metabolites.[78] In light of these observations and the fact that biotransformation rates vary considerably among individuals,[79, 80] dosage requirements should not be predicted arbitrarily, but titrated against clinical effects. Analogous pharmacodynamic considerations apply to clorazepate, which is absorbed after acid hydrolysis in the stomach as desmethyldiazepam.[67] That inhibition of clorazepate absorption may occur when antacids are coadministered will be discussed below in the section devoted to gastrointestinal disorders. Prazepam also has its clinical activity primarily determined by this same active metabolite, desmethyldiazepam.

In clinical practice, diazepam and chlordiazepoxide are frequently administered by the intramuscular route despite convincing evidence that their absorption from intramuscular sites may be slow and unpredictable.[67, 81, 82] One recent study, however, found that when diazepam was injected into the thigh (vastus lateralis muscle), a site rarely chosen either for clinical purposes or bioavailability studies, absorption over three hours was about as complete and rapid as via the oral route.[83] This finding is difficult to interpret since it contradicts previous evidence which indicated that the thigh offers no special advantage as a site for intramuscular absorption of either diazepam or other drugs.[84] Our position is that the oral or intravenous route should be employed whenever possible.

In contrast to these four benzodiazepines, oxazepam and lorazepam are rapidly biotransformed through glucuronide formation, and active metabolites are not produced.[85] Accordingly, the problems of long half-life, drug accumulation, and the putatively related hostility-excitability response appear less frequent with these agents. As a result of such pharmacokinetic characteristics, oxazepam may be the preferred benzodiazepine for elderly patients.[86, 87] However, its use is limited by the lack of a parenteral preparation. Lorazepam, although available in both oral and parenteral forms, may cause anterograde amnesia when administered parenterally at only slightly greater than therapeutic doses.[88] This may restrict the usefulness of the parenteral forms to special situations (e.g., as an adjunct to anesthesia, for cardioversion, etc.).

Flurazepam is marketed as a benzodiazepine hypnotic, although its sleep-inducing properties may not differ significantly from other benzodiazepines if they are used in appropriate bedtime dosages.[89, 90] Flurazepam undergoes very rapid hepatic degradation. The resulting active metabolite is then slowly biotransformed and may accumulate with repeated flurazepam administration.[91] Although the clinical significance of accumulating flurazepam-active metabolites is still not established, it is possible that hangover and/or other CNS effects which correlate with the presence of active metabolites may increase with repeated flurazepam use. Thus, cumulative clinical effects may occur with all *commonly used* benzodiazepines except oxazepam and lorazepam.

### Antipsychotic Drugs (Major Tranquilizers, Neuroleptics)

Neuroleptic drugs can produce appreciable improvement in the disordered thought, perception, and behavior of psychotic patients. These drugs produce an unusually diverse variety of additional pharmacologic effects, however, involving the central and peripheral nervous systems as well as most major organ systems. Generalized anticholinergic and antiadrenergic action are particularly troublesome in the physiologically impaired patient. Therefore, before using these agents in a medical setting, the prescribing physician must be familiar with their protean pharmacological properties. This subject is comprehensively reviewed elsewhere.[92, 93]

Of the five classes of antipsychotic (neuroleptic) drugs currently available for clinical use (Table 7-2), only the phenothiazines and butyrophenones will be considered here. The other classes have many similar characteristics, but their use with medical patients has been limited. Loxapine, a recently introduced dibenzoxazepine derivative, may prove useful in the medical setting because it appears to possess the most potent antiemetic effect of all neuroleptic drugs.[94]

Phenothiazines are subdivided according to whether they have aliphatic, piperidine, or piperazine side chains added to their basic three-ring structure. The nature of the side chain greatly influences the differences among these compounds in their neurotransmitter blocking effects, and accordingly, in their predominant autonomic side effects.

Patients who tolerate postural hypotension poorly should be spared the potent alpha-adrenergic blocking effects of the piperidine and aliphatic phenothiazines. It also is possible that adrenergic blockade induced by drugs like reserpine, methyldopa, phentolamine, or phenoxybenzamine could be potentiated by aliphatic

**Table 7-2**
Antipsychotic Drugs

| | |
|---|---|
| I.  *Phenothiazines* | II.  *Butyrophenones* |
|     *Aliphatic Phenothiazines* |     Haloperidol |
|         Chlorpromazine |     Droperidol |
|         Promazine | |
|         Trifluopromazine | III.  *Thioxanthenes* |
|     *Piperidine Phenothiazines* |     *Aliphatic thioxanthenes* |
|         Thioridazine |         Chlorprothixene |
|         Mesoridazine |     *Piperazine Thioxanthenes* |
|         Piperacetazine |         Thiothixene |
|     *Piperazine Phenothiazines* | |
|         Prochlorperazine | IV.  *Dihydroindolones* |
|         Trifluoperazine |     Molindone |
|         Butaperazine | |
|         Perphenazine | V.  *Dibenzoxazepines* |
|         Fluphenazine |     Loxapine |
|         Acetophenazine | |
|         Carphenazine | |

and piperidine phenothiazines. These two subclasses, especially the piperidines, have significant antimuscarinic side effects, and would represent irrational choices for patients with untreated glaucoma, intestinal obstruction, or urinary outlet obstruction. They may potentiate the anticholinergic effects of other drugs, and accordingly should not be used to treat anticholinergic delirium or hyperpyrexia.[95, 96]

Impaired hypothalamic temperature regulation can be demonstrated in laboratory animals receiving phenothiazines, and severe hyperpyrexia has been reported in patients treated with phenothiazines during hot weather or exercise.[97-101] Hypothermic states have also been reported, associated with cold weather[102] and myxedema.[103] Again, elderly patients are a high-risk group who may show increased sensitivity to these thermal dysregulation effects.[104] The unusual cases of bone marrow depression, skin reactions, hepatotoxicity, and lenticular changes seem to occur more frequently with aliphatic phenothiazines, while pigmentary retinopathy occurs almost exclusively with the piperidines. Cardiotoxic effects of these drugs will be considered in more detail in the section devoted to heart disease.

Unlike the piperidine and aliphatic derivatives, piperazines are less sedating, have less potent autonomic effects, but more frequently cause unwanted extrapyramidal reactions. Their use with patients manifesting Parkinsonian symptoms is ill-advised. These drugs are particularly effective antiemetics for nausea and vomiting of nonvestibular origin.

The butyrophenones, despite a unique chemical structure, are pharmacologically similar to the piperazine phenothiazines. Extensive experience with haloperidol, the most widely used butyrophenone, confirms the infrequency of serious autonomic nervous system and cardiovascular side effects,[105, 106] rendering this drug especially safe for medical patients. As with the piperazine phenothiazines, extrapyramidal reactions are common.

Dosage of all antipsychotic drugs must be individually tailored to the particular medical condition. Their sedative effects may potentiate other CNS-depressant influences, whether from exogenous substances like sedative-hypnotics, methyldopa, propranolol, etc.; or disease states like myxedema, uremia, hypoxia, etc. Furthermore, since less than five percent of the circulating drug exists in a free form (i.e., not bound to serum proteins),[107] hypoproteinemic states may necessitate considerably less total drug for a desired effect.

Whether certain disease states or other drugs alter the bioavailability of antipsychotics is uncertain. Several reports suggest that in the presence of antacids, bioavailability of chlorpromazine is reduced.[16, 108, 109] These studies dealt with rate, however, not completeness of absorption.

In certain individuals major tranquilizers appear to lower seizure threshold.[92] However, the clinical significance of this, especially for the medical patient with a preexisting seizure disorder, is still unclear and will be considered in more detail below.

## Antidepressants

Tricyclic antidepressants are the preferred pharmacological agents for the treatment of depression. Three chemical classes are currently available for clinical use: dibenzazepine derivatives (imipramine, desipramine); dibenzocycloheptene derivatives (amitriptyline, nortriptyline, protriptyline); and dibenzoxepines (doxepin). Since these drugs have relatively long half-lives, and yield long-lived active metabolites, single daily dosage regimens generally are effective and rational.[110-112] An exception may apply to certain cardiac patients in whom a smoother blood level should be maintained by using three to four divided doses per day.

Antidepressants cause significant autonomic effects which may pose serious hazards to physiologically compromised patients. Orthostatic hypotension often occurs, especially in the early phases of treatment. The mechanism of this effect is unclear. Anticholinergic actions are particularly potent and should be carefully considered in patients with myxedema, glaucoma, intestinal obstruction, or micturition difficulties. Animal studies suggest that amitriptyline and nortriptyline possess the strongest antimuscarinic properties, and desipramine and doxepin the weakest.[113] These findings support the general clinical impression that amitriptyline and nortriptyline are unrivaled in peripheral anticholinergic activity. According to several reports, doxepin in standard dosage elicits the lowest incidence of autonomic side effects,[114-116] and may, therefore, represent the safest tricyclic antidepressant for medical patients. Clinical experience with doxepin is limited, however, compared to other tricyclics. Data in support of its superior safety are tempered by unresolved questions concerning its relative therapeutic potency.

Autonomic side effects are of obvious concern for patients with heart disease. The cardiotoxic effects of these drugs represent their greatest potential hazard and will be considered in detail in the section devoted to heart disease.

Atropine-like delirium is not an uncommon event in the course of treatment with these drugs, particularly if other anticholinergic agents are coadministered.[117] In elderly patients, lower dosage is advisable since, as a group, older persons are more susceptible to toxic as well as therapeutic effects.

Considerations relating to other drugs with sedative properties are equally important with the antidepressants. Nonspecific sedative effects are strongest with amitriptyline and weakest with protriptyline.

Numerous drug interactions have been associated with tricyclic antidepressant treatment. Phenylbutazone[118] and levodopa[119] absorption are delayed and possibly reduced as a result of the anticholinergic effects on gastrointestinal motility. Absorption of other drugs may be similarly influenced or perhaps even enhanced by this mechanism, since diminished gut motility may make some drugs more available for absorption while leaving others more susceptible to gut metabolism. This requires further study. Several drugs appear to alter tricyclic metabolism. Phenothiazines,[120] estrogens,[121] and methylphenidate[122] all raise antidepressant blood levels, probably by inhibiting microsomal enzymes in the liver. In contrast, barbiturates lower blood levels apparently by stimulating antidepressant drug metabolism.[49-51] An interesting report found significantly decreased tricyclic blood levels in depressed patients who smoke,[123] but the interaction mechanism is as yet unknown. Thyroid hormone in small doses appears to enhance the antidepressant effects of these drugs, even in euthyroid patients.[124-128] Higher doses, however, may enhance tricyclic toxicity.

Plasma protein binding is another significant factor in the pharmacology of these drugs. One study demonstrated that interindividual variation in plasma proteins can account for as much as a fourfold difference in blood levels of the active, unbound drug.[129] This may be an important clinical consideration if, as current research suggests, toxic and therapeutic effects correlate positively with plasma levels in many patients.

Hypertension, although conceivable in view of the noradrenergic potentiating effect of these drugs, is an unusual occurrence. In only one reported case was hypertension convincingly attributed to a tricyclic.[130] It has also been suggested that other sympathomimetic drugs may potentiate the adrenergic effects of tricyclics,[131] but the clinical significance of this is not established.

Monoamine oxidase (MAO) inhibitors are currently employed in the United States as secondline antidepressant drugs because of unresolved questions about their efficacy in relationship to their greater hazards. Orthostatic hypotension can be severe, while the opposite extreme, hypertensive crisis, may present an even greater threat. Recent reports suggest, however, that the newer generation of MAO inhibitors can be used safely by responsible patients even in combination with tricyclics, and that past risks may have been exaggerated.[132] Before prescribing one of these agents, however, a careful review of their well-known adverse interactions with various drugs affecting the sympathetic nervous system and tyra-mine-containing food substances, as well as their multisystem side effects, cannot be overlooked.

### Lithium

Lithium carbonate has unique mood stabilizing effects. It is the treatment of choice in the acute management of the manic and hypomanic phases of manic-depressive illness and for long-term prophylaxis against the recurrence of either phase.[133] For patients with recurrent "unipolar" depressions, it appears to have significant prophylactic value in preventing relapses and/or diminishing their severity.[133] As an antidepressant for the acute treatment of depression its value remains controversial, but it is generally considered inferior to tricyclics.

Lithium has attracted a great deal of medical attention not only because of its unique therapeutic profile, but also because it affects numerous physiological systems. Lithium pharmacology has been extensively studied.[134-136] The serious toxic manifestations seen with excessive plasma and intracellular levels are the major hazards of lithium use. The toxic-to-therapeutic dose ratio is small, with therapeutic blood levels customarily in the 0.7 to 1.5 mEq/liter range, and toxic effects common at blood levels approaching 2 mEq/liter. Therefore, dosage must be guided by closely monitored plasma levels, clinical effects, and toxic symptoms.

For medical patients with physiological imbalances, lithium therapy requires particularly assiduous management. Fluid and electrolyte balance, and cardiovascular, renal, thyroid, and CNS function, are the primary areas of concern.

Changes in fluid and sodium balance influence lithium blood levels, since ion transport systems (e.g., renal tubular and gastrointestinal) accept sodium and lithium interchangeably. Therefore, patients on low sodium diets, sodium-depleting diuretics, or in dehydrated or hypovolemic states will reabsorb a greater amount of lithium relative to sodium from the renal tubular lumen and elevate their lithium blood level proportionally. Elevated body temperature and excessive sweating will likewise predispose to potentially toxic lithium blood levels.

Since lithium ion is essentially unbound by serum proteins and excreted unchanged by the kidney, lithium clearance is directly proportional to creatinine clearance, and is approximately one-fifth of creatinine clearance in most individuals. There is no *a priori* reason that lithium cannot be used in the presence of impaired renal function or even during dialysis, provided stable lithium balance is achieved. Dosage must be adjusted to maintain safe plasma levels similar to other drugs, such as digoxin or gentamicin, whose clearance depends on renal excretion.

Lithium also influences renal function directly. Reversible defects in tubular concentrating mechanisms occur in approximately 30 percent of lithium-treated patients. The nephrogenic diabetes insipidus syndrome that results has been attributed to inhibition of ADH-induced adenyl cyclase.[136] This is rarely a significant clinical problem provided water is available and thirst mechanisms are intact.

In the therapeutic dose range, lithium does not appear to impair cardiac function significantly. Nonspecific ST- and T-wave electrocardiographic (EKG) changes may occur,[137, 138] however; and, according to one study of nine patients,[139] can be demonstrated universally if repeated EKG's with precordial leads are taken. These changes, although similar to hypokalemic effects, seem unrelated to normal variation in serum electrolytes, and possibly are independent of changes in lithium plasma levels within the therapeutic range.[140] Such benign lithium effects may reflect unmeasured shifts in intracellular ion concentrations. In cases of lithium overdosage, however, serious EKG effects and arrhythmias have occasionally been reported.[141, 142]

The appearance of subtle "organic" mental status symptoms, such as confusion, disorientation, or inattentiveness, may be easily overlooked or misinterpreted, especially in elderly patients, and not recognized as manifestations of lithium neurotoxicity. Since 1959, there have been reports of variable changes in CNS function in patients taking lithium; changes that might be expected from toxic blood levels were found in a few patients with lithium levels in the therapeutic range.[143, 144] It has been proposed that this reflects an idiosyncratic intolerance or hypersensitivity to lithium effects.[137] EEG abnormalities are the most consistent laboratory finding, and closely parallel mental status changes. That lithium neurotoxicity may be a reflection of toxic intracellular lithium concentration was suggested by a report which documented a correlation between neurotoxic symptoms, EEG changes, and red blood cell (RBC) lithium ion concentration in the face of low normal plasma levels.[145] Subsequent reports have confirmed that RBC lithium concentration, and more specifically the RBC-to-plasma lithium ratio, is a more sensitive indicator of incipient toxicity.

Other lithium effects which can be problematic in the treatment of medical patients include coarse resting tremor, a frequent dose-related neuromuscular symptom occasionally ameliorated by propranolol or a benzodiazepine, reversible glucose intolerance similar to chemical diabetes, and dose-independent, reversible leukocytosis. A variety of dermatitides have been attributed to lithium carbonate therapy.[146, 147] Most of these (e.g., localized papular eruptions, folliculitis, acneiform dermatitis) resemble inflammatory reactions of nonallergic origin and do not necessarily require termination of drug treatment. One recent anecdotal case report described a patient with myasthenia gravis who suffered exacerbation of his neuromuscular symptoms coincident with lithium carbonate treatment.[148] Interactions with thyroid function will be considered below.

## Drugs for Senile Mental Changes

This is a heterogeneous group of pharmacologically active agents, including papaverine, cyclandelate, and dihydrogenated ergot alkaloids (Hydergine[R], DEA), promoted by their manufacturers as effective in the management of the cognitive, emotional, and behavior changes associated with senility. The validity of these claims is still under review. Most studies have been criticized because of their methodological inconsistencies and contradictory findings.[149, 150] Nevertheless, some reports suggest that subtle changes, particularly mood elevation, may occur in certain patients after 6 to 8 weeks of treatment, while serious adverse effects are rare. Whether a tricyclic antidepressant in low dosage would be equally, or perhaps more, effective and as safe as the above agents has not been established.

## INDICATIONS FOR PSYCHOTROPIC DRUGS IN MEDICAL PATIENTS

Signs and symptoms generally imputed to emotional distress or illness are frequently seen in medical patients. Before considering treatment with psychotropic drugs, these findings must be assessed with the same circumspection applied to dyspnea or other symptoms generally imputed to organic disease. It is a longstanding paradox of medical practice, stemming from archaic mind-body paradigms, that emotional symptoms are regarded as "organ-specific" while dyspnea or the like is related to a number of possible etiologies. Before treating such symptoms in medical patients, or anyone for that matter, a search for organic factors must be undertaken—organic factors which may cause the symptoms, result from the symptoms, or relate coincidentally. Only then is the physician able to rationally consider the questions "will a psychotropic drug help?" and "what are the hazards?" Although the questions may still resolve into a therapeutic trial, the likelihood for a positive outcome is certainly greater.

### Insomnia

Insomnia is a common complaint among medical patients, especially when hospitalized. It is a potentially serious oversight to dismiss this symptom lightly or to prescribe a hypnotic drug automatically. Often, the source of insomnia is readily attributable to environmental factors such as intensive care unit noise, nursing intervention, nocturnal procedures like intravenous changes or medication administration, or to increased anxiety about the hospital setting, impending surgery, or the prospect of serious organic disease. Even in such cases, empathic understanding and discussion of the patient's fears may be all that is necessary.

In many instances, insomnia may result from some aspect of a disease process or its therapy. In such cases, treatment of the underlying cause is preferred. Examples include physical discomforts, pain, hypoxia, fever, asthma attacks, nocturnal angina, endocrinopathies, etc. Table 7-3 lists other medical conditions which may cause insomnia. Clearly, many of these conditions can be exacerbated by misapplied sedation. Psychotic or depressed patients often sleep poorly and respond better to treatment of their primary disorder. In senile or demented patients, increased agitation and confusion may occur at night ("sundowning") and respond best to small doses of an antipsychotic.[151] Sedative-hypnotics may make "sundowners" worse.[8] Likewise, certain patients with rare sleep-related respiratory

**Table 7-3**
Some Conditions that may Present with Insomnia or
Prominent Anxiety Symptoms

---

Angina
Aspirin Intolerance
Drug Intoxications
Behavioral Toxicity from Drugs
Caffeinism
Cerebral Arteriosclerosis
Epilepsy (especially psychomotor)
Hyperdynamic Beta-Adrenergic Circulatory State (Hyperventilation)
Hypoglycemia; Hyperinsulinism
Hypoxic States
Pain
Paroxysmal Tachyarrhythmias
Pheochromocytoma
Premenstrual Tension
Pulmonary Embolism
Hyperthyroidism
Withdrawal from CNS Depressant Drugs

---

Reproduced in modified form with permission from Shader RI (Ed.): Manual of Psychiatric Therapeutics. Boston, Little Brown, 1975.

difficulties (e.g., Ondine curse syndrome[152] and sleep-induced airway obstruction[153]) may seek treatment for insomnia; use of hypnotics with such patients has in some instances proven fatal.[152]

In most medical patients, insomnia results from a combination of emotional and organic factors. Pharmacotherapy offers a high likelihood of success with few hazards, provided the nature of the target symptoms and the pharmacology of the hypnotic agents are understood.[154] Numerous clinical studies confirm the effectiveness of most commonly available hypnotics in inducing and maintaining sleep.[155-161] On the basis of flurazepam's greater safety, and findings indicating that little or no tolerance to its hypnotic effects develops even after several weeks of repeated use,[156, 162, 163] flurazepam is generally preferred over other hypnotics currently marketed in the United States. This should not suggest, however, that chronic administration of flurazepam is totally benign. Hangover and other CNS effects may become more frequent with prolonged use, possibly correlating with the accumulation of active metabolites. Furthermore, other benzodiazepines are probably equally effective hypnotic agents when prescribed in an appropriate bedtime dosage (e.g., oxazepam, 45 mg).[90] When chronic treatment is unavoidable, lorazepam, which lacks accumulation effects, may provide a more rational alternative. Nevertheless, the pharmacotherapy of insomnia is best formulated as a short-term, intermittent treatment.

Recent progress in sleep research has raised many questions about the effect of sleep on certain medical conditions. For example, angina, tachyarrhythmias, and gastric hyperacidity have been correlated with REM activity during sleep.[157] Whether REM-suppressing pharmacotherapy would alter the natural history of these conditions is unknown, and deserves further investigation. The possibility of REM breakthrough or, more seriously, REM rebound when the drug is discontinued may offset any potential benefit derived from REM suppression.

Other sleep-related disorders such as somnambulism, enuresis, and night terrors (pavor nocturnus) may occur specifically during stage IV slow-wave sleep. Although controlled studies are lacking, some preliminary evidence suggests that diazepam and flurazepam, perhaps because of their stage IV sleep-suppressing effect, may be helpful in the treatment of such conditions.[67]

## Anxiety

Medical patients frequently describe symptoms which may be manifestations of anxiety. Excessive worry, fearfulness, overconcern, irritability, tension, and difficulty concentrating are common signs associated with the psychic component of anxiety. As a reaction to medical illness, such psychic distress is often appropriate and not necessarily an indication for pharmacotherapy. Some medical patients manifest anxiety more as a disproportionate sense of impending doom, a fear of dying, or a morbid preoccupation with certain illnesses. At times, the patient's anxiety can obstruct his own participation in medical treatment or create major problems in ward management. Anxiety of such proportions is generally maladaptive, particularly for a medical patient.

Most anxious patients also evince somatic manifestations which present problems for differential diagnosis (e.g., agitation, insomnia, tremor, breathlessness, tachycardia, palpitations, diaphoresis, headache, chest pain, nausea, diarrhea, or urinary frequency). Such somatic manifestations may simulate, complicate, or obscure other medical problems. Moreover, as already mentioned, some medical conditions (see Table 7-3) present with nonspecific anxiety symptoms which can dangerously obfuscate the true nature of the underlying illness. Clearly, dramatic feelings of anxiety or even panic should not distract the treating physician from a search for possible organic etiologies (e.g., hypoglycemia, hypoxia, thyrotoxicosis, pheochromocytoma, etc.).

The decision to treat anxiety with pharmacotherapy involves many factors. The nature of the symptoms, their psychological and medical context, and their severity all must be carefully evaluated. Placebo effects, the importance of the physician's attention and reassurance, and at times the ephemeral nature of anxiety itself, are other significant aspects of the treatment and its results. Finally, rational selection and administration of antianxiety drugs requires an understanding of their pharmacology.

In numerous controlled studies, the antianxiety effects of benzodiazepines have been demonstrated; for anxiety symptoms associated with cardiovascular, gastrointestinal, dermatological, or gynecological disorders, the degree of symptomatic benefit approximates that seen in anxious patients without organic disease.[164-170] Because anxiety symptoms tend to fluctuate, appropriate dosage will vary considerably from one individual to another or in the same individual over time. In addition to the considerations already discussed for benzodiazepine therapy, it must be remembered that oversedation and ataxia are more likely to occur when these drugs are used chronically than as an intermittent or bedtime medication. Therefore, antianxiety pharmacotherapy is best conceived as a short-term and intermittent treatment program.

Physicians commonly prescribe antianxiety agents as a part of the long-term management of certain medical conditions thought to be adversely effected by anxiety-related autonomic nervous system hyperactivity. Accordingly, many patients with peptic ulcer disease, inflammation bowel disease, asthma, heart disease, and hypertension receive adjunctive antianxiety therapy, occasionally in the absence of overt anxiety. Whether such treatment actually influences the natural course or progression of the disease remains obscure and merits controlled investigation. The use of antianxiety pharmacotherapy in specific disease states will be discussed below.

Recently, beta-adrenergic blocking agents like propranolol have proven effective in treating certain somatic anxiety symptoms, particularly tachycardia, palpitations, tremulousness, diaphoresis, and hyperventilation.[171-176] Although this form of treatment is less effective for the psychic manifestations of anxiety and generally inferior to benzodiazepines in controlled trials, it may be useful in carefully selected patients whose anxiety is experienced primarily as peripheral somatic symptoms which interfere with certain performance tasks, such as examinations, public speeches, or other settings typical of situational anxiety.[176-178] The usual contraindications for propranolol (e.g., asthma, diabetes, heart failure, etc.) must be observed. Anxiety is not an FDA-approved indication for propranolol or other $\beta$-adrenergic blocking agents, however, at the present time.

Antidepressant drugs and major tranquilizers have also been promoted for antianxiety therapy. In the absence of serious depression or psychosis, respectively, these drugs are more hazardous and no more effective than a benzodiazepine. In only two situations where anxiety appears to be the primary psychological symptom is pharmacotherapy with nonsedative-hypnotic agents possibly preferred. As mentioned, neuroleptics often ameliorate agitation, anxiety, and assaultiveness in elderly patients with signs of dementia who may do worse with sedative-hypnotics. In certain patients who manifest agoraphobic anxiety with spontaneous attacks of extreme anxiety or panic, tricyclic antidepressants have been demonstrated in several controlled studies to be the therapy of choice.[178] MAO inhibitors, although more hazardous, may also be effective for panic attacks. Unfortunately, the use of antidepressants to control such attacks is not an FDA-approved indication at the present time.

## Depression

The current system for classifying depression and depressive disorders is egregiously confused.[179] Many situational, characterological, or reactive depressions are often best treated by nonpharmacological therapies.[180] In medical patients without prior history of depression who seem depressed as a reaction to their illness, response to antidepressant drugs is generally poor. In fact, only in the treatment of so-called "endogenous depressions" is drug therapy consistently superior to placebo, psychotherapy, or antianxiety agents.[180-183] Thus, administration of tricyclic antidepressants generally follows a diagnosis of endogenous depression. This diagnostic label can be misleading. It refers to a clinical syndrome, defined by certain signs and symptoms, which does not necessarily develop "endogenously" in the sense of being unrelated to external circumstances. The diagnosis depends on certain core clinical criteria: psychic retardation, anergy, anhedonia or apathy, decreased productivity, diuvinal variation (worse in the morning), and autonomy of the depressive syndrome.[180, 181] Sad affect, sleep disturbances, anorexia, agitation, decreased libido, suicidal preoccupation, etc., may be present but are not generally required for the diagnosis and do not discriminate between endogenous depression and other depressive illnesses.

The presence of a clear precipitant, such as a medical illness, although usually associated with situational depressions, occasionally presages a serious, prolonged depressive illness having the clinical characteristics of an endogenous depression. In such cases, antidepressant pharmacotherapy is indicated unless an organic cause of the depression exists. Obviously, many of the characteristics of an endogenous depression can be confused with other factors affecting the medical patient, particularly if he is hospitalized. Sleep or appetite may be curtailed by the hospital routine. Weight loss may result from a prescribed dietary change. Listlessness, anergy, etc., result from many systemic therapies. The patient may be so weakened that he barely responds to the environment. Thus, seriously ill medical patients may appear endogenously depressed according to the strict criteria and indeed may be affectively troubled, and yet lack a discrete affective disorder. In such cases, therapy should be postponed until the patient can be evaluated in a more favorable environment.

When depression is a manifestation of an organic disturbance, treatment should be directed at the primary disorder. Patients with Parkinson's disease or apathetic hyperthyroidism often appear depressed because of their predominant symptoms,[184] yet, their symptoms do not have their etiologies in a depressive disorder. Many other diseases, however, are responsible for organically-determined depressive syndromes including anemia, uremia, carcinomatosis or occult carcinoma, acute intermittent porphyria, various endocrinopathies, systemic lupus erythematosus, parathyroid disease, etc.

Numerous drugs have also been implicated as causes of depression and should be used with caution in patients with a prior history of affective disorders. These include reserpine,[185] oral contraceptives,[186] methyldopa,[187] propranolol,[188] clonidine,[189] corticosteroids,[190] possibly diazepam,[191] and various antineoplastic agents.[192]

In elderly patients, the manifestations and/or etiology of depression may be even more obscure. Many depressed geriatric patients fail to describe the typical mood changes. Some individuals with impaired mental functioning evince marked cognitive deteriorations as their major response to depression. Others who show little evidence of cognitive impairment beforehand, appear "pseudo-demented" when depressed.[193] When depression is responsible for such mental deterioration, antidepressant drugs may appear to have a surprising effect on cognition. Therefore, the possibility of a depressive disorder should not be overlooked in geriatric patients, because appropriate pharmacotherapy yields impressive results.[151]

The role of MAO inhibitors in the pharmacotherapy of depression is still unresolved. They are generally less effective than the tricyclics. Several recent controlled studies suggest, however, that in certain patients with chronic depressive and anxiety symptoms, hypersomnia and hyperphagia, and with hypochondriacal complaints, who are resistant to conventional treatment, MAO inhibitors may be worthy of a trial.[194-196]

Antidepressants have also been tried in a large number of unrelated chronic illnesses. Anecdotal reports appear in the literature alleging symptomatic benefit from tricyclic antidepressants in the treatment of various chronic pain syndromes, headaches, and musculoskeletal disorders.[197] The clinical significance of these reports is difficult to assess, since tricyclics have no established analgesic action and such syndromes are known to respond to a wide variety of other therapies. Nevertheless, chronic pain, headache, muscle aches, etc., may represent depressive somatic equivalents or manifestations of an occult depression in some patients.[198] These presently are not FDA-approved indications for antidepressants.

Once the decision to prescribe an antidepressant is made, certain guidelines must be followed. Adequate dosage of tricyclics usually means a minimum of 150 mg per day of imipramine or its equivalent for most patients. Geriatric patients usually need one-half to one-third this dose. Because of individual variations in metabolism, protein binding, etc., some patients will require considerably higher doses. As already mentioned, determination of plasma drug levels may simplify therapy in the future if the pattern of findings from contemporary studies is confirmed. Improvement in mood seldom results in less than seven days of treatment, and dosage adjustments should be made gradually.

## Psychosis

In some medical patients with no prior history of psychosis, schizophrenia-like symptoms—hallucinations, delusions, inappropriate or labile effect, impaired reality sense, feelings of depersonalization, and psychotic agitation or terror—appear during the course of a medical illness or its treatment. In almost all cases, an underlying organic cause can be identified. A careful mental status examination will usually reveal varying degrees of disorientation, memory impairment, and other indicators of cognitive dysfunction. If the patient is delirious, his level of arousal may fluctuate. Such organic mental states tend to vacillate from hour to hour, or from evaluator to evaluator.

The list of possible organic etiologies for psychotic behavior in medical patients is lengthy. Common causes include: hypoxia, impaired CNS perfusion, increased intracranial pressure, hepatic or renal decompensation, almost any known primary brain disease, numerous alterations in electrolytes and endocrine balance, as well as hypoglycemia, dehydration, and fever.[199] Withdrawal from addictive drugs (e.g., ethanol, barbiturates, opiates) causes psychotic agitation and other symptoms in many hospitalized patients. Other drugs may cause psychosis by direct action. These include amphetamines, hallucinogens, tricyclic antidepressants, MAO inhibitors, other CNS stimulants, corticosteroids, lidocaine, pentazocine, digitalis, anticholinergic drugs, isoniazid, cycloserine, etc.[190]

In certain hospital settings, such as intensive care units (ICUs), burn units, surgical wards, etc., psychotic behavior, feelings of unreality or depersonalization, and intermittent delirium are especially common. The syndrome of "ICU psychosis," suggestive of a reaction to "environmental shock," sleep deprivation, and other nonspecific factors, probably does not exist as such, but represents the cerebral effects of cumulative physiological and metabolic stresses experienced by critically ill patients. Where cerebral function is already diminished, psychosis may result from only minimal physiological disturbances.

Clearly, if psychotic symptoms arise, treatment should follow an exhaustive search for an underlying organic etiology. Only when no specific remedial cause can be found or when the patient's behavior is unmanageable by other means, should antipsychotic agents be prescribed. The choice of a specific drug must depend on the clinical setting and the pharmacological properties of the various agents. It should also be remembered that delirium due to anticholinergic agents or to withdrawal from addictive drugs is best treated with a sedative-hypnotic (e.g., a benzodiazepine) rather than with antipsychotic agents whose intrinsic anticholinergic properties may add to the patient's symptomatology.

## USE OF PSYCHOTROPIC DRUGS IN SPECIFIC DISEASE STATES

### Hypertension

Many physicians prescribe antianxiety agents for their hypertensive patients. An obvious and important question is whether anxiety in these patients, particularly when inapparent, adversely effects their underlying hypertensive disease. Although antianxiety pharmacotherapy may be a useful treatment for their overt anxiety symptoms, there is no evidence that supports the value of such therapy as an adjunct to, or substitute for, antihypertensive drugs in the long-term management of hypertension and its complications. Benzodiazepines have no known anti-hypertensive effects of their own, and there are no data currently available to suggest that hypertensive patients are intrinsically "hyper-tense." On the other hand, benzodiazepines have no known interactions with other antihypertensive treatments. It is conceivable, however, that any sedative-hypnotic might potentiate the depression occasionally caused by reserpine, methyldopa, or clonidine. Furthermore, barbiturate and chloral hydrate sedative effects have been allegedly potentiated by propranolol.[200, 201] Whether sedative-hypnotic drug use alters the natural course of hypertensive disease deserves further investigation.

Guanethidine sulfate, a potent antihypertensive agent in use for over a decade, is partially or completely antagonized by coadministration of certain psychotropic drugs. Tricyclic antidepressants, probably because they inhibit the active transport mechanism responsible for guanethidine entry into adrenergic neurons,[202] will gradually reverse its antihypertensive action. This has been demonstrated in several clinical reports.[203-206] Preliminary observations suggested that doxepin did not cause this effect;[115] subsequent reports revealed that the antagonism is less potent but will result when higher doses are used.[207] The same interaction seems to occur with bethanidine[208] and clonidine,[209] similar antihypertensive agents. Recently, chlorpromazine has been implicated as another guanethidine antagonist.[210]

In light of these observations, concurrent therapy with antidepressants or chlorpromazine and guanethidine-like drugs is ill-advised.

## Thyroid Disease

The sedating properties of any psychotropic drug may be strikingly severe in patients with hypothyroidism. Anticholinergic effects also may be exaggerated. In addition, hypothyroid patients seem especially sensitive to the temperature dysregulation effects of phenothiazines.[103] These hazards are further compounded because various drug-metabolizing systems may be depressed in myxedematous states, and the presence of hypoproteinemia will increase the fraction of circulating active (unbound) drug at any given total drug serum level. Thus, psychotropic agents must be used cautiously in patients with hypothyroidism.

Since lithium inhibits the release of thyroid hormone from the thyroid gland,[211-214] thyroid disorders occur in some patients receiving this drug. Nontoxic goiters appear in approximately four percent of lithium treated patients, and clinical hypothyroidism occasionally develops.[215-219] Other patients may have abnormal thyroid function tests during their course of treatment. Coadministration of lithium and an iodine preparation may further predispose to hypothyroidism.[220] Irreversible changes caused directly by lithium have not been reported, but the possibility that lithium may unmask clinically latent Hashimoto's thyroiditis has been suggested.[221] These observations indicate that thyroid function should be monitored at regular intervals in patients treated with lithium. Internists who use lithium to treat thryotoxicosis should be wary of the possible neurotoxic effects of the drug which may further complicate the clinical picture.[222]

## Seizure Disorders

Psychosis or depression requiring psychopharmacological intervention is not an infrequent event in the life of an epileptic. Caution has been advised in the use of psychotropic drugs with such patients since some antipsychotic agents and antidepressant drugs lower the seizure threshold. Most clinical reports of this phenomenon have been anecdotal, and many of the patients involved had no prior history of a seizure disorder.[223-227] The clinical implications of these observations are unclear, since they have shed no light on how one identifies the susceptible patient. No prospective controlled study exists. Furthermore, literally hundreds of thousands of patients have received psychotropic drugs while being treated concurrently with anticonvulsants without evidence of increased seizure activity. The only convincing data from which treatment guidelines can be drawn involve withdrawing alcoholics. Several well-controlled trials indicate that alcohol withdrawal seizures occur more frequently in patients treated with certain phenothiazines than with placebo or sedative-hypnotics.[228-231] Of the phenothiazines implicated, chlorpromazine and promazine appear to be primary offenders, but this may reflect their more extensive use rather than a specific pharmacological property. Clinical experience with haloperidol and piperazine phenothiazines, in general, suggests that they may be safer alternatives.

Seizure activity is an occasional manifestation of lithium neurotoxicity.[134] Whether patients with preexisting seizure disorders are more sensitive to this effect is unresolved.

## Pulmonary Disease

Any CNS depressant is potentially hazardous in patients with minimal pulmonary reserve. The possibility of precipitating respiratory failure must be considered. Barbiturates are well-known offenders. Anecdotal case reports[232] and studies of pulmonary function[233-236] have demonstrated increased hypoxia, hypercapnia, and respiratory acidosis in patients with unstable obstructive airway disease treated with benzodiazepines. The clinical significance of these findings is questionable, however, since the magnitude of the reported changes is small, and in some instances, equal only to the normal variations found with sleep.[235, 236] Furthermore, most of these studies used a benzodiazepine via the intravenous route. Insufficient data exist to indicate how serious the threat of respiratory depression is with oral administration of these drugs. In two trials with oral medication, insignificant changes in respiratory function occurred.[237, 238] Even intravenous use has yielded benign results in some other reports.[239, 240] Although the effects of benzodiazepines on pulmonary function appear variable, clinicians should respect the possibility of diminished respiratory function while using these drugs in patients with serious respiratory disease, especially if other CNS-active drugs are coadministered.

Sedative-hypnotic agents are frequently combined with xanthine derivatives and sympathomimetic amines in various antiasthmatic preparations. There is little evidence to suggest that the antianxiety agent contributes additional clinical benefit. The possible adverse effect of prescribing phenobarbital for steroid-dependent asthmatics is discussed above.

### Renal Disease

Since hepatic enzyme systems detoxify most psychopharmacological agents, changes in renal function seldom effect the clinical use of these drugs. In the late stages of renal failure hepatic function may also be impaired, however. As in other hypoproteinemic states, patients with the nephrotic syndome may show greater effects from psychotropic drugs even at normal dosage because of decreased availability of serum protein binding sites. Dialysis can be expected to have little effect on the clearance of most psychotropic drugs because of their poor dialyzeability. By contrast, renal excretion is responsible for the removal of lithium and for approximately 30 percent of phenobarbital clearance, both of which may require dosage adjustments in patients with renal disease. The relationship between lithium and renal function was considered above.

A recent report implicated flurazepam and diazepam as causes of a reversible encephalopathy in three patients on chronic dialysis.[241] The mechanism of this effect was not determined, but this report should prompt further investigation since patients on chronic hemodialysis occasionally manifest nonuremic encephalopathies which defy the usual etiological determinations. The pharmacokinetic profiles of both diazepam[242] and lorazepam[243] in patients with poor renal function do not appear to be significantly altered, however.

### Gastrointestinal Disorders

Recent evidence indicates that changes in the intraluminal gastrointestinal contents can affect the absorption of psychotropic drugs. Food delays the absorption of pentobarbital.[244] Antacids reduce the rate and possibly completeness of chlorpromazine absorption when the two are coadministered.[108, 109] A similar effect has been observed with chlordiazepoxide.[245] Clorazepate absorption may be greatly inhibited by coadministered antacids which neutralize the gastric acidity required for the intragastric hydrolysis of clorazepate to desmethyldiazepam.[246] Such findings are relevant to the clinical use of these drugs in patients receiving antacid treatment and possibly also in patients with achlorhydria.

The potent anticholinergic effects of antipsychotic drugs and antidepressants were described above. Significant reduction in gastrointestinal motility caused by these drugs may affect absorption of unrelated pharmacological agents, such as phenylbutazone and levodopa (discussed above), and augment preexisting gastric or bowel obstruction.

The metabolism of various drugs depends on normal hepatic function. In the presence of parenchymal liver disease, notably cirrhosis and hepatisis, altered drug biotransformation occurs. This has been demonstrated for many pharmacological agents, and seems to involve several factors, including changes in hepatic enzymes, protein synthesis, and general nutritional status.[247] Clearance of barbiturates and meprobamate is prolonged in patients with chronic liver disease;[247-249] phenobarbital clearance, perhaps because of a concomitant increase in renal excretion, is prolonged the least. Since excessive sedation or respiratory depression are potential precipitants of hepatic coma, barbiturate use is dangerous in susceptible patients.

Chlorpromazine clearance studies have shown that removal of the parent compound proceeds normally despite severe hepatic disease.[247, 250, 251] Nevertheless, increased CNS depression and EEG changes have been observed in chronic liver disease patients receiving chlorpromazine, particularly patients with a past history of hepatic coma.[250, 251] The factors contributing to this effect are unclear, but may involve changes in the degradation of chlorpromazine's active metabolites or in drug-protein binding. Neither of these possibilities has been evaluated.

Diazepam pharmacokinetics are dramatically altered in the presence of cirrhosis or hepatitis. Half-life of the parent compound may be prolonged several-fold[247] and protein-binding diminished significantly.[252] The appearance of desmethyldiazepam, the first metabolic product, was delayed in one study, suggesting that impaired demethylation accounts for reduced diazepam clearance.[252]

Chlordiazepoxide half-life appears to be prolonged also, and perhaps in predictable proportion to certain clinical parameters of hepatic dysfunction.[253] The clinical significance of these findings is uncertain. Obviously, the major concern in using any sedatives with liver disease patients is CNS depression and hepatic coma. Whether impaired hepatic metabolism or protein-binding predisposes to excessive benzodiazepine sedation or drug-precipitated hepatic coma remains unresolved. In one prospective report, patients with a history of hepatic coma remained stable on oral diazepam.[254] Retrospective studies, however, have implicated diazepam and chlordiazepoxide as causes of excessive sedation and hepatic coma.[255, 256] An epidemiological survey indicated that patients with low serum albumin appear to be at highest risk.[255]

In the absence of more conclusive reports, diazepam and chlordiazepoxide should be considered potentially hazardous in patients with severe liver disease, especially in those patients who are hypoalbuminemic. Oxazepam, because it is detoxified by glucuronide formation, appears to be a safer alternative. Preliminary observations with cirrhotic patients have found no impairment in oxazepam clearance.[257] Thus, based on both clinical and pharmacological evidence, oxazepam at present is the benzodiazepine of choice for the anxious patient with chronic liver disease who cannot be managed by nonpharmacotherapeutic means.

Hepatic encephalopathy is an excellent example of a metabolic disorder which presents with primarily psychiatric or mental status disturbances. As in all such conditions, treatment should be directed toward the underlying disorder. In the case of hepatic encephalopathy, the recent introduction of lactulose, a poorly absorbed synthetic disaccharide, represents a significant addition to the treatment armamentarium. Apparently by lowering intraluminal gut pH, lactulose indirectly effects a significant reduction in blood ammonia levels, improvement in mental symptoms, prevention of recurrence, and increased protein tolerance.[258-263] Although considerably less toxic than neomycin, its relative clinical superiority is still debated. (See addendum).

## Heart Disease

Many physicians prescribe antianxiety drugs as part of a treatment plan for patients with various cardiac disorders. When anxiety is evident, benzodiazepines can be expected to provide benefit similar to their effects with other patients. In the absence of overt anxiety, however, the usefulness of these drugs is controversial. Questions still to be resolved include whether anxiety, overt or inapparent, has greater physiological significance for patients having a particular medical illness, and whether pharmacotherapy with antianxiety drugs can influence the eventual outcome of the cardiac disorder.

Anxiety has been implicated as a factor in potentially lethal cardiac arrhythmias, even in the absence of preexisting coronary vascular disease.[264-266] Although antianxiety therapy has been advocated, evidence for its long-term value in such cases is only anecdotal. In patients with acute myocardial infarction (MI), anxiety is common and usually responsive to treatment with benzodiazepines.[170, 267] An important question is whether such anxiety plays a significant role in the post-MI pattern of arrhythmias. A positive correlation between endogenous epinephrine excretion and ventricular arrhythmias has been demonstrated in some patients.[268] One "controlled" study evaluated the effects of high dose diazepam therapy in acute MI.[269] Endogenous epinephrine levels, usually elevated in the post-MI period, were significantly lower in the sedated patients, who also experienced significantly fewer episodes of ventricular arrhythmias. The clinical importance of this study is uncertain, however, because patients were heavily sedated (45 mg/day orally, following a 10-mg intravenous dose on admission) and other clinical parameters, such as enzyme levels and ultimate outcome, did not differ significantly between groups. Even imputing the lower incidence of arrhythmias to the treatment of anxiety *per se* is inferential, since other reports have suggested that diazepam may have some direct antiarrhythmic activity.[270, 271] Thus, benzodiazepine therapy though an effective treatment for anxiety symptoms often seen in patients with various cardiac disorders, has no established impact on the morbidity or mortality secondary to heart disease.

Both phenothiazines and tricyclic antidepressants appear to manifest potentially serious cardiotoxicity in certain individuals. It is likely that the reported adverse effects result from one or more of several pharmacological properties attributed to both classes of drugs, specifically hypotensive effects, direct effects on cardiac tissue, and indirect actions mediated via the autonomic nervous system.

Several reports implicate phenothiazines as the cause of unexplained sudden deaths in previously healthy individuals.[272-275] The exact nature of these events is unclear, but other reports have noted delayed repolarization,[276-280] tachyarrhythmias,[277, 281-286] EKG changes,[277, 287-292] and congestive heart failure[277] in some patients taking these drugs. Based on these reports thioridazine appears to be the most frequent cause of EKG changes and serious arrhythmias. ST- and T-wave abnormalities, similar to hypokalemic effects and generally reversible with administration of potassium, may occur even with therapeutic doses of thioridazine. In addition, a prolonged QT-interval is often seen. Taken together, these effects have earned thioridazine the label "quinidine-like." Whether such actions or EKG changes predispose to life-threatening events or select those at high risk is uncertain. Furthermore, there is insufficient evidence to assess how these effects might interact with those of other cardioactive drugs.

Although it is difficult to draw any definitive clinical guidelines from these reports, several observations are worth noting. Most cases of serious cardiotoxicity have involved the two phenothiazines possessing the most potent autonomic nervous system effects, namely thioridazine and chlorpromazine. It would seem wise to minimize the use of these agents in patients with heart disease. Furthermore, such potentially lethal cardiac effects have not been reported with haloperidol, or with high-milligram-potency piperazine phenothiazines (e.g., fluphenazine), drugs with relatively weak autonomic effects. These drugs may, therefore, represent the safer choices for cardiac patients. Haloperidol seems quite popular at present, receiving considerable use (both oral and parenteral) in coronary and intensive care units without reported untoward cardiac effects.

Serious cardiotoxicity has also been reported with tricyclic antidepressants. In overdosage, conduction disturbances, tachyarrhythmias, and congestive heart failure are not uncommon.[277, 293-304] Amitriptyline appears to be the most cardiotoxic. Animal studies have shown that tricyclics generally produce dose-dependent conduction and rhythm disturbances and diminished myocardial contracility.[305-307]

EKG abnormalities and conduction disturbances also occur in certain individuals taking these drugs in therapeutic dosages. Patients with preexisting cardiac disease are probably more susceptible,[308] but serious effects have been reported in individuals with a negative cardiac history.[309-313] In most cases, EKG changes include reversible prolongation of PR interval and QRS complex, nonspecific T-wave changes, and supraventricular tachycardia. These hazards may be potentiated if amine-depleting drugs like guanethidine are coadministered.[302] Complete heart block has also been reported.[309] Most of these changes have correlated with serum drug levels.[309, 314-316]

Recent investigations using *his*-bundle recordings in patients overdosed with nortriptyline reveal selective prolongation of the H-V interval.[315] *His*-bundle recordings in patients on therapeutic doses of nortriptyline also indicate prolonged H-V conduction time, with normal A-H conduction.[315] These changes resemble the antiarrhythmic effects of quinidine and procainamide, prompting some investigators to advise against the use of these antiarrhythmics in the treatment of tricyclic-induced arrhythmias.[314, 316] Even in the absence of heart block or arrhythmias, concurrent treatment with tricyclics and quinidine-like drugs should be carefully supervised, if not avoided. Physostigmine, a centrally active anticholinesterase agent, is useful in reversing many of the toxic CNS manifestations of tricyclic overdose.[317, 318] It may also potentiate heart block in such patients and must be administered cautiously, however. The cardiac effects of tricyclics may not prove exclusively deleterious in all patients with heart disease. One recent study suggested that these quinidine-like properties may actually be exploitable for antiarrhythmic purposes.[316]

In terms of cardiac toxicity, doxepin has proved considerably less problematic in many of these reports. In overdosage,[315] and in normal doses,[310, 315] doxepin appears to cause fewer alterations in rhythm or conduction. *His*-bundle recordings, again in toxic and therapeutic doses, show fewer significant changes in patients taking this tricyclic.[315] The incidence of hypotension and supraventricular tachycardia is also reportedly lower.[114, 310] Even nonspecific T-wave changes appear less common in doxepin-treated patients.[115, 116, 310]

The likelihood that a given patient will experience clinically significant cardiac effects is difficult to predict. The fact that drug serum levels show considerable interindividual variation is a further complication. Certain conclusions seem warranted, however. Tricyclic antidepressants have a potent cardiotoxic potential and should be used with extreme caution in patients with a history of cardiac disease. Careful EKG monitoring and possible drug serum levels are important clinical parameters. Although there is less clinical experience with doxepin, and doubts exist as to its therapeutic potency, the prevailing evidence suggests that it may be the safest antidepressant for such patients.

Finally, electroconvulsive therapy (ECT) is still recognized as an unusually effective treatment for endogenous depressive disorders.[319] Some authors suggest that in delusional depressions it may be the therapy of choice.[53, 320] This treatment modality deserves consideration for medical patients suffering severe morbidity from a depressive illness, particularly if pharmacotherapy presents significant hazards. The risk of ECT for cardiac patients is small, and they can be carefully monitored throughout their relatively brief course of treatment.

### Addendum

Morgan et al[321] have recently reported the use of bromocriptine, a long-acting dopamine agonist,[322] in the treatment of a patient with chronic hepatic encephalopathy. The rationale for attempting this form of treatment stems from previous suggestions that dopamine neurotransmission is altered in hepatic encephalopathy[323] and that levodopa is helpful in some cases.[324, 325] Morgan describes dramatic improvement in cognitive motor and social function in their patient without adverse pharmacological side effects. The use of bromocriptine is still experimental at this time.

## References

1. Greenblatt DJ, Shader RI, Koch-Weser J: Psychotropic drug use in the Boston area: a report from the Boston Collaborative Drug Surveillance Program. Arch Gen Psychiatry 32:518–521, 1975

2. Gottschalk LA, Bates DE, Fox RA, et al: Psychoactive drug use. Patterns found in samples from a mental health clinic and a general medical clinic. Arch Gen Psychiatry 25:395–397, 1971

3. Parry HJ, Balter MB, Mellinger GD, et al: National patterns of psychotherapeutic drug use. Arch Gen Psychiatry 28:769–783, 1973

4. Stolley PD, Becker MH, McEvilla JD, et al: Drug prescribing and use in an American community. Ann Intern Med 76:537–540, 1972

5. Miller RR: Drug surveillance utilizing epidemiological methods—a report from the Boston Collaborative Drug Surveillance Program. Am J Hosp Pharm 30:584–592, 1973

6. May FE, Stewart RB, Cluff LE: Drug use in the hospital: evaluation of determinants. Clin Pharmacol Ther 16:834–845, 1974

7. Balter MB, Levine JO: The nature and extent of psychotropic drug usage in the United States. Psychopharmacol Bull 5:3–13, (October), 1969

8. Greenblatt DJ, Shader RI: Psychotropic drugs in the general hospital. In Shader RI (Ed.): Manual of Psychiatric Therapeutics. Boston, Little, Brown and Company, 1975, pp 1–26

9. Greenblatt DJ, Shader RI: The clinical choice of sedative-hypnotics. Ann Intern Med 77:91–100, 1972

10. Hartmann E: The effect of four drugs on sleep patterns in man. Psychopharmacologia 12:346–353, 1968

11. Kales A, Bixler EO, Tan T-L, et al: Chronic hypnotic-drug use. Ineffectiveness, drug-withdrawal, insomnia, and dependence. JAMA 227:513–517, 1974

12. Conney AH: Pharmacological implications of microsomal enzyme induction. Pharmacol Rev 19:317–366, 1967

13. Kuntzman R: Drugs and enzyme induction. Annu Rev Pharmacol 9:21–36, 1969

14. Remmer H: Induction of drug metabolizing enzyme systems in the liver. Eur J Clin Pharmacol 5:115–136, 1972

15. Koch-Weser J, Sellers EM: Drug interactions with coumarin anticoagulants. N Engl J Med 285:487–498, 547–558, 1971

16. Forrest FM, Forrest IS, Serra MT: Modification of chlorpromazine metabolism by some other drugs frequently administered to psychiatric patients. Biol Psychiatry 2:53–58, 1970

17. Curry SH, Davis JM, Janowsky DS, Marshall JHL: Factors affecting chlorpromazine plasma levels in psychiatric patients. Arch Gen Psychiatry 22:209–215, 1970

18. Alexanderson B, Evans DAP, Sjöqvist F: Steady-state plasma levels of nortriptyline in twins: influence of genetic factors and drug therapy. Br Med J 4:764–768, 1969

19. Burrows GD, Davies B: Antidepressants and barbiturates. Br Med J 3:113, 1971

20. Vesell ES, Page JG: Genetic control of the phenobarbital-induced shortening of plasma antipyrine half-lives in man. J Clin Invest 48:2202–2209, 1969

21. Kater RMH, Tobon F, Iber FL: Increased rate of tolbutamide metabolism in alcoholic patients. JAMA 207:363–365, 1969

22. Kater RMH, Roggin G, Tobon F, et al: Increased rate of clearance of drugs from the circulation of alcoholics. Am J Med Sci 258:35–39, 1969

23. Solomon HM, Abrams WB: Interactions between digitoxin and other drugs in man. Am Heart J 83:277–280, 1972

24. Nitti V, Ninni A, Meola G, et al: Comparative investigations of the enzyme-inducing activity of rifampicin and barbiturates in man. Chemotherapy 19:206–210, 1973

25. Neuvonen PJ, Penttila O: Interaction between doxycycline and barbiturates. Br Med J 1:535–536, 1974

26. Greenwood RH, Prunty FTG, Silver J: Osteomalacia after prolonged glutethimide administration. Br Med J 1:643–645, 1973

27. Correy AH, Jacobson M, Schneidman K, et al: Induction of liver microsomal cortisol 6 β-hydroxylase by diphenylhydantoin or phenobarbital: an explanation for the increased excretion of 6-hydroxycortisol in humans treated with these drugs. Life Sci 4:1091–1098, 1965

28. Burns JJ, Conney AH, Koster R: Stimulating effect of chronic drug administration on drug metabolizing enzymes in liver microsomes. Ann NY Acad Sci 104:881–893, 1963

29. Misra PS, Lefevre A, Ishii H, et al: Increase of ethanol, meprobamate, and pentobarbital metabolism after chronic ethanol administration in man and rats. Am J Med 51:346–351, 1971

30. Cucinell SA, Conney AH, Sansur M, et al: Drug interactions in man. I. Lowering effect of phenobarbital on plasma levels of bishydroxycoumarin (Dicumarol) and diphenylhydantoin (Dilantin). Clin Pharmacol Ther 6:420–429, 1965

31. Buchanan RA, Heffelfinger JC, Weiss CF: The effect of phenobarbital on diphenylhydantoin metabolism in children. Pediatrics 43:114–116, 1969

32. Kristensen M, Hansen JM, Skovsted L: The influence of phenobarbital on the half-life of diphenylhydantoin in man. Acta Med Scand 185:347–350, 1969

33. Sotaniemi E, Arvela P, Hakkarainen H, et al: The clinical significance of microsomal enzyme induction in the therapy of epileptic patients. Ann Clin Res 2:223–227, 1970

34. Morselli PL, Rizzo M, Garattini S: Interaction between phenobarbital and diphenylhydantoin in animals and in epileptic patients. Ann NY Acad Sci 179:88–107, 1971

35. Kaldor A, Juvancz P, Demeczky M, et al: Enhancement of methyldopa metabolism with barbiturate. Br Med J 3:518–519, 1971

36. O'Reilly RA, Aggeler PM: Determinants of the response to oral anticoagulant drugs in man. Pharmacol Rev 22:35–96, 1970

37. Hansten PD: Drug Interactions, (3rd ed.). Philadelphia, Lea and Febiger, 1975, p 201

38. Evaluations of Drug Interactions, (2nd ed.). American Pharmaceutical Association, Washington, D.C. 1976

39. Goss JE, Dickhaus DW: Increased bishydroxycoumarin requirements in patients taking phenobarbital. N Engl J Med 273:1094–1095, 1965

40. Corn M, Rockett JF: Inhibition of bishydroxycoumarin activity by phenobarbital. Med Ann DC 54:578–579, 1965

41. Robinson DS, MacDonald MG: The effect of phenobarbital administration on the control of coagulation achieved during warfarin therapy in man. J Pharmacol Exp Ther 153:250–253, 1966

42. MacDonald MG, Robinson DS: Clinical observations of possible barbiturate interference with anticoagulation. JAMA 204:97–100, 1968

43. Levy G, O'Reilly RA, Aggeler PM, Keech GM: Pharmacokinetic analysis of the effect of barbiturate on the anticoagulant action of warfarin in man. Clin Pharmacol Ther 11:372–377, 1970

44. van Dam FE, Gribnau-Overkamp MJH: The effect of some sedatives (phenobarbital, gluthetimide, chlordiazepoxide, chloral hydrate) on the rate of disappearance of ethyl biscoumacetate from the plasma. Folia Med Neerl 10:141–145, 1967

45. MacDonald MG, Robinson DS, Sylwester D, Jaffe JJ: The effects of phenobarbital, chloral betaine, and glutethimide administration on warfarin plasma levels and hypoprothrombinemic responses in man. Clin Pharmacol Ther 10:80–84, 1969

46. Corn M: Effect of phenobarbital and glutethimide on biological half-life of warfarin. Thromb Diath Haemorrh 12:606–612, 1966

47. Starr KJ, Petrie JC: Drug interactions in patients on long-term oral anticoagulant and antihypertensive adrenergic neuron-blocking drugs. Br Med J 4:133, 1972

48. Brooks SM, Werk EE, Ackerman SJ, et al: Adverse effects of phenobarbital on corticosteroid metabolism in patients with bronchial asthma. N Engl J Med 286: 1125–1128, 1972

49. Hammer W, Ideström C-M, Sjöquist F: Chemical control of antidepressant drug therapy. In Garattini S, Dukes MNG (Eds.), Proceedings of the First International Symposium on Antidepressant Drugs. Excerpta Medica International Congress Series No. 122, 1967, pp 301–310

50. Asberg M, et al: Relationship between plasma level and therapeutic effect of nortriptyline. Br Med J 3:331–334, 1971

51. Kragh-Sorensen P, Hansen CE, Asberg M: Plasma levels of nortriptyline in the treatment of endogenous depression. Acta Psychiatr Scand 49:444–456, 1973

52. Kane J, Rifkin A, Quitkin F, Klein DF: Antidepressant drug blood levels, pharmacokinetics and clinical outcome. In Klein DF, Gittelman-Klein R (Eds.), Progress in Psychiatric Drug Treatment, 2. New York, Brunner/Mazel, 1976, p 136

53. Glassman A, Perel J, Shostak M, et al: Clinical implications of imipramine plasma levels for depressive illness. Arch Gen Psychiatry 34(2):197–204, 1977

54. Gibson IIJM: Barbiturate delirium. Practitioner 197:345–347, 1966

55. Dawson-Butterworth K: The chemopsychotherapeutics of geriatric sedation. J Am Geriatr Soc 18:97–114, 1970

56. Lamy PP, Kitler ME: Drugs and the geriatric patient. J Am Geriatr Soc 19:23–33, 1971

57. Goldstein L, Graedon J, Willard D, et al: A comparative study of the effects of methaqualone and glutethimide on sleep in male chronic insomniacs. J Clin Pharmacol 10:258–268, 1970

58. Robinson DS, Sylwester D: Interaction of commonly prescribed drugs with warfarin. Ann Intern Med 72:853–856, 1970

59. Sellers EM, Lang M, Koch-Weser J, Colman RW: Enhancement of warfarin-induced hypoprothrombinemia by triclofos. Clin Pharmacol Ther 13:911–915, 1972

60. Sellers EM, Koch-Weser J: Potentiation of warfarin-induced hypoprothrombinemia by chloral hydrate. N Engl J Med 283: 827–831, 1970

61. Lunde PKM, Anders R, Summer JY: Plasma protein binding of diphenylhydantoin in man. Clin Pharmacol Ther 11: 846–855, 1970

62. Solomon HM, Schrogie JJ: The effect of various drugs on the binding of $^{14}C$ to human albumin. Biochem Pharmacol 16: 1219–1226, 1967

63. Kramer CH: Methaqualone and chloral hydrate: preliminary comparison in geriatric patients. J Am Geriatr Soc 15:455–461, 1967

64. Kales J, Tan T-L, Swearingen C, et al: Are over-the-counter sleep medications effective? All-night EEG studies. Curr Ther Res 13:143–151, 1971

65. Shader RI, Greenblatt DJ: Uses and toxicity of belladonna alkaloids and synthetic anticholinergics. Semin Psychiatry 3: 449–476, 1971

66. Greenblatt DJ, Shader RI, Koch-Weser J: Flurazepam hydrochloride. Clin Pharmacol Ther 17:1–14, 1975

67. Greenblatt DJ, Shader RI: Drug therapy. Benzodiazepines. N Engl J Med 291: 1011–1015; 1239–1243, 1974

68. Greenblatt DJ, Shader RI: Meprobamate: a study of irrational drug use. Am J Psychiatry 127:1297–1303, 1971

69. Laites VG, Weiss B: A critical review of the efficacy of meprobamate (Miltown, Equanil) in the treatment of anxiety. J Chronic Dis 7:500–519, 1958

70. Hunninghake DB, Azarnoff DL: Drug interactions with warfarin. Arch Intern Med 121:349–352, 1968

71. Udall JA: Warfarin therapy not influenced by meprobamate. A controlled study. Curr Ther Res 12:724–728, 1970

72. Shelton J, Hollister LE: Simulated abuse of tybamate in man. JAMA 199:338–340, 1967

73. Greenblatt DJ, Shader RI: Rational use of psychotropic drugs. II. Antianxiety agents. J Maine Med Assoc 65(9):225–229, 1974

74. Shader RI, Greenblatt DJ, Salzman C, et al: Benzodiazepines: safety and toxicity. Dis Nerv Syst 36(2):23–26, 1975

75. Zbinden G, Bardon RE, Keith EF, et al: Experimental and clinical toxicity of chlordiazepoxide (Librium$^R$). Toxicol Appl Pharmacol 3:619–637, 1961

76. Carroll BJ: Attempted suicide: hypnotics and sedatives. Med J Aust 2:806, 1970

77. Greenblatt DJ, Allen MD, Noel BJ, et al: Acute overdosage with benzodiazepine derivatives. Clin Pharmacol Ther 21: 497–514, 1977

78. Greenblatt DJ, Shader RI: The pharmacologic release of hostility? In, Benzodiazepines in Clinical Practice. New York, Raven Press, 1973, p 85

79. Schwartz MA, Postma E, Gaut Z: Biological half-life of chlordiazepoxide and its metabolite, demoxepam, in man. J Pharm Sci 60:1500–1503, 1971

80. Kaplan SA, Jack ML, Alexander K, et al: Pharmacokinetic profile of diazepam in man following single intravenous and oral and chronic oral administration. J Pharm Sci 62:1789–1796, 1973

81. Baird ES, Hailey DM: Plasma levels of diazepam and its major metabolite following intramuscular administration. Br J Anaesth 45:546–548, 1972

82. Kanto J: Plasma concentrations of diazepam and its metabolites after peroral intramuscular, and rectal administration. Int J Clin Pharmacol Biopharm 12(4): 427–432, 1975

83. Korttila K, Sothman A, Anderson P: Polyethylene glycol as a solvent for diazepam: bioavailability and clinical effects after intramuscular administration. Acta Pharmacol Toxicol 39:104–117, 1976

84. Greenblatt DJ, Koch-Weser J: Drug therapy: intramuscular injection of drugs. N Engl J Med 295:542–546, 1976

85. Greenblatt DJ, Shader RI, Koch-Weser J: Pharmacokinetics in clinical medicine: oxazepam versus other benzodiazepines. Dis Nerv Syst 36(2):6–13, 1975

86. Ayd FJ: Oxazepam: an overview. Dis Nerv Syst 36(2):14–16, 1975

87. Merlis S, Koepke HH: The use of oxazepam in elderly patients. Dis Nerv Syst 36(2):27–29, 1975

88. Blitt C, Petty WC, Wright WA, et al: Clinical evaluation of injectable lorazepam as a premedicant: the effect on recall. Anesth Analg 55(4):522–525, 1976

89. Drugs for anxiety and insomnia. Med Lett Drugs Ther 18(22):Oct. 22, 1976

90. Greenblatt DJ, Shader RI, Koch-Weser J: Flurazepam hydrochloride, a benzodiazepine hypnotic. Ann Intern Med 83: 237–241, 1975

91. Kaplan SA, DeSilva JAF, Jack ML, et al: Blood level profile in man following chronic oral administration of flurazepam hydrochloride. J Pharm Sci 62:1932–1935, 1973

92. Shader RI, DiMascio A (Eds.): Psychotropic Drug Side Effects: Clinical and Theoretical Perspectives. Baltimore, Williams & Wilkins, 1970

93. Greenblatt DJ, Shader RI: Rational use of psychotropic drugs, III. Major tranquilizers. Am J Hosp Pharm 31:1226–1331, 1974

94. Loxitane[R], Loxapine Succinate. Pearl River, New York, American Cyanimid Company, 1975, p 15

95. Greenblatt DJ, Shader RI: Drug therapy—anticholinergics. N Engl J Med 288: 1215–1219, 1973

96. Gershon S, Neubauer H, Sundland DM: Interaction between some anticholinergic agents and phenothiazines. Clin Pharmacol Ther 6:749–756, 1965

97. Ayd FJ: Fatal hyperpyrexia during chlorpromazine therapy. J Clin Exp Psychopathol 17:189–192, 1956

98. Ford WL: Heat stroke with mepazine therapy. Am J Psychiatry 116:357, 1959

99. Shapiro MF: Despair, trifluoperazine, exercise and temperature of 108 F. Am J Psychiatry 124:704–707, 1967

100. Zelman S, Guillan R: Heat stroke in phenothiazine-treated patients: a report of three fatalities. Am J Psychiatry 126: 1787–1790, 1970

101. Greenblatt DJ, Greenblatt GR: Chlorpromazine and hyperpyrexia. Clin Pediatr 12:504–505, 1973

102. Sharma NGK, Tikare SK: Accidental hypothermia following chlorpromazine ingestion. J Assoc Physicians India 19: 879–881, 1971

103. Jones IH, Meade TW: Hypothermia following chlorpromazine therapy in myxoedematous patients. Gerontol Clin 6:252–256, 1964

104. Exton-Smith AN: Phenothiazines in cold weather. Br Med J 1:441, 1972

105. DiMascio A, Shader RI (Eds.): Butyrophenones in Psychiatry. New York, Raven Press, 1972

106. Ayd FJ: Haloperidol: fifteen years of clinical experience. Dis Nerv System 33:459–468, 1972

107. Curry SH, Davis JM, Janowsky DS, et al: Factors affecting chlorpromazine plasma levels in psychiatric patients. Arch Gen Psychiatry 22:209–215, 1970

108. Fann WE, Davis JM, Janowsky DS, et al: The effects of antacids on the blood levels of chlorpromazine. Clin Pharmacol Ther 14:135, 1973

109. Fann WE, Davis JM, Janowsky DS, et al: Chlorpromazine: effects of antacids on its gastrointestinal absorption. J Clin Pharmacol 13:388–390, 1973

110. Alexanderson B: Pharmacokinetics of desmethylimipramine and nortriptyline in man after single and multiple oral doses—a cross-over study. Eur J Clin Pharmacol 5:1–10, 1972

111. Saraf K, Klein DF: The safety of a single daily dose schedule for imipramine. Am J Psychiatry 128:483–484, 1971

112. Ayd FJ: Rational pharmacotherapy: once-a-day dosage. Dis Nerv Syst 34:371–378, 1973

113. Ayd FJ: Central anticholinergic activity and tricyclic antidepressant efficacy. International Drug Therapy Newsletter. 10(6): June, 1975

114. Pitts NE: The clinical evaluation of doxepin—a new psychotherapeutic agent. Psychosomatics 10:164–171, 1969

115. Sinequan (Doxepin HCL). A Clinical Appraisal, New York, Pfizer Laboratories, 1971

116. Ayd FJ: Long-term administration of doxepin. Dis Nerv Syst 32:617–622, 1971

117. Ballin JC: Toxicity of tricyclic antidepressants (editorial). JAMA 231:1369, 1975

118. Consolo S, Morselli PL, Zaccalea M, et al: Delayed absorption of phenylbutazone caused by desmethylimipramine in man. Eur J Pharmacol 10:239–242, 1970

119. Messiha FS, Morgan JP: Imipramine-mediated effects on levodopa metabolism in man. Biochem Pharmacol 23:1503–1507, 1974

120. Gram LF, Overo KF: Drug interaction: inhibitory effect of neuroleptics on metabolism of tricyclic antidepressants in man. Br Med J 1:463–465, 1972

121. Khurana RC: Estrogen-imipramine interaction. JAMA 222:702–703, 1972

122. Zeidenberg P, Perel JM, Kanzler M et al: Clinical and metabolic studies with imipramine in man. Am J Psychiatry 127: 1321–1326, 1971

123. Perel JM, Shostak M, Gann E, et al: Pharmacodynamics of imipramine and clinical outcome in depressed patients. In Gottschalk LA, Merlis S (Eds.), Pharmacokinetics of Psychoactive Drugs: Blood Levels and Clinical Response. New York, Spectrum, 1976.

124. Prange AJ, Wilson IC, Rabon AM, et al: Enhancement of imipramine antidepressant activity by thyroid hormone. Am J Psychiatry 126:457–469, 1969

125. Earle BV: Thyroid hormone and tricyclic antidepressants in resistant depressions. Am J Psychiatry 126:1667–1669, 1970

126. Prange AJ, Wilson IC, Knox A, et al: Enhancement of imipramine by thyroid stimulating hormone: clinical and theoretical implications. Am J Psychiatry 127: 191–199, 1970

127. Wilson IC, Prange AJ, McClane TK, et al: Thyroid-hormone enhancement of imipramine in nonretarded depression N Engl J Med 282:1063–1067, 1970

128. Prange AJ, Wilson IC, Knox AE, et al: Thyroid-imipramine clinical and chemical interaction: evidence for a receptor deficit in depression. J Psychiatry Res 9:187–205, 1972

129. Glassman AH, Hurwic MJ, Perel JM: Plasma binding of imipramine and clinical response. Am J Psychiatry 130: 1367–1369, 1973

130. Hessov J: Hypertension during chlorimipramine therapy. Br Med J 1:406, 1971

131. Boakes AJ, Laurence DR, Teoh PC, et al: Interactions between sympathomimetic amines and antidepressant agents in man. Br Med J 1:311–315, 1973

132. Spiker DG, Pugh DD: Combining tricyclic and monoamine oxidase inhibitor antidepressants. Arch Gen Psychiatry 33: 828–830, 1976

133. Davis JM: Overview: maintenance therapy in psychiatry, II. Affective disorders. Am J Psychiatry 133:1–13, 1976

134. Gershon S, Shopsin B (Eds.): Lithium: Its

Role in Psychiatric Research and Treatment. New York, Plenum Press, 1973

135. Bunney WE, Murphy DL: The neurobiology of lithium. Neurosci Res Program Bull 14:2, 1976

136. Singer I, Rottenberg D: Mechanisms of lithium action. N Engl J Med 289: 254–206,1973

137. Schou M: Lithium in psychiatric therapy. Psychopharmacologia 1:65–78, 1959

138. Schou M: Electrocardiographic changes during treatment with lithium and with drugs of the imipramine-type. Acta Psychiatr Scand 39(169):258–259, 1963.

139. Demers RG, Heninger GR: Electrocardiographic changes during lithium treatment. Dis Nerv System 33:674–679, 1970

140. Demers RG, Heninger GR: Electrocardiographic T-wave changes during lithium carbonate treatment. JAMA 218:318–386, 1971

141. Verbov JL, Phillips JD, Fife DG: A case of lithium intoxication. Postgrad Med 41: 190–192, 1965

142. Horowitz LC, Fisher GU: Acute lithium toxicity. N Engl J Med 281:1369, 1969

143. Gershon S, Shopsin B (Eds.): Lithium: Its Role in Psychiatric Research and Treatment. New York, Plenum Press, 1973, pp 110–113

144. Gershon S: The treatment of manic-depressive states. In Shader RI (Ed.), Manual of Psychiatric Therapeutics. Boston, Little, Brown and Company, 1975, p 101

145. Elizur A, Shopsin B, Gershon S: Intracellular lithium ratios and clinical course in affective states. Clin Pharmacol Therap 13:947–953, 1972

146. Kurtin S: Lithium carbonate dermatitis. JAMA 223:802, 1973

147. Ruiz-Maldonado R, Perez deFrancisco C, Tamayo L: Lithium dermatitis. JAMA 224:1534, 1973

148. Neil JF, Himmelbach J, Licata S: Emergence of myasthenia gravis during treatment with lithium carbonate. Arch Gen Psychiatry 33:1090–1092, 1976

149. Drugs for improvement of cerebral function in the elderly. Med Lett Drugs Ther 18(9):April 23, 1976, pp 38–39

150. Shader RI, Goldsmith GN: Dihydrogenated ergot alkaloids and papaverine: a status report on their effects in senile mental deterioration. In Klein DF, Gittelmann-Klein R (Eds.), Progress in Psychiatric Drug Treatment, 2. New York, Brunner/Mazel, 1976, pp 540–554

151. Salzman C, van der Kolk B, Shader RI: Psychopharmacology and the geriatric patient. In Shader RI (Ed.): Manual of Psychiatric Therapeutics. Boston, Little, Brown and Company, 1975, p 171

152. Fruhman G: Hypersomnia with primary hypoventilation syndrome and following cor pulmonale. Bull Physiopathol Respir (Nancy) 8:1173–1179, 1972

153. Guilleminault C, Eldridge FL, Phillips JR, et al: Two occult causes of insomnia and their therapeutic problems. Arch Gen Psychiatry 33:1241–1245, 1976

154. Greenblatt DJ, Shader RI, Lofgren S: Rational psychopharmacology for patients with medical diseases. Annu Rev Med 27:407–420, 1976

155. Kales A, Kales JD: Recent advances in the diagnosis and treatment of sleep disorders. In Usdin G (Ed.), The Relevance of Sleep Research to Clinical Practice. New York, Brunner/Mazel, 1972, pp 61–94

156. Kales A, Allen C, Scharf MB, et al: Hypnotic drugs and their effectiveness: all night EEG studies of insomniac subjects. Arch Gen Psychiatry 23:226–232, 1970

157. Kales A, Kales J: Sleep disorders. Recent findings in the diagnosis and treatment of disturbed sleep. N Engl J Med 290: 487–499, 1974

158. Rickels K, Bass H: A comparative controlled clinical trial of seven hypnotic agents in medical and psychiatric inpatients. Am J Med Sci 245:142–159, 1963

159. Brown WT: A comparative study of three hypnotics: methyprylon, glutethimide, and chloral hydrate. Can Med Assoc J 102: 510–511, 1970

160. Jick H, Slone D, Shapiro S, et al: Clinical effects of hypnotics, I. A controlled trial. JAMA 209:2013–2015, 1969

161. LeRiche WG, van Belle G: Clinical and statistical evaluation of six hypnotic agents. Can Med Assoc J 88:837–841, 1963

162. Kales J, Kales A, Bixler EO, et al: Effects of placebo and flurazepam on sleep patterns in insomniac subjects. Clin Pharmacol Ther 12:691–697, 1971

163. Kales A, Kales JD, Leo LA, et al: Evaluation of the effectiveness of hypnotic drugs under conditions of prolonged use (abstract). Sleep Res 2:157, 1973.

164. Baume P, Cuthbert J: The effect of medazepam in relieving symptoms of functional gastrointestinal distress. Aust NZ J Med 3:457–460, 1973

165. Hagermark O: Influence of antihistamines, sedatives, and aspirin on experimental itch. Acta DermaVenereol 53:363–368, 1973

166. Deutsch E: Relief of anxiety and related emotions in patients with gastrointestinal disorders. Amer J Dig Dis 16:1091–1094, 1971

167. Calvert A, Mitchell AS, Sinclair G: A double-blind evaluation of diazepam and amylobarbutone in acute myocardial infarction. Med J Aust 2:624–627, 1974

168. Benson WH: Comparative evaluation of diazepam (Valium) and phenobarbital. J Med Assoc Ga 60:276–278, 1971

169. Kasich AM: Clorazepate dipotassium in the treatment of anxiety associated with chronic gastrointestinal disease. Curr Ther Res 15:83–91, 1973

170. Hackett TP, Cassem NH: Reduction of anxiety in the coronary care unit: a controlled double-blind comparison of chlordiazepoxide and amobarbital. Curr Ther Res 14:649–656, 1972

171. Granville-Grossman KL, Turner P: The effect of propranolol in anxiety. Lancet 1:788–790, 1966

172. Wheatley D: Comparative effects of propranolol and chlordiazepoxide in anxiety states. Br J Psychiatry 115:1411–1412, 1969

173. Tyrer PJ, Lader MH: Response to propranolol and diazepam in somatic and psychic anxiety. Br Med J 2:14–16, 1974

174. Bonn JA, Turner P, Hicks DC: Beta-adrenergic blockade with practolol in treatment of anxiety. Lancet 1:814–815, 1972

175. Tyrer PJ, Lader MH: Effects of beta-adrenergic blockade with sotalol in chronic anxiety. Clin Pharmacol Ther 14:418–426, 1973

176. Shader RI, Good MI, Greenblatt DJ: Anxiety states and beta-adrenergic blockade. In Klein DF, Gittleman-Klein R (Eds.), Progress in Psychiatric Drug Treatment, 2. New York, Brunner/Mazel, 1976, pp 509–528

177. Lader M: The peripheral and central role of catecholamines in the mechanisms of anxiety. Int Pharmacopsychiatry 9:125–137, 1974

178. Shader RI, Greenblatt DJ: The psychopharmacologic treatment of anxiety states. In Shader RI (Ed.), Manual of Psychiatric Therapeutics. Boston, Little, Brown and Company, 1975, p 27

179. Kendall RE: The classification of depressions: a review of contemporary confusion. Br J Psychiatry 129:15–28, 1976

180. Schildkraut JJ, Klein DF: The classification and treatment of depressive disorders. In Shader RI (Ed.), Manual of Psychiatric Therapeutics. Boston, Little, Brown and Company, 1975, p 39

181. Greenblatt DJ, Shader RI: Rational use of psychotropic drugs. IV. Antidepressants. J Maine Med Assoc 65(11):283–288, 1974

182. Morris JB, Beck AT: The efficacy of antidepressant drugs. Arch Gen Psychiatry 30:667–674, 1974

183. Raskin A: A guide for drug use in depressive disorders. Am J Psychiatry 131(2):181–185, 1974

184. Thomas FB, Mazzaferri EL, Shillman TG: Apathetic thyrotoxicosis: a distinctive clinical and laboratory entity. Ann Intern Med 72:679–684, 1970

185. Goodwin FK, Ebert MH, Bunney WE: Mental effects of reserpine in man: a review. In Shader RI (Ed.), Psychiatric Complications of Medical Drugs. New York, Raven Press, 1972, pp 73–101

186. Smith SL: Mood and the menstrual cycle. In Sachar EJ, Topics in Psychoendocrinology. New York, Grune and Stratton, 1975, pp 19–58

187. Prichard BNC, Johnston AW, Hill ID, et al: Bethanidine, guanethidine, and methyldopa in treatment of hypertension: a within-patient comparison. Br Med J 1:134–144, 1968

188. Waal HJ: Propranolol-induced depression. Br Med J 2:50, 1967.

189. MacDougal AI, Addis GJ, MacKay N, et al: Treatment of hypertension with clonidine. Br Med J 3:440–442, 1970

190. Shader RI (Ed.): Psychiatric Complications of Medical Drugs. New York, Raven Press, 1972

191. Hall RWC, Jaffe JR: Aberrant response to

diazepam: a new syndrome. Am J Psychiatry 126:738–742, 1972

192. Weiss HD, Walker MD, Wiernik PH: Neurotoxicity of commonly used antineoplastic agents. N Engl J Med 291:75–81; 127–133, 1974

193. Post F: Dementia, depression and pseudodementia. In Benson DF, Blummer D (Eds.), Psychiatric Aspects of Neurologic Desease. New York, Grune and Stratton, 1975, pp 99–120

194. Pollit J, Young J: Anxiety state or masked depression? a study based on action of monoamine oxidase inhibitors. Br J Psychiat 119:143–149, 1971

195. Raviris CL, Nies A, Robinson D, et al: A multiple-dose controlled study of phenelzine in depression—anxiety states. Arch Gen Psychiatry 33:347–350, 1976

196. Robinson DS, Nies A, Ravaris L, et al: The monoamine oxidase inhibitor phenelzine, in the treatment of depressive-anxiety states. a controlled clinical trial. Arch Gen Psychiatry 29:407–413, 1973

197. Greenblatt DJ, Shader RI: Psychotropic drugs, medical disease, and other medical therapies. In Greenblatt M (Ed.), Drugs in Combination with Other Therapies. New York, Grune and Stratton, 1976

198. Singh G, Verma HC: Drug treatment of chronic intractable pain in patients referred to a psychiatry clinic. J Indian Med Assoc 56:341–345, 1971

199. Detre MP, Jarecki HG: Modern Psychiatric Treatment. Philadelphia, J.P. Lippincott Company, 1971, Chapter 11

200. Leszkovsky G, Tardos L: Some effects of propranolol on the central nervous system. J Pharm Pharmacol 17:518–519, 1965

201. Singh KP, Bhavdari DS, Mahawaler MM: Effects of propranolol (a beta-adrenergic blocking agent) on some central nervous system parameters. Indian J Med Res 59:786–794, 1971

202. Mitchell JR, Oates JA: Guanethidine and related agents, I. Mechanisms of the selective blockade of adrenergic neurons and its antagonism by drugs. J Pharmacol Exp Ther 172:100–107, 1970

203. Leishman AWD, Matthews HL, Smith HL: Antagonism of guanethidine by imipramine. Lancet 1:112, 1963

204. Mitchell JR, Arias L, Oates JA: Antagonism of the antihypertensive action of guanethidine sulfate by desipramine hydrochloride. JAMA 202:973–976, 1967

205. Meyer JF, McAllister K, Goldberg LI: Insidious and prolonged antagonism of guanethidine by amitriptyline. JAMA 213:1487–1488, 1970

206. Mitchell JR, Cavanaugh JH, Arias L, et al: Guanethidine and related agents, III. Antagonism by agents which inhibit the norepinephrine pump in man. J Clin Invest 49:1596–1604, 1970

207. Fann WE, Cavanaugh JH, Kaufman JS: Doxepin: effects on transport of biogenic amines in man. Psychopharmacologia 22:111–125, 1971

208. Ober KF, Wang RIH: Drug interactions with guanethidine. Clin Pharmacol Ther 14:190–195, 1973

209. Briant RH, Reid JL, Dollerty CT: Interaction between clonidine and desipramine in man. Br Med J 1:522–523, 1973

210. Janowsky DS, El-Yousef MK, Davis JM: Antagonism of guanethidine by chlorpromazine. Am J Psychiatry 130:808–812, 1973

211. Shopsin B: Effects of lithium on thyroid function (a review). Dis Nerv Syst 31: 237–244, 1970

212. Rifkin A, Quitkin F, Blumberg AG, et al: The effect of lithium on thyroid functioning: a controlled study. J Psychiatr Res 10:115–120, 1974

213. Spaulding SW, Burrow GN, Bermudez F, et al: The inhibitory effect of lithium on thyroid hormone release in both euthyroid and thyrotoxic patients. J Clin Endocrinol Metab 35:905–911, 1972

214. Burrow GN, Burke WR, Himmelhoch JM, et al: Effect of lithium on thyroid function. J Clin Endocrinol Metab 32:647–652, 1971

215. Schou M, Amdisen A, Jensen SE, et al: Occurence of goitre during lithium treatment. Br Med J 3:710–713, 1968

216. Villeneuve A, Gautier J, Jus A, et al: The effect of lithium on thyroid in man. Int J Clin Pharmacol 9:75–80, 1974

217. Crowe MJ, Lloyd GG, Bloch S, et al: Hypothyroidism in patients treated with lithium: a review and two case reports. Pyschol Med 3:337–342, 1973

218. Rogers MP, Whybrow PC: Clinical hypothyroidism occurring during lithium treatment: two case histories and a review of thryoid function in 19 patients. Am J Psychiatry 128:158–163, 1971

219. Lindstedt G, Lundberg P-A, Tofft M, et al: Serum thyrotropin and hypothyroidism during lithium therapy. Clin Chim Acta 48:127–133, 1973

220. Shopsin B, Shenkman L, Blum M, et al: Iodine and lithium-induced hypothyroidism. Am J Med 55:695–699, 1973

221. Edhag O, Swahn A, Wester PO: Hypothyroidism following lithium treatment. Acta Med Scand 193:553–555, 1973

222. Temple R, Berman M, Carlson HE, et al: The use of lithium in the treatment of thyrotoxicosis. J Clin Invest 51:2746–2756, 1972

223. Lomas J, Boardman RH, Markowe M: Complications of chlorpromazine therapy in 800 mental-hospital patients. Lancet 1:1144–1147, 1955

224. Shaw EB: Convulsive seizures following phenothiazine tranquilizers. Pediatrics 22:175–176, 1958

225. Dallos V, Heathfield K: Iatrogenic epilepsy due to antidepressant drugs. Br Med J 4:80–82, 1969

226. Betts TA, Kalra PL, Cooper R, et al: Epileptic fits as a possible side-effect of amitriptyline. Report of seven cases. Lancet 1:390–392, 1968

227. Brown D, Winsberg BG, Bialer I, et al: Imipramine therapy and seizures: three children treated for hyperactive behavior disorders. Am J Psychiatry 130:210–212, 1973

228. Chambers JF, Schultz JD: Double-blind study of three drugs in the treatment of acute alcoholic states. Q J Stud Alcohol 26:10–18, 1965

229. Sereny G, Kalant H: Comparative clinical evaluation of chlordiazepoxide and promazine in treatment of alcohol-withdrawal syndrome. Br Med J 1:92–97, 1965

230. Golbert TM, Sanz CJ, Rose HD, et al: Comparative evaluation of treatments of alcohol withdrawal syndromes. JAMA 201:99–102, 1967

231. Kaim SC, Klett CJ, Rothfeld B: Treatment of the acute alcohol withdrawal state: a comparison of four drugs. Am J Psychiatry 125:1640–1646, 1969

232. Model DG: Nitrazepam induced respiratory depression in chronic obstructive lung disease. Br J Dis Chest 67:128–130, 1973

233. Gaddie J, Legge JS, Palmer KN, et al: Effect of nitrazepam in chronic obstructive bronchitis. Br Med J 2:688–689, 1972

234. Catchlove RFH, Kafer ER: The effects of diazepam on respiration in patients with obstructive pulmonary disease. Anesthesiology 34:14–18, 1971

235. Denault M, Yernault JC, DeCoster A: Double-blind comparison of the respiratory effects of parenteral lorazepam and diazepam in patients with chronic obstructive lung disease. Curr Med Res Opinion 2:611–615, 1975

236. Rao S, Sherbaniuk RW, Prasad K, et al: Cardiopulmonary effects of diazepam. Clin Pharmacol Ther 14:182–189, 1973

237. Kronenberg RS, Cosio MG, Stevenson JE, et al: The use of oral diazepam in patients with obstructive lung disease and hypercapnia. Ann Intern Med 83:83–84, 1975

238. Model DG, Berry DJ: Effects of chlordiazepoxide in respiratory failure due to chronic bronchitis. Lancet 2:869–870, 1974

239. Pearce C: The respiratory effects of diazepam supplementation of spinal anesthesia in elderly males. Br J Anasth 46:439–441, 1974

240. Greenblatt DJ, Koch-Weser J: Adverse reactions to intravenous diazepam: a report from the Boston Collaborative Drug Surveillance Program. Am J Med Sci 266:261–266, 1973

241. Taclob L, Needle M: Drug-induced encephalopathy in patients on maintenance haemodialysis. Lancet 2:704–705, 1976

242. Kangas L, Kanto J, Forsström J, et al: The protein binding of diazepam and N-methyl diazepam in patients with poor renal function. Clinical Nephrology 5:114–118, 1976

243. Verbeeck R, Tjandramaga R, Verberckmoes R, et al: Biotransformation and excretion of lorazepam in patients with chronic renal failure. Br J Clin Pharmacol 3:1033–1039, 1976

244. Smith RB, Dittert LW, Griffen WO, et al:

Pharmacokinetics of pentobarbital after intravenous and oral administration. J Pharmacokin Biopharm 1:5–16, 1973

245. Greenblatt DJ, Shader RI, Harmatz JS, et al: Influence of magnesium and aluminum hydroxide mixture on chlordiazepoxide absorption. Clin Pharmacol Ther 19: 234–239, 1976

246. Shader RI, Georgotas A, Greenblatt DJ: Influence of magnesium and aluminum hydroxide on clorazepate absorption. Unpublished data

247. Schenker S, Hoyumpa AM, Wilkinson GR: The effects of parenchymal liver disease on the disposition and elimination of sedatives and analgesics. Med Clin North Am 59:587–596, 1975

248. Mawer GE, Miller NE, Turnberg LA: Metabolism of amyolbarbitone in patients with chronic liver disease. Br J Pharmacol 44:549–560, 1972

249. Alvin J, et al: The effect of liver disease in man on the disposition of phenobarbital. J Pharmacol Exp Ther 192:224–235, 1975

250. Read AE, Laidlaw J, McCarthy CF: Effects of chlorpromazine in patients with hepatic disease. Br Med J 3:497–499, 1969

251. Maxwell JD, Carbella M, Parkes JD, et al: Plasma disappearance and cerebral effects of chlorpromazine in cirrhosis. Clin Sci 43:143–151, 1972

252. Klotz U, Avant GR, Hoyumpa A, et al: The effects of age and liver disease on the disposition and elimination of diazepam in adult man. J Clin Invest 55:347–359, 1975

253. Mendenhall CL, Robinson JD, Morgan DD: Chlordiazepoxide, Librium (L), therapy in hepatic insufficiency. Gastroenterology 69:845, 1975

254. Murray-Lyon IM, Young J, Parkes JD, et al: Clinical and electroencephalic assessment of diazepam in liver disease. Br Med J 4:265–266, 1971

255. Greenblatt DJ, Koch-Weser J: Clinical toxicity of chlordiazepoxide and diazepam in relation to serum albumin concentration: a report from the Boston Collaborative Drug Surveillance Program. Eur J Clin Pharmacol 7:259–262, 1974

256. Fessel JM, Conn HO: An analysis of the causes and prevention of hepatic coma. Gastroenterology 62:191, 1972

257. Schenker S, Breen KG, Hoyumpa AM: Hepatic encephalopathy: current status. Gastroenterology 66:121–151, 1974

258. Jacobsen S, Bell B: Recognition and management of acute and chronic hepatic encephalopathy. Med Clin North Am 57:1569–1577, 1973

259. Agnosti L, Down PF, Murison J, et al: Faecal ammonia and pH during lactulose administration in man: comparison with other cathartics. Gut 13:859–866, 1972

260. Avery GS, Davies EF, Brogden RN: Lactulose: review of its therapeutic and pharmacological properties with particular reference to ammonia metabolism and its mode of action in portal systemic encephalopathy. Drugs 4:7–48, 1972

261. Elkington SG: Lactulose. Gut 11: 1043–1048, 1970

262. Brown H, Trey C, McDermott WV: Lactulose treatment of hepatic encephalopathy in out-patients. Arch Surg 102:25–27, 1971

263. Kosman ME: Lactulose (Cephulac) in portosystemic encephalopathy. JAMA 236:2444–2445, 1976

264. Bishop LF, Reichert P: The interrelationship between anxiety and arrhythmias. Psychosomatics 4:330–334, 1970

265. Engel GL: Sudden and rapid death during psychological stress: folklore or folk wisdom? Ann Intern Med 74:771–782, 1971

266. Lown B, Tempte JV, Reich P, et al: Recurring ventricullar fibrilation in the absence of coronary heart disease. N Engl J Med 294:623–629, 1976

267. Hackett TP, Cassem NH, Wishnie H: Detection and treatment of anxiety in the coronary care unit. Am Heart J 78: 727–730, 1969

268. Jewett DE, Mercer CJ, Reid O, et al: Free noradrenaline and adrenaline excretion in relation to the development of cardiac arrhythmias and heart failure in patients with acute myocardial infarction. Lancet 1, 635, 1969

269. Melsom M, Andreassen H, Melsom H, et al: Diazepam in acute myocardial infarction. Clinical effects and effects on catecholamines, free fatty acids and cortisol. Br Heart J 38:804–810, 1976

270. Van Loon GR: Ventricular arrhythmias treated by diazepam. Can Med Assoc J 98:785, 1968

271. Papp C: New Look at arrhythmias. Br Heart J 31:267, 1969

272. Hollister LE, Kosek JC: Sudden death during treatment with phenothiazine derivatives. JAMA 192:1035–1038, 1965

273. Moore MT, Book MH: Sudden death in phenothiazine therapy. Psychiatr Q 44:389–402, 1970

274. Leestma JE, Koenig KL: Sudden death and phenothiazines. A current controversy. Arch Gen Psychiatry 18:137–148, 1968

275. Cancro R, Wilder R: A mechanism of sudden death in chlorpromazine therapy. Am J Psychiatry 127:368–371, 1970

276. Madan BR, Pendse VK: Antiarrhythmic activity of thioridazine hydrochloride (Mellaril). Am J Cardiol 11:78, 1963

277. Fowler NO, McCall D, Chou T, et al: Electrocardiographic changes and cardiac arrhythmias in patients receiving psychotropic drugs. Am J Cardiol 37:233–230, 1976

278. Alexander CS, Nino A: Cardiovascular complications in young patients taking psychotropic drugs. Am Heart J 78: 757–769, 1969

279. Guillan RA, Smalley RL, Zelman S: Electrocardiographic and ultrastructural cardiac effects of phenothiazine in rabbits. Chest 62:62–65, 1972

280. Santos-Martinez J, Laboy-Torres JA, Aviles TA, et al: Electrocardiographic changes induced by some phenothiazine derivatives. Res Commun Chem Pathol Pharmacol 5:345–358, 1973

281. Ayd FJ: Cardiovascular effects of phenothiazines. Int Drug Ther Newslett 5:1–8, 1970

282. Fletcher GF, Kazamias TM, Wenger NK: Cardiotoxic effects of Mellaril: conduction disturbances and supraventricular arrhythmias. Am Heart J 78:135–138, 1969

283. Giles TD, Modlin RK: Death associated with ventricular arrhythmia and thioridazine hydrochloride. JAMA 205:108–110, 1968

284. Sydney MA: Ventricular arrhythmias associated with the use of thioridazine hydrochloride in alcohol withdrawal. Br Med J 4:467, 1973

285. Tranum BL, Murphy ML: Case report: successful treatment of ventricular tachycardia associated with thioridazine (Mellaril). South Med J 62:357–358, 1969

286. Schoonmaker FW, Osteen RT, Greenfield JC: Thioridazine (Mellaril[R])-induced ventricular tachycardia controlled with an artifical pacemaker. Ann Intern Med 65: 1076–1078, 1966

287. Wendkos MH: Cardiac changes related to phenothiazine therapy, with special reference to thioridazine. J Am Geriatr Soc 15:20–28, 1967

288. Wendkos MH: The significance of electrocardiographic changes produced by thioridazine. J New Drugs 4:322–332, 1964

289. Lapierre YD, Lapointe L, Bordeleau JM, et al: Phenothiazine treatment and electrocardiographic abnormalities. Can Psychiatr Assoc J 14:517–523, 1969

290. Alexander S, Shader R, Grinspoon L: Electrocardiographic effects of thioridazine hydrochloride (Mellaril). Lahey Clin Found Bull 16:207–215, 1967

291. Thornton CC, Wendkos MH: EKG T-wave distortions among thioridazine-treated psychiatric inpatients. Dis Nerv Syst 32:320–323, 1971

292. Alvarez-Mena SC, Frank MJ: Phenothiazine-induced T-wave abnormalities. JAMA 224:1730–1733, 1973

293. Davis JM, Bartlett E, Termini BA: Overdosage of psychotropic drugs: a review. Dis Nerv Syst 29:157–164, 246–256, 1968

294. Freeman JW, Mundy GR, Beattie RR, et al: Cardiac abnormalities in poisoning with tricyclic antidepressants. Br Med J 2: 610–611, 1969

295. Sedal L, Korman MG, Williams PO, et al: Overdosage of tricyclic antidepressants. Med J Aust 2:74–79, 1972

296. Thompson GA: Amitriptyline overdose. Drug Intel Clin Pharm 7:451–458, 1973

297. Nobel J, Matthew H: Acute poisoning by tricyclic antidepressants: clinical features and management of 100 patients. Clin Toxicol 2:403–421, 1969

298. Fouron J-C, Chicoine R: ECG changes in fatal imipramine (Tofranil) intoxication. Pediatrics 48:777–781, 1971

299. Sueblinvong V, Wilson JF: Myocardial damage due to imipramine intoxication. J Pediatr 74:475–478, 1969

300. Hong WK, Mauer P, Hochman R, et al: Amitriptyline cardiotoxicity. Chest 60: 304–306, 1974

301. Thorstrand C: Cardiovascalar effects of poisoning with tricyclic antidepressants. Acta Med Scand 195:505–514, 1974

302. Williams RB, Sherter C: Cardiac complications of tricyclic antidepressant therapy. Ann Intern Med 74:395–398, 1971

303. Robinson DS, Barker E: Tricyclic antidepressant cardiotoxicity. JAMA 236: 2089–2090, 1976

304. Raisfeld IH: Cardiovascular complications of antidepressant therapy. Am Heart J 83:129–133, 1972

305. Langslet A, Johansen WG, Ryg M, et al: Effects of dibenzepine and imipramine on the isolated rat heart. Eur J Pharmacol 14:333–339, 1971

306. Baum T, Shopshire AJ, Rowles G, et al: Antidepressants and cardiac conduction: iprindole and imipramine. Eur J Pharmacol 13:287–291, 1971

307. Buckley JP, Steenberg ML, Jandhyala BS, et al: Effects of imipramine, desmethylimipramine and their 2-OH metabolites on hemodynamics and myocardial contractility. Fed Proc 34:450, 1975

308. Jefferson J: A review of the cardiovascular effects and toxicity of tricyclic antidepressants. Psychosom Med 37:160–179, 1975

309. Kantor SJ, Bigger JT, Glassman AH, et al: Imipramine-induced heart block. JAMA 231:1364–1366, 1975

310. Vohra J, Burrows GD, Sloman G: Assessment of cardiovascular side effects of therapeutic doses of tricyclic antidepressant drugs. Aust NZ J Med 5:7–11, 1975

311. Ramanathan KB, Davidson C: Cardiac arrhythmias and imipramine therapy. Br Med J 1:661–662, 1975

312. Scollins MJ, Robinson DS, Nies A: Cardiotoxicity of amitriptyline. Lancet 2:1202, 1972

313. Moir DC, Crooks J, Cornwell WB, et al: Cardiotoxicity of amitriptyline. Lancet 2:561–564, 1972

314. Ziegler VE, Co BT, Biggs JT: Plasma Nortriptyline levels and ECG findings. Am J Psychiatry 134:441–443, 1977

315. Vohra J, Burrows G, Hunt D: The effect of toxic and therapeutic doses of tricyclic antidepressants on intra-cardiac conduction. Eur J Cardiol 3:219–227, 1975

316. Bigger JT, Giardina EGV, Perel J, et al: Cardiac antiarrhythmic effect of imipramine. N Engl J Med 296:206–207, 1977

317. Granacher RP, Baldessarini RJ: Physostigmine. Arch Gen Psychiatry 32: 375–380, 1975

318. Holinger PC, Klawans HL: Reversal of tricyclic-overdosage-induced central anticholinergic syndrome by physostigmine. Am J Psychiatry 133:1018–1023, 1976

319. Salzman C: Electroconvulsive therapy. In Shader RI (Ed.), Manual of Psychiatric Therapeutics. Boston, Little, Brown and Company, 1975, pp 115–124

320. Glassman A, Kantor S, Shostak M: Depression, delusions and drug response. Am J Psychiatry 132:716–719, 1975

321. Morgan MY, Jakobovits A, Elithorn A, et al: Successful use of bromocriptine in the treatment of a patient with chronic portasystemic encephalopathy. N Engl J Med 296:793–794, 1977

322. Hökfelt T, Fuxe K: Effects of prolactin and ergot alkaloids on the tuberoinfundibular dopamine (DA) neurons. Neuroendocrinology 9:100–122, 1972

323. Fischer JE, Baldessarini RJ: False neurotransmitters and hepatic failure. Lancet 2:75–79, 1971

324. Parkes JD, Sharpstone P, Williams R: Levodopa in hepatic coma. Lancet 2: 1341–1343, 1970

325. Lunzer M, James IM, Weinman J, et al: Treatment of chronic hepatic encephalopathy with levodopa. Gut 15: 555–561, 1974

Solomon S. Steiner
Arthur M. Arkin

# 8
# Biofeedback in the Treatment of Mental Illness

## INTRODUCTION

Writing a chapter on biofeedback in the treatment of medical illness is somewhat akin to writing a chapter on drugs in the treatment of medical illness. Like drugs, there are many different kinds of biofeedback which can be applied in many different ways to a variety of different disorders. One can push the analogy with drugs even further in that the "dose" of biofeedback, that is, the frequency and duration of the practice of a particular form of biofeedback is an important parameter in determining its efficacy. Furthermore, like drugs, biofeedback has frequently been applied to apparently well-functioning individuals to produce a state presumed to be more desirable or to further enhance normally functioning processes.

Biofeedback is a wide variety of techniques which have in common the detection and amplification of information derived from specific physiological processes which are then transformed into a modality readily discriminable by the subject (sometimes patient). The subject is then taught how to use this information to influence the physiological process in the desired fashion. (If someone can be taught to play tennis, why can he not be taught to regulate his blood pressure?) Frequently the physiological process is presumed to be influenced by the nervous system, and the specific physiological response generally eludes clear or accurate perception. This is not always the case; in a very real sense, when one gets on a bathroom scale to measure one's weight, one is using a biofeedback technique. Large changes in weight are directly perceivable by the subject. Small day to day fluctuations of weight are generally not accurately perceived by most subjects, however. The bathroom scale detects small changes in weight, amplifies these changes, and transduces them to a visual display readily perceived and understood by the subject (number of pounds and ounces or kilograms). It should be further noted that in this example, one need not assume the weight gain or loss is under direct control of the nervous system. The indirect control, by altering feeding behavior, suffices quite well in a well-motivated subject, to produce the desirable outcome of weight loss. This is a particularly important point when one is attempting to evaluate the efficacy of biofeedback as a *treatment* because at present, there is a great deal of apparent disagreement or contradiction in the literature.[1, 2] The discrepencies, we feel, are more apparent than real, because often many very different questions are being addressed which appear to be the same to the uninitiated. In order to develop this point, we must first make some distinctions between different paradigms of learning and their relationship to biofeedback.

Historically, there are two major models of conditioning and hence learning: the classical or respondent model, and the operant or instrumental model.[3] In classical conditioning, one takes advantage of an already existing innate relationship between a particular stimulus or set of stimuli and a particular response or set of responses. By definition, any stimulus which reliably elicits a response, in the absence of a conditioning history, is called the unconditioned stimulus and the response which it elicits is the unconditioned response. By temporarily pairing a previously neutral stimulus (a stimulus not capable of eliciting the response prior to conditioning) with the unconditioned stimulus, the previously neutral stimulus develops the power or the ability to elicit the response in question. Once this has taken place, the previously neutral stimulus becomes the conditioned stimulus and the response which it elicits is called the conditioned response. For example, when a little baby receives an injection for the first time, he tightens up and cries. The injection is the unconditioned stimulus, the baby's tightening up and crying is the unconditioned response. Prior to this, entering the doctor's office meant nothing to the child. With repetition, merely entering the waiting room elicits the crying and tightening. The waiting room has now become a conditioned stimulus, because by repetitive pairing with the injection (unconditioned stimulus) it is now capable of eliciting the crying and tightening in the absence of the unconditioned stimulus. Notice that this type of conditioning is most affected by stimuli or events which precede the presentation of the stimulus and are little affected by events which follow the response. This paradigm is the classical conditioning paradigm first developed by Pavlov with the now famous example of conditioning a dog to salivate to the sound of a bell. A distinctive feature of respondent conditioning is that the conditioned response occurs only after presentation of the conditioned stimulus. Thus, the frequency of the conditioned response is determined mainly by the frequency of its eliciting conditioned stimulus (the stimulus or events that *precede* it). In the absence of eliciting stimuli, the respondent behavior is either absent or infrequent. In addition, responses mediated wholly or in part by the automatic system are most readily conditioned by this procedure.

The term "Operant Conditioning" was introduced by B. F. Skinner in 1938, and is historically similar to instrumental conditioning.[3] Operant conditioning relies on responses that are already in the organism's repertoire and which are occuring "spontaneously," and which occur frequently enough to allow the therapist or experimenter to reinforce them. A reinforcer is defined as any stimulus or event which when made contingent upon a response, increases the probability of that response. For example, if we wished to operantly condition a rat to press a lever at a high rate, we would first place the animal in an environment where the response was: (1) possible and (2) likely to occur. Following these principles, the rat would be placed in a small chamber containing a lever and little else. This gives the organism the opportunity to make the response and increases the probability that the response will occur frequently because we have purposely restricted the environment so there is little to compete with it. Notice that the response (pressing the lever) is already in the animal's repertoire. Sooner or later, in this restricted environment, the rat will press the lever in its meanderings around the cage and the therapist will immediately provide a suitable reinforcer. By virtue of its having been reinforced, the response is more likely to occur again, and is again followed by reinforcement. In this fashion, a response with a relatively low rate of occurence is now occuring at a high rate because it has been suitably reinforced.

### Reinforcers

A reinforcer, in a strict operant sense, is a stimulus or event which, when made contingent upon a response, increases the probability of that response.[4] This definition, while sounding tautological, is really extremely empirical because it defines a reinforcer in terms of the *consequences* of its application on observable behavior in a specific environment. Getting back to our example of a rat learning to press a lever, a pellet of food might be a suitable reinforcer if the rat were hungry and the food were palatable and recognized by the rat as edible. When working with human beings in a biofeedback situation, simply providing information that the correct or desired response has occurred serves as a sufficient reinforcer. Reinforcers are further divided into two broad categories: positive reinforcers and negative reinforcers. All reinforcers, both positive and negative, increase the probability of a response upon which they have been made contingent. The distinction is that positive reinforcers do so when their *presentation* is made contingent upon a response, while negative reinforcers do so when their *removal* is made contingent upon a response. For example, in a biofeedback situation, if one is attempting to teach a patient to relax a group of muscles and the biofeedback device produces a high pitched tone while the muscles are tense, the high pitch tone is a negative reinforcer because it increases the probability of relaxing these muscles when its removal is made contingent upon relaxing these muscles. Negative reinforcers, while frequently aversive stimuli, are not to be confused with punishers which tend to suppress responding.

## Shaping

Operant conditioning techniques would not be nearly as useful as they are if all they did was to increase the probability of a response already in the organism's repertoire. In fact, by employing a technique called "shaping" by the method of successive approximations, it is possible to condition a response to occur at a high rate which before conditioning was not in the organism's repertoire. For example, we might wish, using electro-myographic (EMG) biofeedback techniques, to condition a patient who had suffered a stroke, to contract a group of muscles so that he could lift his leg. Initially, the patient is not able to produce sufficient tension in the muscles to accomplish the response; however, some small degree of muscle tension is present. We would first establish the range of muscle tension present and then only reinforce the subject (with a tone) when the muscle tension was in the top 20 percent of the range. After some practice, those higher muscle tensions would be occurring much more frequently than 20 percent of the time and we would then have a new distribution of muscle tension, containing at its upper end tensions which were not at first present. We then change our criterion for reinforcement in the sense that we now only reinforce the top 20 percent of this new distribution of muscle tensions. By repeating this procedure again and again, we achieve a state where the patient is now reliably producing muscle tensions which were totally absent at the beginning of the training procedure and which are sufficiently high to achieve the desired movement. In this way, by the method of successive approximations, we have used an operant technique with biofeedback to achieve a desired response that was not in the organism's repertoire at the beginning of training. It has frequently been found that unlike classical conditioning, operant conditioning is most effective with responses mediated by the somatic rather than the autonomic nervous system.

The pairing of operant conditioning with the somatic nervous system, and classical conditioning with the autonomic nervous system, has led to considerable ongoing research; the results of which directly affect, and in our opinion, unnecessarily cloud and confound the use and acceptance of biofeedback techniques as a treatment modality. At this point some historical perspective seems in order. From the inception of the concepts of operant and classical conditioning until the 1960s, most research involving classical conditioning dealt with responses believed to be autonomically mediated, while operant conditioning dealt with responses believed to be somatically mediated.[3] In the 1960s, a number of investigators, most notably Neil Miller and his associates attempted to apply operant conditioning techniques to a variety of responses mediated by the autonomic nervous system.[5] Their initial attempts met with considerable success, and clinical implications became immediately apparent. In a very real sense, this success served as the stimulus for the very rapid growth and application of biofeedback to a wide variety of clinical problems. In recent years, these,[6] and other investigators, have begun to question their original theoretical interpretation as to whether operant conditioning techniques could directly influence autonomically mediated responses to a clinically significant degree. Although research on this issue continues, the doubts raised as to the theoretical correctness of the interpretations have cast a serious, and in our opinion, unwarranted pale on the clinical application of biofeedback. There are actually a number of issues that must first be separated. The first is whether or not operant conditioning procedures can directly affect autonomically mediated responses. Although this is an important scientific and theoretical question, it is of limited relevence to the clinical application of biofeedback procedures to autonomically mediated responses. From a clinical point of view, what is of relevence is the efficacy with which these procedures alter the response in question in a desired direction. Whether or not the mechanism is by direct conditioning of the autonomic nervous system, or through an indirect and more circuitous route in which one operantly conditions a somatic response which, as a sequella, produces an autonomically mediated response in a desired direction, is important theoretically. In addition, this information may be useful clinically in that it could help us to refine and perhaps make more efficient our procedures. From a clinical standpoint, however, it is illogical to cast out the use of a procedure which produces the desired effect only because we change our ideas as to the mechanisms of action. If an objectively stated set of procedures can be demonstrated to efficaciously change a pathological state to a clinically significant degree without producing unwanted effects, then that would warrant its continued usage despite questions as to the nature of the precise mechanisms by which these changes are accomplished.

In recent years, we have seen a number of research papers on the efficacy of biofeedback treatment. For example, it has been reported as being possibly valuable in the treatment of a variety of disorders including: headache syndromes (both tension[7] and migraine,[8] Raynaud's disease,[9] cardiac arrythmias,[10] hypertensive[11] and hypotensive[12] states, muscular spastic conditions,[13] epileptic seizures,[14] insomnia,[15] neurological problems requiring muscle retraining,[16] control over penile erection,[17] dysmenorrhea,[18] spastic colon,[19] rectal incontinence,[20] generalized anxiety,[21] asthma,[22] alcoholism,[23] obsessive-compulsive behavior,[24] phobic behavior,[25] pain syndrome,[26] and stuttering.[27] Despite this impressive list of applications, research in the clinical efficacy of biofeedback at the present time is in considerable flux. This should not be surprising considering the newness of the field and the diversity of both procedures and clinical applications that currently exist. At this point, it seems useful to discuss an ideal set of criterion that must be fulfilled in order to demonstrate the efficacy of a particular form of biofeedback and a particular regimen of therapy for a particular disorder. As of this writing, some forms and some regimens of biofeedback, for some specific disorders have been extensively researched, and there is relatively good agreement as to the efficacy of the particular treatment and regimen for the specific disorder. At the other extreme, the research basis for some biofeedback applications and regimens to some specific disorders is based on nothing more than a few case history reports.

Melzack, in an article entitled "The Promise of Biofeedback: 'Don't Hold the Party Yet,'"[1] has stated four criterion which must be fulfilled before one may validly establish biofeedback treatment as effective and useful:

1.  There must be *placebo effect* controls in clinical research studies. Among the factors involved in placebo effects one must include patients' desires to please the therapist, beliefs in magic, suggestion, anticipation of relief, decreased anxiety and arousal of hope—all of these and more are likely to ameliorate any disease process. In addition, Neil Miller has stated that most chronic syndromes undergo spontaneous ebbs and flows in severity. It is reasonable to expect that patients will more often seek out therapeutic help as the crest of exacerbation approaches, and that almost anything the therapist does is likely in many cases to be followed by a spontaneous recession from the exacerbation; the reduction in intensity of the clinical condition is then likely to be ascribed to whatever the therapist has prescribed, be it magic spell or authentic active therapy.

2.  The treatment must be shown capable of *significant effect production*: that is, the changes for which biofeedback is specifically responsible must be of sufficient magnitude to have clinical, rather than only statistical, significance. Thus, if diastolic blood pressure in hypertensive patients can be reliably reduced but only by 5mm Hg, or blood flow to specific areas can be reliably increased but insufficient in amount to affect local pathological processes, the therapy has either limited or no value, even if the target effects are the result of biofeedback and not placebo factors.

3.  It must be possible to demonstrate *transferability of effects from the laboratory or hospital setting to everyday life*. What if dramatic specific favorable effects from biofeedback are demonstrable in the laboratory or hospital setting but are not sustained while at home or work? If such is the case, then the value of the treatment is again highly questionable. In this connection, Neil Miller recently expressed the concern that, in some instances, we might succeed in training patients and physicians to acquire a false sense of security; that is, patients would learn how to reduce their blood pressures at the time of examinations but only have it become elevated after leaving the doctor's office. Under such circumstances, antihypertensive medication would not be used even though indicated. It is possible, of course, to develop portable biofeedback devices but, again, it must be shown that these are as effective in the patient's normal environment as in the laboratory.

4.  The treatment must be shown to possess *durability of results*. That is, what if well-controlled studies show that biofeedback exceeds a placebo in effectiveness and is also capable of doing so in the patient's normal environment outside the laboratory, but that a few weeks after treatment termination, symptoms and signs return? Results must be durable to be clinically meaningful; or at least be capable of providing some relief where all previous treatment methods have failed, that is, even without tightly controlled experiments, a therapy is clinically important when it is reliably associated with relief in a condition previously not responsive to a variety of interventions, even if the results lack durability. How many studies in the clinical biofeedback literature meet these stringent criteria?—precious few!

Of course, in terms of maintaining a reasonable clinical perspective, one must also ask, "How many treatments outside of biofeedback that occupy a standard and accepted place in the clinical armamentarium have fulfilled and met these same criteria that Melzack suggests be applied to biofeedback therapies?" We think the answer to this question too, would be "precious few." Perhaps a more judicious approach to deciding when to apply a new biofeedback technique and regimen to a clinical disorder would be to maintain a position of skeptical optimism. Rather than wait for rigorously controlled scientific studies to demonstrate the efficacy of a particular biofeedback approach to a disorder beyond reasonable doubt, we would ask the following clinically relevant questions: (1) Is there another treatment for the disorder which is believed to be more demonstrably efficacious than the proposed biofeedback treatment? (2) Is this other treatment as safe?. (One must also consider the possibility that both treatments may be applied simultaneously if they are not incompatable, and in situations where quick alleviation of the condition is an important requirement, this might prove to be the more conservative approach.) In addition, the costs of the treatment may be a factor, as well as a patient's preference for a particular treatment and the likelihood that the patient will accept and carry out the treatments considered. Possibly because biofeedback therapies have their inceptions in the experimental laboratory and came quite quickly to be used as therapeutic procedures, there has been a tendency to apply the rigorous scientific criteria to the clinical application of biofeedback therapies while not applying these same criteria to other forms of therapy when choosing between them.

## DIFFERENT KINDS OF BIOFEEDBACK

### Electro-Myographic Biofeedback (EMG)

All muscles generate electrical activity, most readily measured as voltage, when they contract. The heart, a large muscle that contracts rhythmically, generates a characteristic charge in voltage with respect to time, which is the basis for the electrocardiogram (EKG). In some sense, the EKG is a special case of an EMG signal. Skeletal muscles generate a voltage which is proportional to the degree of contraction. Therefore, the higher the voltage, the more contracted the muscle is; and the lower the voltage, the more relaxed the muscle is. EMG biofeedback records the voltage produced by a muscle or muscle group, amplifies this voltage, and transduces it into some readily discernible signal, most typically a tone, whose frequency and/or amplitude varies with the amplitude of the voltage recorded. Commonly, these voltages are detected by surface electrodes attached to the skin and positioned over the muscle or muscles to be monitored. (In special cases, for very precise work with small muscle groups, needle electrodes which actually pierce the skin, are sometimes employed; however, for most clinical applications, surface electrodes suffice.)

In addition to the degree of contraction or relaxation, the amplitude of the EMG signal recorded is dependent on a number of factors such as (1) the size of the muscle group (larger muscles generally yielding higher amplitude voltages than smaller muscles); (2) the proximity of the electrodes to the muscle; (3) the electrical impedance between muscle and electrode (which in itself is a function of a wide variety of factors); (4) the position of the electrodes with respect to the muscles (greater voltages will be recorded when the electrodes are positioned across the greatest length of the muscle); (5) the type of recording employed (such as peak to peak, root mean square, average voltage); and (6) the signal-to-noise ratio in the entire system.[28] For these reasons, it is frequently difficult, if not impossible, to compare absolute EMG values (expressed in microvolts) between research studies. One must take special care in the clinical application of biofeedback to scrupulously adhere to the details of measurement if one is attempting to use absolute level of EMG as a criterion for therapeutic outcome. Fortunately, in most clinical applications of EMG biofeedback, the relative EMG level is sufficient as a criterion; and so long as one reliably adheres to the same method of measurement from session to session, suitable results are achievable.

EMG biofeedback is generally used to (1) decrease the tension in a muscle group or groups which are chronically or periodically overly tense; or (2) in the case of muscle reeducation, to increase or restore tones in functionally impaired muscles. The former goal can be used for specific muscle groups, as in the treatment of Bruxism, tempro mandibular joint disorder, and neck and back pains due to periodic severe contractions of specific muscle groups; or presently, more frequently used, as an adjunct in the treatment of general and nonspecific anxiety and tension, desensitization procedures, and tension headaches.

Although in theory this EMG biofeedback can be applied to any muscle group(s) for purposes of relaxation and as an adjunct to psychotherapy, the most commonly monitored muscle group is the frontalis (forehead) because of its accessibility, ease of measurement, and because it is purported to be a good general indicator of muscle tension and concomitant stress.

## Skin Temperature and Biofeedback

Surface skin temperature in the periphery fluctuates as a function of a number of variables such as core body temperature, ambient environmental temperature, and vasomotor activity. Under most circumstances, core body temperature remains relatively constant, and the ambient environmental temperature can be made to do so. Therefore, measurement of surface skin temperature can be conveniently used as an indication of vasodilatation and vasoconstriction. Although other more direct measures of vasomotor activity exist, they tend to be more intrusive and less sensitive. In addition, through recent advances in instrumentation, relatively inexpensive (under $1000) instruments have been devised which are capable of measuring relative differences of $0.01°F$, and absolute differences of $0.05°F$.

Peripheral vasomotor activity is influenced by a variety of neurochemical, neuropharmacological, physiological, environmental, and psychophysiological factors.[29] The primary clinical use of skin temperature biofeedback is to provide information and control over a number of psychophysiological factors in an environment where the other variables are essentially constant. In general, stress and anxiety produce peripheral vasoconstriction which is most apparent in the extremities (fingertips and toes). For this reason, clinicians who use skin temperature biofeedback as an adjunct to psychotherapy in behaviorally oriented desensitization procedures and general reduction of anxiety, tend to use skin temperature biofeedback from the fingers and toes. Very similar procedures employing skin temperature biofeedback from the periphery have also been used to very different clinical ends: peripheral vasodilation has been used as a specific treatment for Raynaud's disease[9] and migraine headaches.[8] Although the procedures employed are similar, the patient population and the specific goals to which they are addressed are markedly different.

Skin temperature biofeedback involves the measurement (usually by means of a sensitive thermistor) of small fluctuations as little as 0.01°F in surface skin temperature, and displays these changes to the individual. Although some controversy still exists as to the exact mechanism by which subjects can achieve control over skin temperature, a number of studies have clearly demonstrated that biofeedback procedures are effective in teaching human subjects to alter peripheral skin temperature[30-32]—in some cases as much as 10°F.

## Galvanic Skin Response Biofeedback (GSR) or Electrodermal Biofeedback

The term "Galvanic Skin Response" (GSR) while being almost 100 years old, remains probably the most misunderstood and misapplied concept in biofeedback in particular, and electrophysiology in general. More recently, many attempts have been made to update and systematize terminology of a variety of electrodermal characteristics and responses. First we must distinguish between skin conductance, its reciprocal, skin resistance, and electrical potential differences (voltage), detected across portions of the skin.

The skin has certain characteristics with respect to its ability to conduct electricity. If one were to apply either a fixed voltage or a fixed current across some area of the skin, one could measure how much of that current or voltage the skin conducts; or conversely, how much resistance or impedance the skin offers to the passage of electricity. The unit of resistance to the flow of electricity is the "ohm," and its reciprocal, the unit of conductance is the "mho." The outside applied source of electricity can either be DC (direct current) or AC (alternating current). Each has its own particular advantages and sources of artifact when measuring skin resistance or conductance. While the correlations between DC and AC measurements of resistance or conductance are extraordinarily high (r = +0.97), the absolute values achieved by these different measures will differ. Furthermore, if one uses AC, the frequency at which the current alternates is an important variable in determining the impedance (resistance in an AC circuit) or conductance measured. To further complicate matters, one may choose to apply a constant current and measure the voltage in order to ascertain the resistance or its reciprocal conductance. Since voltage, resistance, and current are related by Ohm's law (voltage = current × resistance), one could also choose to apply a fixed voltage and measure the current to ascertain the resistance or conductance. Since all of these procedures have been used in various research studies, it is not surprising that absolute values differ markedly from study to study, and general confusion tends to plague the uninitiate to the field. Fortunately, relative differences, rather than absolute values, in skin conductance or skin resistance suffice for most clinical applications.

Skin conductance shows both slow and rapid pertabations which are on a continuum. Many clinicians are primarily concerned with the relatively rapid fluctuations in skin conductance and skin resistance which are labeled "skin conductance response" and "skin resistance response." The basal levels, i.e. the relatively slow fluctuations, are defined as "skin conductance level" or its reciprocal "skin resistance level." As we pointed out earlier, pertabations in skin conductance and resistance are really on a continuum from very slow to relatively rapid, and the distinction between the two is somewhat arbitrary.

An entirely different phenomenon, sometimes called "Galvanic skin potential," is a difference in electrical potential, i.e. voltage, which can be recorded from the surface of the skin. This is frequently termed "skin potential" or "electrodermal potential." The "skin potential level" denotes the basal skin potential, while the term "skin potential response" refers to relatively rapid changes in skin potential and is usually elicited by some stimulus, thought, or feeling.

Most biofeedback clinicians who use electrodermal biofeedback employ some measurement of skin conductance and skin resistance to (1) aid in the achievement of a state of relaxation to reduce stress and anxiety, or (2) as an adjunct to psychotherapy, both as an indicator of internal states (e.g., in desensitization procedures) and a means of making a patient more aware of his feelings. Although a considerable amount of research has been done with electrodermal changes and their psychophysiological concomittance in general, and electrodermal biofeedback in particular, most investigators accept the phenomenon without understanding exactly what it reflects.[33] Furthermore, unlike EMG, EEG, or skin temperature biofeedback, at this point, we are not aware of any definitive study which demonstrates the clinical efficacy of electrodermal biofeedback for any specific clinical disorder.

## Electroencephalographic (EEG) Biofeedback

Electroencephalographic biofeedback involves the recording of a relatively narrow band of frequencies of electrical activity measured at the scalp and presumably generated by the brain. The goal of this type of feedback is to allow the subject to gain voluntary control of his EEG. The basic rationale for many, but not all, of EEG biofeedback procedures is that specific EEG patterns are known to correlate with various mental states. The logic is that by altering the EEG pattern, one should be capable of altering or enhancing a particular mental state.

EEG biofeedback is at one and the same time the most popularly renown, misunderstood, and artifact-prone of the biofeedback procedures. With one important exception, at this time, it has very little demonstrable clinical efficacy for any disorder. Despite its drawbacks, it has captured the imagination of the general press, the public, and a good portion of the scientific community, as well; and holds out promise for some of the most exciting possibilities for application in psychiatry and psychology.

In the great majority of cases, EEG, for purposes of biofeedback, is recorded from surface electrodes on the scalp. This electrical activity is the averaged and distorted signal produced by the underlying neural tissue. In addition, the EEG apparatus, itself, limits the range of frequencies which are recorded. Most EEG biofeedback machines are only sensitive to frequencies from a 0.5 Hz (cycles per second) to 40–50 Hz.

Despite these limitations, in normal human adults, different EEG patterns, which are characterized by their dominant frequency, are correlated with arousal level. Classically, four EEG rhythms are commonly distinguished: delta (0.5 - 4 Hz), seen in deep dreamless sleep; theta (4–8 Hz), seen in sleep, associated with hypnogogic and hypnopompic imagery; alpha (8–14 Hz), relaxed, drowsy, unfocused attention; and beta (14–30+ Hz), active concentration, focused attention, and a general high level of mental arousal.[28]

It should be understood that these EEG rhythms are not pure frequencies. In any 30 seconds of EEG, one is likely to see a number of these frequencies occurring at different amplitudes. The EEG rhythm is designated by the dominant frequency seen during an arbitrary period of time. The dominant frequency is the most commonly occurring frequency at an *amplitude* sufficient to be discriminated by the EEG machine. Therefore, we can see that amplitude, as well as frequency, determines the EEG rhythm; and amplitude can be a source of considerable artifact with some biofeedback devices. The earliest EEG biofeedback devices worked in the following fashion: A set of electronic filters attenuated the amplitude of any signal outside of a band of frequencies. For example, if one wished to train for the alpha rhythm, one would first set the filters such that frequencies between 8 and 14 Hz would pass unattenuated, while any signal lower than 8 Hz, or greater than 14 Hz, would be attenuated. The EEG signal so modified, would then be fed into an amplitude-level detector. Signals greater than an arbitrarily specified value (e.g., 20 microvolts) would turn on a tone, indicating to the subject that he was producing alpha. In theory, since only the 8–14 Hz signal (alpha rhythm) would pass unattenuated, the subject would receive feedback only when his dominant frequency was 8–14 Hz, because all frequencies outside of this band would be sufficiently attenuated so that they would be incapable of exceeding the arbitrary level set on the level detector.

Unfortuately, electronic filters are not perfect, and the degree of attenuation is greatest the further the frequency is from the designated band, and very little attenuation (in some systems) occurs at frequencies close to the band. Furthermore, other biological and nonbiological signals picked up by the machine, if of sufficient amplitude, will trigger the level detector even if their frequency is far removed from the band. For example, with EEG electrodes placed on the forehead, a 250 microvolt signal readily obtainable from the frontalis muscles, even if attenuated by a factor of 10, will still be sufficient to trigger the level detector (set at 20 microvolts) and provide false feedback that the subject is producing alpha when in fact he is simply furrowing his brow. One of us (S.S.) would occasionally gain a form of perverse pleasure by going around to EEG biofeedback equipment manufacturers' displays at conventions, and with eyes closed, have the machine indicate that he was producing continuous alpha while subtracting serial sevens outloud. Common wisdom was that this was impossible, but it was accomplished by the simple expedient of rolling his eyeballs back in his head. More sophisticated equipment now available controls for such simple artifacts; however, EEG biofeedback is fraught with a number of potential artifacts that even the most sophisticated equipment cannot entirely rule out. In our opinion, people employing EEG biofeedback should have considerable familiarity and training with the EEG, because false feedback, which would lead the patient to do just the opposite of what is desirable, is a distinct possibility. Furthermore, when given EEG biofeedback to control seizures, Sterman has demonstrated that the wrong biofeedback can worsen the condition.[14] When dealing with patients who are either seizure prone or who suffer from seizures, EEG biofeedback should best be left to a highly trained professional.

At present, alpha and theta biofeedback are clinically employed to aid in states of relaxation and in facilitating sleep in insomniacs. Currently, EEG has very limited clinical usefulness with one major exception. Sterman[14] and others[34] have been able to demonstrate that EEG biofeedback can be clinically effective in reducing or entirely eliminating seizures in selected populations of subjects, some of whom were refractive to pharmacotherapy.

At present, a number of studies suggest that subjects can be trained with the use of differential hemispheric EEG biofeedback to suppress beta acticity from one hemisphere while enhancing it from the other hemisphere. The potential for this technique as a research tool to explore differential hemispheric function, and as a clinical technique to enhance psychological states which may be more conducive to various forms of psychotherapy, has yet to be exploited.

## Blood Pressure Biofeedback (BPF)

A number of studies have demonstrated that direct feedback of systolic blood pressure can produce small, but statistically significant changes in normotensive subjects and somewhat larger (17–20 mm Hg) in hypertensive subjects. [11, 35] Direct measurement of blood pressure is difficult in humans, and techniques which involve inflating and deflating a blood pressure cuff produce delay in feedback and consequently obviate the major advantage of biofeedback technique: immediate feedback. Clinically, equivalent or superior results in lowering blood pressure in hypertensive patients have been achieved with the use of relaxation procedures and/or EMG and skin temperature biofeedback.[36-38]

A recent innovation in blood pressure biofeedback is the "pulse wave velocity" technique, which measures the velocity of the pulse and is believed to be linearly correlated with blood pressure changes. The major advantages of this technique is that (1) it does not require an inflatable cuff, and (2) can give much more immediate feedback (beat-to-beat). Although this technique seems promising, a great deal more research is necessary to establish clinical efficacy; and in addition, it would be necessary to demonstrate superiority over other biofeedback techniques used in the treatment of hyper- and hypo- tensive patients.

### Heart Rate Biofeedback

A variety of relatively simple sensors (electronic, mechanical, plethesmographic, and auditory) have been employed to provide feedback information about heart rate. It is quite clear that subjects can use this information to alter their heart rate to both increase and decrease it.[39] Most studies find that it is easier to train increases. At present, research into the efficacy of using heart rate biofeedback in the treatment of cardiac arrhythmias continues.

### Bowel Sounds Biofeedback

With the use of an electronic amplification stethescope, direct monitoring and display of bowel sounds can be provided. The patient can hear his own bowel sounds, and, in a relaxed state, learns to reduce them. In principle, the amplified audio signal, once converted into an electrical signal, could be used to provide any type of feedback to the patient; however, most (few) studies use the amplified sounds themselves as the feedback.

### Penile Erection Biofeedback

It is possible to directly measure penile tumescence and detumescence by placing an elastic cuff, in which a mercury strain gauge loop is embedded, directly around the penis. The strain gauge gives off an electrical signal which is proportional to tumescence, and which can be used to control any appropriate feedback stimulus. This form of biofeedback can be used for either the reduction of erections or for the increase of erections.

### CLINICAL APPLICATIONS

Our limited goal at this point is to summarize and critique in depth a number of selected research studies which demonstrate clinical efficacy for a number of biofeedback procedures used with a variety of clinical disorders.

### Tension Headache Treated by EMG Biofeedback[7]

Out of a large pool of nonpaid volunteer patients suffering chronically from severe frequent headaches, 18 were selected whose clinical picture was typical of the muscular tension headache syndrome qualities, or by other organic pathology. Typically, the headaches were experienced in the occipital region bilaterally as dull and "bandlike" and also occurred in the frontal area. Although gradual in onset, they might last from hours to weeks to months. The mean age was 36 years—2 males and 16 females. Occupations included secretaries, teachers, housewives, graduate students, nurses, and a writer. The mean duration of the headache syndrome was 7.7 years. Dropouts were replaced from a similar subject pool.

DESIGN

*Baseline.* All 18 subjects received a 2-week pretreatment baseline during which daily, hour-by-hour records were kept by the patients for headache activity. These records were kept similarly throughout the entire study period.

*Subject group assignment.* Next, on a random basis, subjects were assigned to one of three groups:

1. Group A. Receiving EMG biofeedback (BF) to the frontal muscle area.
2. Group B. Receiving pseudo-EMG BF to the frontal muscle area.
3. Group C. Receiving no EMG training, but asked to record their headache activity (HA) daily for two months at which time they would begin to receive EMG BF.

*The treatment procedure.* Sixteen approximately twice weekly, 30-minute BF sessions. EMG BF consisted of a series of clicks heard through headphones; the rate of clicks was proportional to frontal are muscle activity, becoming slower with muscular relaxation. Subjects were told to observe themselves, what makes the click rate slow down and what makes it speed up, and to sustain whatever inner conditions were associated with the slowest rate. As mentioned, Group B was given pseudoauditory BF (tape recordings of the Group A patients' clicks).

In addition, *both* groups were told that their headaches were produced by sustained muscular tension and that they were told to practice such relaxation at home just as they did in the laboratory for two 15–20 minute intervals daily.

*Follow-up studies.* The next phase of the design consisted of two follow-up studies as follows:

1. The EMG and HA levels were assessed three months after treatment termination.
2. The HA levels of group A patients were assessed 18 months after treatment termination. Four out of the original six Group A patients were available at this time for this procedure.

RESULTS

*EMG levels.*

1. *Baseline.* The baseline two week average was 10 microvolts (mv), which was at least twice as great as that of normal headache-free subjects in their

laboratory. No significant differences were observed across Groups A, B, and C.

2. *Effects of EMG BF training.* Group A showed significantly lower levels of muscle activity than B throughout, once training began (2.95 mv versus 6.8 mv, $p < 0.05$).
3. *Three month follow-up results.* At this time, the average EMG level for Group A = 3.9 mv, whereas that for Group B = 8.4 mv. This difference was markedly significant ($p < 0.01$).

HEADACHE ACTIVITY (HA)

1. *Baseline HA* was not significantly different across groups. The mean HA for all groups equalled 0.65 hours HA per day.
2. *Mean HA* at the end of the 8-week training period -

        Group A = 0.15 hours per day
        Group B = 0.63 hours per day
        Group C = 0.65 hours per day

   With Group A, the decrease of HA in comparison to baseline levels was markedly significant ($p < 0.001$).
3. *Assessment of HA changes by subject.* In Group A, 4 out of 6 subjects experienced a significant reduction of HA in comparison to the baseline levels. In Group B, 1 out of 6 subjects experienced a significant decrease of HA. In Group C, 0 out of 6 had a decrease of HA.
4. *Three month follow-up data.* Group A as a whole had very little HA (0.04 hours per day), whereas Group B became stabilized at a mean of 0.53 hours per day spent with headaches. None in Group C showed any significant change. (A versus B: $p < .001$.)

*Correlation between EMG levels and HA.* The correlation between HA and EMG levels in Group A throughout was +0.90, whereas it was -0.05 or essentially no correlation in Group B.

*Subjective reports.* The patients' spontaneous comments at each treatment session were recorded in a log book. Analysis of this data revealed four states in the development of their ability to use a "cultivated" relaxation response to reduce HA outside the clinic setting.

1. Patient is unable to prevent or abort HA.
2. Patient is aware of tension preceding HA, can relax to some degree with conscious effort but cannot abort HA.
3. Patient has increasing awareness of tension and is better able to relax and abort light to moderate HA. Frequency and severity of HA now decreasing.

4. Patient is now able to relax automatically without conscious effort in the face of stress and experiences a reduction in overreactions to stress in general. HA is now appreciably reduced or even eliminated.

*Further follow-up data.*

1. At three months posttreatment, all Group A and B patients were required to complete an extensive questionnaire enabling assessment of drug use, mood and behavior changes, interpersonal relationships, and evidence of symptom substitution.

   In general, both groups showed some improvement, but Group A more so. Specifically, Group A patients registered larger decreases in tiredness, apathy, fear of crowds, and compulsive behavior. Group A patients also experienced a dramatic decrease of drug use (analgesics and antianxiety agents). Also, favorable psychological test changes were significantly greater in Group A.

   The importance of daily relaxation practice at home was indicated by the observation that the two patients in Group A who did not significantly improve found it difficult to carry out the exercises because of domestic turmoil.
2. At the 18 month follow-up of Group A patients, four of the original six patients were available. Three of these four who had shown significant declines in HA during the training, had maintained their gains. There was no sign of new symptom substitution throughout.
3. "Real" BF was administered to members of Groups B and C after the first experiment was over. Two out of three Group B and four out of five Group C members then showed significant declines in HA during training.

In summary, patients suffering from chronic severe tension headaches can learn to decrease their forehead EMG levels by 50 to 75 percent, and with this, experience a significant reduction in HA. The improvement in both is durable and maintainable in real life, and is accompanied by increased tolerance to stress and reduction in drug use, with no evidence of symptom substitution.

CONCLUSIONS

This study, as well as a number of more recent reports,[40, 41] clearly demonstrate that EMG biofeedback in combination with relaxation procedures can produce clinically significant and long-term reduction (and in some cases total alleviation) of tension headaches.

## Biofeedback Treatment of Severe Fecal Incontinence due to Organic Impairment[20]

The patient population consisted of seven ambulatory patients with 5–8-year histories of chronic daily severe fecal incontinence, all due to organic impairments associated with such conditions as a prostatectomy for a tumor, hemmorrhoidectomy, diabetic neuropathy, a laminectomy, and an anal fissurectomy. One patient was a 6-year-old child who had never had normal defecation; her incontinence was episodic and was associated with surgery for a meningomyelocoele. All patients went through three phases of study and treatment. In Phase 1, the severity of impairment of the recto-sphincteric reflexes was objectively determined by a double balloon manometer device making possible separate evaluation of the internal and external anal sphincters.

In normal subjects, momentary inflation of the rectal balloon causes reflex relaxation of internal sphincters and reflex contraction of the external sphincters. By contrast, in the patient population, the external sphincter response was either diminished or absent. After completion of the diagnostic studies, all patients except the 6-year-old child received a detailed explanation of normal recto-sphincteric action and the way in which their responses differed from the normal.

In Phase 2 (the initial stage of training), immediate biofeedback (BF) was provided the patient by means of displaying to him the polygraphic tracings of his sphincteric responses as they were being recorded. Patients were reminded of the differences between their responses and those of normals. They were encouraged to attempt to modify their responses and make them appear normal. They were praised whenever they produced a normal-appearing response and informed whenever responses were poor. Verbal reinforcement was gradually decreased when patients gave evidence that they knew what what was expected of them, and as it became clear that they were acquiring influence over their sphincteric responses. Each patient was able to sense the rectal distension, and each patient knew that this stimulus was the cue to initiate sphincter control.

Phase 3 was the final stage of laboratory training. Two goals were set. The first goal involved refinement of sphincteric responses such that the normal response amplitude was approximated and the external sphincter contraction coincided with internal sphincter relaxation. These refinements utilized BF with verbal reinforcement.

The second goal entailed the gradual weaning of the patient away from dependency on the apparatus. This involved periodic withholding of the visual BF and, after a series of trials, permitting patients to observe their performances.

Each laboratory session occupied two hours during each of which patients received 50 training trials. About three weeks elapsed between each session, during which time practice was recommended. No patient required more than four sessions.

RESULTS

Six of the seven patients completed the treatment. All learned to produce external sphincter contraction in synchrony with internal sphincter relaxation. During follow-up periods ranging from six months to five years, four of the patients remained completely continent, and the other two were definitely improved. The 6-year-old child not only achieved continence but also normal defecation for the first time in her life.

## The Overall Clinical Effectiveness of
## Biofeedback—Current Assessment

This section briefly summarizes the conservative conclusions of Blanchard and Young[42] regarding the effectiveness of the different types of BF, and cites a few other papers as well.

### EMG BF

EMG BF for muscle retraining has definitely established the therapeutic effect of BF. Perhaps the most dramatic example is the report of Andrews on a series of 20 patients suffering from hemiplegia.[16] They had shown no return of function in one year after the onset, nor had they responded to traditional neuromuscular rehabilitation procedures. A necessary condition for inclusion in the study was residual ability to produce *some* EMG. When such patients received auditory EMG BF, they were instructed to generate the biofeedback sound, and, with this, initiate movement. Seventeen patients learned smooth, strong, well-modulated, voluntary movements in previously paralyzed muscles in one trial. Similar results have been obtained by Johnson and Garton with a large proportion of 10 patients with hemiplegic lower extremity residuals such as foot drop, and who required a foot brace.[13] Five patients attained dorsiflexion of the foot and could dispense with the brace. Significant therapeutic benefits have also been demonstrable for Bell's Palsy and other types of neuromuscular disorders.

EMG BF derived from speech musculature has been shown effective in eliminating subvocal speech associated with slow reading. It has not yet been difinitely established, however, whether reading efficiency is thereby improved.

EMG BF assisted general relaxation and home practice has been shown to be useful especially in reduction of anxiety-related condition. The best study is that of Raskin et al., in which 10 young adult subjects with anxiety and other symptoms for at least three years, and who were unresponsive to psychotherapy for two years, received EMG BF and home relaxation.[21] Although only 4 out of 10 experienced improvement of their anxiety, 5 of 6 with insomnia and 4 of 4 with tension headaches improved considerably.

Townsend et al. compared results of two weeks of EMG BF self-practice, with group psychotherapy on 30 patients with anxiety reactions—15 patients in each group.[43] At the end of three weeks, two BF and seven group therapy patients dropped out. Of those remaining, significant decreases were found in the BF group in EMG levels, mood disturbance, and anxiety measures, whereas no such decreases were observed in the control group during the three-week study period. Only two BF patients were available for a six-month follow-up and they reported improvement maintenance.

As described, EMG BF according to several studies, is useful in tension headaches.

As a general criticism, however, inasmuch as all of these studies used self-practice in relaxation in addition to EMG BF, it is not known whether EMG BF is the crucial factor or whether general relaxation training instructions and practice would be as good. It does appear, according to Budzynski et al., that patients who practice assiduously on their own do better with EMG BF than those who use EMG BF alone, suggesting a synergistic effect.[7]

## Cardiovascular Responses to Biofeedback

HEART RATE AND RHYTHM

Weiss and Engel showed that in five of nine patients, beat-by-beat BF showed significant decrease of premature ventricular contractions with improvement maintained up to five years afterward.[10] Three of the failures had severely damaged hearts. In addition, there are a number of single case reports of improvements with a variety of arrhythmias and tachycardias. These studies as a group have been criticized by Blanchard and Young as lacking in strictly adequate controls, e.g., in some cases, baseline data were inadequate.[42] Despite this, results show promise.

BLOOD PRESSURE

Although several studies appear to indicate that it is possible to lower systolic and, to a lesser degree, diastolic blood pressure, both to a significant degree; none of the studies with the best results have averaged better than the 25mm Hg systolic and 15 mm diastolic drop found with placebo medication over a seven-week period,[11, 37] as reported by Greenfell et al.[44]

PERIPHERAL VASODILATATION

Surwit reported four of five cases of Raynaud's disease responded well to skin temperature BF.[9] The failure was an ambivalent patient who discontinued treatment prematurely. Surwit could not ascribe benefits solely to BF, however, because relaxation and autogenic imagery were also used.

## EEG Biofeedback

It is an easy matter with EEG BF to seemingly maximize the amount of alpha rhythm that an individual is capable of producing, but this has not resulted in any clearly demonstrable therapeutic benefit except for the possible synergism with hypnotic relaxation techniques as described by Melzack.[1] In this study, 24 patients with chronic, severe, continuous intractable pain due to a variety of organic causes were treated either by alpha BF alone, alpha BF and hypnotic relaxation training, or hypnotic relaxation training alone. The results were: (1) patients on alpha training *alone* showed virtually no change or else a slight increase of pain toward the end of the procedure; (2) alpha BF plus hypnotic training was capable of reducing pain by at least 33 percent in 58 percent of subjects; (3) hypnotic training alone was likewise effective in relieving pain but to a lesser degree than when combined with alpha BF. The difference between alpha BF plus hypnotic training and hypnotic training alone was not statistically significant, however. Nevertheless, the trend suggests a possible synergism of the two combined.

A most important EEG BF study first reported by Sterman,[14] and presently updated,[4] that BF given for 12–14 Hz rhythm (sensorimotor rhythm—SMR) over the sensorimotor cortex is capable of reducing the frequency of a variety of severe seizure disorders. Prior evidence revealed that in animals this rhythm appeared over sensorimotor cortex during voluntary suppression of movement, suggesting that it was a sign of motor inhibition. In four of five cases, there was decided clinical improvement concurrent with increased emission of SMR. In three of the cases, cessation of training after six months led to exacerbations of seizure activity within four to six weeks, and subsequent reintroduction of BF led to restoration of the former improvement level. The one case who did not respond throughout showed minimal evidence of learning to increase SMR.

More recently, Sterman and his colleagues demonstrated that seizures were specifically reduced when patients were able to normalize their EEG by decreasing abnormally low frequencies or increasing deficient high frequencies through the use of EEG biofeedback.[34] Furthermore, using a double crossover design, patients showed increases or decreases in seizure activity depending on what EEG frequency band they were rewarded for producing.

## Skin Temperature Biofeedback

Skin temperature BF to increase temperature of the fingers relative to the temperature of the forehead combined with autogenic relaxation training has been said by Sargent et al. to provide improvement in 81 percent of 42 migraine patients followed for more than 150 days.[8] The rationale of the therapy is that increased blood flow to the extremities *by means of BF relaxation* is said to inhibit excessive sympathetic outflow rather than operate via blood volume shifts. It does not help for example, to merely put hands in warm water. In all, 150 patients are in their subject pool, but their data has not yet been completely reported. The degrees of improvement have been slight to dramatic. Of the 42 patients, 19 percent did not improve at all; 21 percent were able to reduce the frequency, duration, and severity of the attacks; 21 percent were able to do this and in addition, abort the headache by relaxation; 24 percent were able in addition to detect preheadache symptoms and avoid the attack by relaxation; and 14 percent were, in addition, virtually able to eliminate drug use for headache relief. In all, 60 percent were able to learn to abort their headaches. Now, although the Menninger group may have discovered a valuable treatment package for migraine, the study has been severely criticized on a number of grounds: neither attention-placebo nor no-treatment control groups were employed; follow-up was not sufficiently long-term; the simultaneous multi-component treatment methods prevent isolation of the relative contributions of each; agreement between three evaluators was not sufficiently consistent (68 to 90 percent were considered improved), and no statistical significance was demonstrable.

## Treatment of Functional Bowel Disorders:
## Irritable Colon Syndromes[19]

The subjects consisted of five chronic cases of varying severity, ranging in age from 15 to 62. BF consisted of amplification of bowel sounds. Subjects were given approval whenever their bowel sounds decreased in intensity. All patients markedly improved symptomatically, including a patient who had never had normal bowel function and who was virtually "toilet bound"; this patient experienced dramatic improvement.

## Treatment of Dysmenorrhea

By providing vaginal temperature biofeedback, Heczey was able to demonstrate that 11 adult females, all suffering form dysmenorrhea, were able to significantly elevate their vaginal temperature.[18] The mean ratio of improvement in dysmenorrhea was 92 percent for the patients receiving BF, 76 percent for the patients receiving autogenic training, and 0 percent improvement in control patients not receiving any treatment. This study is suggestive that vaginal temperature BF may be of considerable utility in the treatment of dysmenorrhea. It is not conclusive, however, because it lacks appropriate placebo controls and sufficient follow-up data.

## CONCLUSIONS

It seems fair to say that a variety of biofeedback procedures in combination with other treatment components have considerable therapeutic utility for a wide range of disorders. This claim seems fairly well substantiated by the results of a number of studies mentioned earlier involving (1) EMG BF in the treatment of tension headaches; (2) Skin temperature BF in the treatment of Raynaud's disease; (3) and EEG BF in control of seizure disorders. Regarding the clinical efficaciousness of other BF therapy, it is necessary to state that there is not as yet, to our knowledge, a definitive study which demonstrates beyond doubt that biofeedback *alone* is capable of producing long-lasting, clinically significant benefits. In other words, we don't know what portion of therapeutic benefit is ascribable to biofeedback alone. Perhaps we will never know exactly.

In agreement with Neil Miller, we believe that the great danger is that a genuine new therapy resource may be lost as a result of mass disillusionment because biofeedback has not turned out to be a panacea as often advertised. If such were to occur, the plodding, careful research work of teasing out the relevant variables may never get done. Even at its present state of early development, biofeedback techniques have already provided a number of clinically useful treatments, and when this work is further along, we may have something valuable.

We should like to point out that biofeedback machines provide a useful tool for trained therapists. Just as the possession of a penicillin-filled syringe or a stethescope does not guarantee that the possessor is an internist or cardiologist, possessing a biofeedback machine does not make one a psychotherapist.

In conclusion, we should like to emphasize that, with the one major exception of seizure-prone patients and EEG biofeedback, it is very difficult to *harm* a patient with biofeedback—one cannot say as much as confidently of other forms of treatment. One should not lose sight of this.

## References

1. Melzack R: The promise of biofeedback: don't hold the party yet. Psychology Today 9 (2):18, 1975
2. Stroebel C, Blueck B: Biofeedback treatment in medicine and psychiatry: an ultimate placebo? Semin Psychiatry 5:379–393, 1973
3. Kimble GA: Hilgard, Marquis: Conditioning and Learning. New York, Appleton-Century-Crofts, 1961
4. Reynold GS: A Primer of Operant Conditioning. Glenview, Ill., Scott, Foresman & view, 1967
5. Miller N: Learning of visceral and glandular responses. Science 163:434–445, 1969
6. Miller NE: Biofeedback: "Evaluation of a New Technic," Biofeedback and Self Control: An Aldine Annual on the Regulation of Bodily Processes and Consciousness. Chicago, Aldine Publ. Co., 1974
7. Budzynski TH, Stoyva JM, Adler CS, Mullaney DJ: EMG biofeedback and tension headache: a controlled outcome study. In Birk L (Ed.), Biofeedback: Behavioral Medicine. New York, Grune and Stratton, 1973
8. Sargent JD, Walters ED, Green, EE: Psychosomatic self-regulation of migraine headaches. In Birk L (Ed.), Biofeedback. New York, Grune and Stratton, 1973, pp. 55–68.
9. Surwit RS: Biofeedback: a possible treatment for Raynaud's disease. In Birk L (Ed.), Biofeedback, New York, Grune and Stratton, 1973, pp. 121–130
10. Weiss T, Engel BT: Operant conditioning of heart rate in patients with premature ventricular contractions. Psychosom Med 33: 301–321, 1971
11. Benson H, Shapiro D, Tursky B, et al.: Decreased systolic blood pressure through operant conditioning techniques in patients with essential hypertension. Science 173: 740, 1971
12. Plumlee LA: Operant conditioning of increases in blood pressure. Psychophysiology 6:283–290, 1969
13. Johnson HE, Garton WH: Muscle reeducation in hemiplegic by use of electromyographic device. Arch Phys Med Rehabil 54:320–323, 1973
14. Sterman MR: Neurophysiology and clinical studies of sensorimotor biofeedback training: some effects on epilepsy. In Birk L (Ed.), Biofeedback: Behavioral Med. New York, Grune and Stratton, pp. 147–165
15. Gershman L, Randall AC: Treating Insomnia with Relaxation and Desensitization in a Group Setting by an Automated Approach; Biofeedback and Self Control. An Aldine Annual on the Regulation of Bodily Processes and Consciousness. Chicago, Aldine Publ. Co., 1974
16. Andrews JM: Neuromuscular reeducation of hemiplegics with the aid of the electromyograph. Arch Phys Med Rehabil 45:530–532, 1964
17. Rosen RC, Shapiro D, Schwartz, GE: Voluntary control over penile tumescence. Psychosom Med 37:479–483, 1975
18. Heczey MD: Unpublished PhD dissertation. City University of N.Y., 1977
19. Furman S: Intestinal biofeedback in functional diarrhea: a preliminary report. J Behav Ther Exper Psychiatry 4:317–321, 1973
20. Engel BT, Nikoomanesh P, Schuster MM: Operant conditioning of rectosphincteric re-

sponses in the treatment of fecal incontinence. N Eng J Med 290:646–649, 1974

21. Raskin M, Johnson G, Rondestvedt JW: Chronic anxiety treated by feedback-induced muscle relaxation. Arch Gen Psychiatry 28: 263–267, 1973

22. Davis M, Saunders DR, Creer TL, Chai H, et al: Relaxation training facilitated by biofeedback apparatus as a supplemental treatment in bronchial asthma. J Psychosom Res 17:121–128, 1973

23. Steffen JJ, et al.: Electromyographically induced relaxation in the treatment of chronic alcohol abuse. J Consult Clin, Psychol 43:2–275, 1975

24. Mills G, Solyom M: Biofeedback of EEG alpha in the treatment of obsessive ruminations: an exploration. Paper presented at Biofeedback Research Society, Denver, 1974

25. Shapiro D, et al.: Operant control of fear-related electrodermal responses in snake phobic subjects. Psychophysiology 9:271 (Abstract), 1972

26. Gannon L, Sternbach RA: Alpha enhancement as a treatment for pain: a case study. Behav Ther Exp Psychiatry 2:209–213, 1971

27. Hanna R, et al: A Biofeedback treatment for stuttering. J Speech Hear Disord 40(2):270–273, 1975

28. Handbook of Physiological Feedback, 3. Berkeley Autogenic Systems Inc., 1976.

29. Sternbach R, Greenfield N: Handbook of Psychophysiology. New York, Holt, Reinhart and Winston, 1973

30. Taub E: Autoregulation of vasomotor tone in peripheral vascular beds, Paper presented at Biofeedback Research Society, San Francisco, 1975

31. Taub E, Emurian CS: Self-regulation of human tissue temperature. In, Biofeedback: Theory and Research, New York, Academic Press, 1978

32. Taub E, Emurian CS: Feedback aided self-regulation of skin temperature with a single feedback locus. 1. Acquisition and reversal training In, Biofeedback and self-regulation 1, 147–168, 1976

33. Hume WI: Electrodermal measures in behavioral research. J Psychosom Res 9:383–391, 1966

34. Sterman MB, Lubar JL, Harper RM: Effects of central cortical EEG feedback training on power-spectral characteristics and seizure incidence in uncontrolled epileptics. Paper presented at Biofeedback Society of America, Orlando, Florida, 1977

35. Elder ST, Ruiz ZB, Deabler HL, Dillenkoffer RL, et al.: Instrumental conditioning of diastolic blood pressure in essential hypertensive patients. J Appl Behav Anal 6:377–382, 1973

36. Love WA et al.: The Treatment of Essential Hypertension with EMG Feedback and Blood Pressure Feedback. Paper presented at Biofeedback Research Society, San Francisco, 1975

37. Montgomery DD, et al.: Effects of electromyographic feedback and relaxation training on blood pressures in essential hypertensives. Biofeedback Research Society, Denver, 1974

38. Russ K: Effect of two different feedback paradigms on blood pressure levels of patients with essential hypertension, Paper presented at Biofeedback Research Society, Denver, 1974

39. Miller N, et al.: Instrumental learning of vasomotor response: a Progress report. Paper presented at Biofeedback Research Society, Denver, 1974

40. Cox DJ et al.: Differential effectiveness of electromyograph feedback, verbal relaxation instructions, and medication placebo with tension headaches, J Consult Clin Psychol 43:6, 1975

41. Otis L, et al.: Voluntary control of tension headaches. Paper presented at Biofeedback Research Society, Denver, 1974

42. Blanchard EB, Young LD: Clinical applications of biofeedback training: a review of evidence. Arch Gen Psychiatry 30: 573–589, 1974

43. Townsend RE, House JF, Addario D: A comparison of biofeedback-medicated relaxation and group therapy in the treatment of chronic anxiety. Am J Psychiatry 132: 598–601, 1975

44. Greenfell RF, Briggs AH, Holland WC: Antihypertensive drugs evaluation in a controlled double-blind study. South Med J 56:1410–1416, 1963

45. Sterman MB: Personal communication

Fred H. Frankel

# 9

# Hypnosis and Altered States of Consciousness in Treatment of Patients with Medical Disorders

We are likely to have little difficulty recognizing the extensive use, through the ages, of hypnosis-like states in the treatment of patients with medical disorders. In any historical review of this subject, no matter how brief, we are obliged to ask how both ancient and modern religious healing rites, many dependent on ambience and incantation as well as on a rhythmic beat or body movement, differ, essentially, from the setting and monotone of a modern hypnotic induction procedure. It seems that one goal, at least, shared by most of the procedures, is the refocusing or redistributing of the subject's attention in a manner which enables him to experience his reality differently—to encourage an altered state of awareness or consciousness.

## HISTORICAL OVERVIEW

The interest of medical science in this experience regarded as equivalent or closely similar to hypnosis, began with the Viennese physician, Franz Anton Mesmer about two centuries ago.[2] Working in Vienna and then in Paris, first with magnets, and later with a wooden tub containing iron filings and protruding metal rods which were applied to the ailing parts by the group of patients surrounding the tub, Mesmer attributed the subjective experiences of his patients, their "convulsions," and the ultimate belief that they were cured, to the effects of an invisible "magnetic fluid." The appropriate redistribution of this fluid by the use of the magnets or the metal rods, or by the intervention of a person, the "animal magnetizer," was held by Mesmer and his followers to be responsible for the dramatic cures of urinary retention, aches and pains, blindness, paralyses, and other ills that had previously been considered incurable.

The theatrical and unscientific, but surprisingly successful system of treatment drew much criticism and hostility from the medical profession. This led, ultimately, to a discrediting of Mesmer and his fluid theory by the findings of two royal commissions.[3] They concluded that no evidence could be found of the physical existence of the magnetic fluid, and ascribed the therapeutic effects to imagination, suggestion, and imitation.

The withdrawal of medical interest from animal magnetism was thus assured by the official disapproval of the scientific world until about the middle of the nineteenth century, roughly fifty years later, when it was reexamined by the English physician, Braid.[4] He relabeled the procedure "hypnosis" because he first believed the experience to be a form of sleep, and emphasized, for the first time in the English language, the primary importance of the psychological factors in the patient that were responsible for the therapeutic effects. Recorded history reveals that the English physician Elliotson and the Scottish surgeon Esdaile fared less well at that time with their colleagues than did Braid.[5] They had failed to recognize the significance of these psychological responses, and were ridiculed for their interest in the subject.

The turn of the century witnessed a remarkable revival of medical interest in hypnosis, with major contributions by prominent clinical investigators such as Charcot,[6] Janet,[7] and Bernheim.[8] Although we might differ today to varying degrees with some of the theoretical concepts they employed in support of their practices, their rich clinical reports bear testimony to the therapeutic impact that is possible with hypnosis in the treatment of patients with medical disorders.

## PAST AND CURRENT OPINIONS

Before we proceed to a description and working definition of hypnosis, it will be useful to touch briefly on various aspects of hypnosis that have been emphasized in the past, or that still are in some quarters held to be true; it will help, too, to report the results of a few relevant studies that have added to our understanding of the nature of the event, as well as a few of the explanatory concepts.

Perhaps because of the unusual subjective experiences that are possible in hypnosis, or perhaps as a result of Mesmer's original dramatization of the uncanny role of the magnetizer, the effects of hypnosis have often been coupled with the supernatural or the quasi-magical. Furthermore, the belief is still frequently expressed that the hypnotist is able to exercise control over the actions of the subject against the latter's will; and that the subject, in some way because of the hypnotist, becomes able, in hypnosis, to transcend his normal physiological limits.

More recently, in attempts to explain hypnosis in terms more suited to the language of modern psychology, phrases and metaphors have been loosely introduced, linking the effects of hypnosis with those of placebo, or ascribing hypnotic behavior to the direct expression of the unconscious.

Although some of the above assertions might border on the truth, it is to the laboratory investigation of recent decades that we look for a clarification of many of the issues. The contribution of the largely anecdotal clinical literature has been limited primarily by its failure to establish the presence or strong likelihood of hypnosis in many of the cases reported, and the tendency to describe as hypnotized, subjects exposed to a hypnotic induction procedure who might merely have been deeply relaxed but not hypnotized because they were not hypnotizable.

These statements are not intended to gainsay the value of the rich accomplishments of clinical hypnosis. Tightly controlled clinical studies are usually extremely difficult if not impossible to do, and the empirical use of the event has added considerably to our general appreciation of its clinical worth and its special qualities. We know from published reports that in the successful treatment of dermatological conditions, for instance, the use of a hypnotic procedure provides access to a psychosomatic interaction in a manner that seems unreachable without it.[9-11] We have also learned from clinical experience that hypnotic procedures facilitate the recall of memories. It is, however, to the experimental research that we must return in order to try to clear up many of the unanswered questions.

## CHARACTERISTICS OF HYPNOSIS

Through the development of standardized scales for the measurement of hypnotizability[12, 13] and an ingenious methodology[14, 15] the essential aspects of hypnosis have become clearer. We can now assert the following:

1. The ability to experience hypnosis is a relatively stable attribute of the person. There is little evidence to indicate that behavioral-situational factors or observational learning procedures can meaningfully enhance hypnotic responsiveness.[16]
2. Hypnotizability is distributed in the population in essentially the same manner as any other skill, along a normal curve, with some positive skew.[17]
3. Not all hypnotic experiences are equivalent. Most people are able to respond to the simple suggestion that the hand and forearm will feel so light that the limb will move in an upward direction, but only some are able to experience compelling positive and negative hallucinations, e.g., that they will hear a fly buzzing, or that they will not be able to see the hour hand on a clock face. We may conclude that a person scoring in the moderate range on the hypnotizability scales will be able to accomplish the simpler suggestions, and will fail to respond to the more difficult ones. In rare instances, however, a person with a low score might be capable of a more difficult response while failing to accomplish the simpler suggestions.
4. There is a growing volume of evidence that hypnosis is not a unitary or homogeneous phenomenon, but that there are several types or clusters of hypnotic phenomena,[18] and that at a given level of hypnotic responsivity not all people can have the same experiences.

5. There are no sex differences in hypnotic responsivity, but there are some changes with age.[17, 19] In general, children are more responsive than adults, a peak of hypnotizability appears in the age interval between nine and twelve years with a gradual decline thereafter; adult levels of responsivity are established by about age sixteen; and responsivity diminishes somewhat in post-middle- and old-age.

6. Hypnotizability is not related to intelligence or cognitive style, and in normal populations the usual personality trait measures have shown no relationships with hypnotizability. In relating the contemporary personality to its longitudinal history and development within the family, however, J. Hilgard points to several influences that affect the development of hypnotizability.[20] These include deep involvement in reading, dramatic art, aesthetic experiences, religious dedication, and adventure. The blurring of fantasy and reality in these activities is intricately bound up with the hypnotic experience.

7. Evidence to support the transcendence of normal physiological and mental capacities in hypnosis is lacking. It appears that, providing the setting is appropriate and the subjects are motivated to carry out the task, they will perform in the waking state to the same degree that they will in hypnosis.[21, 22] This does not entirely eliminate the possibility that hypnosis may actually increase the range of behaviors that people are willing to carry out; it merely demonstrates that subjects tend to do almost anything that might conceivably be required of them in an experimental setting.[23]

8. There is no experimental evidence to support the idea that subjects in hypnosis are more likely to violate their usual moral code than other experimental subjects.[24] A clinician rapidly learns that he can direct the experiences of his patients in hypnosis only to the extent that he remains sensitive to what they communicate they are prepared to follow.

   In the context of medical jurisprudence, opinions differ regarding the more dangerous influence of an unscrupulous operator on the behavior of a deeply hypnotized subject. The logical question seeks to determine whether, under those hypothetical circumstances, the subject could be influenced to commit antisocial acts against his will. Some maintain that if he, in fact, does commit such acts, the hypnotic state cannot be held primarily responsible. The effects of the relationship and the situation in which the request is made must first be ruled out. To examine the question under strictly controlled experimental conditions is, of course, virtually impossible because the experimental situation will immediately generate its own complicating cues.

9. It has been demonstrated that much behavior in hypnosis results from the subject's conception of the role of the hypnotized person as determined by his past experience and learning, and by explicit and implied cues provided by the hypnotist and the situation. Only by being constantly aware of these "demand characteristics" can the investigator prevent them from influencing the subject's behavior. When they do, they create artifacts that have, in the past, confused the understanding of hypnosis. Within the context of a lecture and

demonstration, Orne implied to a group of students that hypnosis was accompanied by catalepsy of the dominant hand.[14] This behavior appeared in some of those students when the group was hypnotized, but failed to appear among any of the members of a control group who had received the identical lecture with no implication that catalepsy of the dominant hand would occur.

10.  There is no evidence that any of the physiological changes occurring in hypnosis are uniquely associated with it.

11.  There is no electroencepholographic evidence that the events in hypnosis are in any way equivalent to those of sleep.[25]

12.  There is evidence that hypnotic analgesia provides a greater tolerance for pain than the effect of placebo when these events are studied in two groups of subjects, one known to be highly hypnotizable, and the other repeatedly unhypnotizable.[15]

## EXPLANATORY CONCEPTS

Among the many theories, some highly involved, that seek to explain the events in hypnosis, space will allow a brief report of a few only. Those that are included are not only broadly representative of the field, but warrant mention because of their relevance or the serious attention they command.

Shor describes hypnosis as having three dimensions.[26, 27] In this manner he disentangles the trance or altered state of consciousness from the remaining aspects of hypnosis. He reminds us that in addition to recognizing the differing abilities of individuals to have an altered subjective experience like the trance, we must acknowledge two additional dimensions, namely, how much trust and confidence the individual feels in the person who is practicing the hypnosis, and how deeply he is motivated to be the subject of a hypnotic encounter at that time. Although Shor goes into considerable and significant detail in describing these aspects, our purposes here will be well served if we recognize that a patient who is capable of an intense trance experience might respond minimally or not at all to the induction procedure if he dislikes or mistrusts the hypnotist. On the other hand, if he has a very limited capacity for experiencing the trance, but is strongly drawn to the personality of the hypnotist and deeply motivated to experience hypnosis, the event for him will have many of the positive aspects of deep hypnosis such as the warm, trusting, relaxed, and agreeable feelings, but will lack the essential subjective blurring of imagination and reality. We will deal later with the relevance of drawing a distinction between these types of responses when we discuss the practical uses of hypnosis.

Support for the emphasis that Shor places on the importance of trance comes from other authors who have attempted to investigate what is described as an altered state of consciousness. Because of the limited interest shown by the Western world in the concept of a nonpathologic altered state of consciousness, we have as yet no dependable definition nor neatly conceptualized notion. Tart strongly encourages the acceptance of the essentially subjective nature of the experience under discussion, in which the individual clearly feels a qualitative shift in his pattern of mental functioning.[28] Ludwig also draws attention to the various agents or maneuvers of a physiological, psychological, or pharmacological kind that can be responsible for such alterations.[29]

Hilgard has recently refocused attention on a form of dissociation which he presents as the probable mental mechanism underlying the subjective experiences in hypnosis.[30]

It is readily seen that the explanations of hypnosis offered above consider the hypnotic state as a special and different psychological event. This concept is challenged by those students of the subject who interpret it within the context of their preferred general psychological theory. They have developed very formalized accounts of hypnosis within the framework of their chosen perspectives. Foremost among these are Sarbin and his co-workers,[31, 32] and the neobehaviorists, whose views are expounded primarily by Barber.[33]

Sarbin's formulation pivots on the concept of role. He sees the role as defined by the instructions and suggestions of the hypnotist, superimposed on the subject's general conception of how a hypnotized person is supposed to behave. The subject strives to take the role of the hypnotized person. Sarbin speaks of the role-playing at a nonconscious level.

Barber and his associates go to great lengths to account for hypnotic behavior in terms of its antecedent events.[33] They cite as important the subject's attitude, expectations, and motivation to cooperate, as well as the tone and wording of the specific suggestions and the tone and wording used to elicit reports of subjective experiences. Barber believes that most of the achievements in hypnosis are within the range of normal human capabilities, and considers as unnecessary the postulate that a person carries out the cognitive processes more proficiently when he is in a hypnotic trance; he claims that individuals can be taught to respond to the suggestions of hypnosis within the context of "training in human potentialities."

This very cursory digression into a few of the theories developed to explain the event of hypnosis has been included not only to whet the appetite of those readers who might be encouraged to pursue the growing literature relating to this fascinating human experience, but because the theories themselves add a perspective to the clinical application of hypnosis. This will become clearer when we grapple in the clinical section with the difference between hypnosis per se and the procedures of hypnosis, namely, with what should be considered hypnosis and what is not necessarily so.

## DESCRIPTION OF HYPNOSIS

Typically, the operator sits by the side of the patient's bed, facing him, or sits opposite or alongside him in the office. When possible, the induction procedure should be preceded by conversation and interaction which encourages the development of a comfortable clinical relationship. A medical history and a psychiatric evaluation when indicated should have been completed; the subject of hypnosis, including the patient's previous experience of it, should have been discussed. For an enriching experience of hypnosis to occur, the patient should be capable of trusting the physician, and willing to be hypnotized. The physician should be sensitive, observant, and supportive. Not all patients are hypnotizable, but most, under appropriate circumstances, can respond to the simpler suggestions.

The induction procedure can be one of many types, ranging from directions to the patient to close his eyes and think of a peaceful scene, to having him gaze at a spot on his hand, a shiny object, or a swinging pendulum until his eyelids become heavy and close.[34] The object is to lead him carefully but confidently, to redistribute his attention so as to withdraw it from his general surroundings and focus it on a circumscribed area. Meanwhile, he is encouraged to relax and let happen what will happen. This induction procedure is sometimes followed, or even replaced, by what are described as deepening techniques. The patient is directed to imagine himself descending gradually on an elevator or staircase, or drifting on a boat past a slowly shifting landscape. Counting forward or backward is another deepening or induction technique. Throughout the procedure the physician fosters the illusions by offering his comments in a slow, repetitive monotone, exhorting the patient to feel relaxed and calm, or to float and drift.

After a period generally lasting from one to several minutes, the physician introduces ideas of a motor or sensory kind. He suggests to the patient, for example, that as he concentrates on the feelings in his fingers and his hand, the small muscles in his fingers will begin to twitch and his hand and forearm will begin to feel light. They will eventually feel so light that they will lift up off the arm-rest of the chair, and continually floating upward, will ultimately reach the side of his face. The physician might add the comment that the higher the hand floats, the deeper will the hypnosis become, and the deeper the hypnosis, the higher the hand will float. He adds, too, that when the hand reaches the side of the face, the patient will be deeply hypnotized.

When this point is reached, and the hand and arm have "levitated," the physician assumes that the patient is hypnotized, and then adds whatever other suggestions are appropriate to the situation.

Before leaving the induction procedure and the introductory phase, it should be emphasized that the initial procedures can be as simple or as complicated as the physician prefers them to be. They can be delivered with a dramatic flourish, or offered very simply. The use of gadgets such as shiny objects, spinning disks, and metronomes is not recommended. The simpler the procedure, the better. The type of suggestions and their sequence is left to the physician's preference. A useful principle, however, is to proceed from the suggestions that are easily experienced to those that are more difficult. Success in the early stages enhances the likely success of the suggestions that follow. As twitching movements in the small muscles of the fingers and hand are more readily experienced in the early stages of hypnosis than levitation of the hand and forearm, the suggestion of the small movements and sensations should precede the other. Failure to experience the suggestions that are offered early in the hypnotizing procedure tends to interfere with its progress. Exhortatory comments are made as the patient progresses from step to step.

Returning now to the point at which the physician considers his patient to be hypnotized, we shall examine some of the possibilities that are available. If the purpose is merely to demonstrate the experience of hypnosis to students, the operator can suggest to the subject that the light feeling in the hand is beginning to fade and is slowly being replaced by a feeling of heaviness that will cause the forearm to lower itself back onto the armrest. The subject is told that at that point he will open his eyes and be wide awake, and that he will notice the usual feelings and control have returned to his hand and forearm. He is told that he will continue to have a comfortable feeling of well-being.

If the purpose of the procedure is to induce dental analgesia, for example, the dentist instructs the patient whose hand is still near his face, to concentrate on the feelings in his fingers, to feel the numb and tingling feelings intensify in his fingertips, and then feel the numb and tingling feelings drain from his fingers into his face and teeth which will then be surrounded and permeated by the numbness. He is then advised that the numb sensation will screen out any hurt or pain from the dental procedures that are about to begin. For the relief of pain in other sites, transferring the numb feeling from the fingertips to other parts of the body is readily accomplished by suggesting that the hand can move to touch the appropriate areas.

Other procedures are, of course, also possible. If the physician is assessing the range of a patient's responsivity, or plans to demonstrate to his patient that he, the patient, does indeed have the capacity to experience hypnosis and therefore to use it in the alleviation of his symptoms, other suggestions can be useful. A relatively simple one is the suggestion that the arm will continue to feel weightless and remain in the levitated position; that when the patient opens his eyes (which he will be instructed to do, shortly) the physician will lower his arm onto the arm-rest; that the arm will then move upward again into the levitated position. Responding to a suggestion as simple as this one is a persuasive experience.

More complex suggestions can be tried with more hypnotizable subjects. In investigative studies, a subject can be encouraged to hear the buzzing of a fly or relive an experience in childhood very vividly; or he can be told that he will not recognize certain letters in the alphabet or that the number five no longer exists—he then finds he cannot comprehend as he tries to read a passage from a book, or he fails to count his fingers correctly. Amnesia for the events in hypnosis can also be suggested.

In the clinical context he can be told that he will have a beautiful dream that is restful, comforting, and totally absorbing; that time will be altered so that a half hour will appear to him as a minute; or that he will be capable, at will, of entering the hypnotic trance at any time in the future by means of a cue or self induction procedure.

He is generally told that when he opens his eyes and awakens he will continue to feel comfortable and relaxed, that he will experience a sense of well-being, and that any unusual sensations created in the hypnosis, such as the tingling in his fingertips, will have disappeared.

The above descriptions are not intended as an exhaustive survey of the experiences possible in hypnosis, but include a sufficiently large number to suggest the variety of clinical uses that can evolve.

## WORKING DEFINITION

Hypnosis is an event developed in the Western world, involving a subject and an operator, and dependent for its occurrence on the trance capabilities of the subject, his or her motivation, the situation, and the relationship between the subject and the operator. When these are appropriate, the subject can be guided or directed to experience reality differently. This experience includes altered or distorted perceptions of various kinds. Unusual achievements of memory such as hypermnesia or amnesia can be part of it. The experience has a beginning and an end, and includes a tolerance for logical inconsistencies. During the event, at some level, an awareness of reality persists, e.g., a subject who is persuaded not to see a chair in the middle of the room, will nevertheless walk around it. The event of hypnosis might include, but is more than, role-playing, suggestibility, deep relaxation, placebo effect, or intense transference. If it is not, we have no need for a separate category or a special concept.

## RELATED STATES

Before proceeding to a consideration of the uses of hypnosis in the treatment of patients with medical disorders, it is important that we briefly direct some attention to the similarities and differences between hypnosis and related states. In other words, we move now from a review of possible constituents of the event to a consideration of its relationships with other similar events. We were reminded, in the introductory comments to this chapter, of the extensive use through the ages of hypnosis-like states in the treatment of patients with medical disorders. During recent years, medical science has focused attention on some of the religious practices designed to lead to altered states of consciousness, experiences of relaxation, and healthier physiological responses. Benson et al have recommended the term relaxation response to describe basic physiological characteristics associated with the experiences of Yoga, Zen, Transcendental Meditation, hypnosis, and other ritualized practices.[36, 37] The technique considered common to them all consists of four basic elements: (1) a mental device such as a fixed gazing or repeating of a phrase, word, or sound silently or audibly; (2) a passive attitude in which distracting thoughts are disregarded; (3) decreased muscle tonus and a comfortable posture; and (4) a quiet environment with decreased environmental stimuli. When the techniques referred to above are practiced, physiological responses alter. In almost all, oxygen consumption, respiratory rate, and heart rate are reported as descreased. Alpha waves are increased, as is skin resistance. Blood pressure shifts may occur.

The relaxation response, stripped of any semblance of a religious ritual, has been offered as a medical prescription;[35] repeating the word "one" is the mental device recommended. One of the aims is improved cardiovascular function.

Formalized studies of Transcendental Meditation have produced reports by individuals practicing the technique that are encouraging. They describe an awareness of a reduction in inner tensions, and demonstrate a more relaxed physiologic state.[37]

Autogenic Training has accomplished impressive shifts in the pathophysiological responses of patients with medical disorders.[38] The technique, which includes the regular practice of exercises in autohypnosis by the patient between visits to the doctor, involves a very relaxed posture, and the focusing of attention on developing specific types of sensations in various parts of the body and limbs.

This brief list of practices conveys some idea of the rituals used to achieve altered physiological states now seriously considered as part of the treatment for medical disorders. Although it cannot be said that they are equivalent to one another, or to hypnosis, there can be little doubt that they are related.

It is possible that once the altered state of consciousness is achieved, each ritualized system proceeds differently. Some intensify the relaxation, firmly establishing the improved physiological response; some concentrate on the religious and mystical qualities of the experience, aiming at deriving benefits from the faith, sense of well-being, and euphoria; hypnosis, and autogenic therapy, which is clearly a derivative of self-hypnosis, concentrate attention on the development of altered bodily perceptions calculated to alter bodily function and even structure. Further investigations of these techniques and their effects are needed. Studies to determine whether success or failure is in any way related to the hypnotizability of the patients involved will help to illuminate the subject.

## CLINICAL USES

Bearing in mind the studies and theory reviewed thus far, we can now develop a series of guidelines to help us in applying hypnosis to the treatment of patients with medical disorders. Knowing the characteristics of hypnosis that have emerged from laboratory studies, and recognizing the complexities involved in trying to understand what belongs to hypnosis and what does not, we can approach the clinical encounter with an evolving basic science to support our assertions. Although we may not infer that what pertains in the experimental area of necessity applies to the clinical situation, we should do well, as we proceed, to examine closely those findings that seem to contradict each other.

Meanwhile, we can enumerate a few principles of therapeutic practice, and thereafter consider them in some detail. We must bear in mind that in the clinical context more than one of them might by active at any given time, especially when the hypnotic situation satisfied the three dimensions of Shor.[27] (I refer here to positive motivation, full trust, and high trance capacity.) The principles provide a useful system for examining the ingredients of they hypnotic procedure.

### Relaxation and the Placebo Effect

The first and probably simplest use of the technique of hypnosis is in the achievement of a state of relaxation. Most induction procedures include suggestions that encourage a feeling of calm and tranquility. Furthermore, the placebo effect, dependent on expectation and faith in the procedure, probably contributes largely to diminishing anxiety.

### Focused Attention

This develops in the context of the induction procedure, and when clinically indicated, is accentuated in the suggestions that follow it. It is the mainstay, for example, in some methods used to eliminate the habit of smoking, where the major thrust depends upon stirring the patient's motivation, and increasing his understanding of the problem.

### Perceptual Alteration

This category is larger than the others, and utilizes an aspect of hypnosis that has been described above as essential to the event as we understand it at this time.

By following suggestions to alter perceptions, the patient might:

1. replace an uncomfortable or unwanted feeling with one that is more comfortable or helpful;
2. shift his attention from the discomfort to a vividly imagined and pleasurable or otherwise demanding situation that becomes more important. This procedure might overlap somewhat with that of the focused attention referred to above. Being able to shift attention from painful feeling relieves the discomfort to some extent, whether or not the patient is able to alter his perception of the pain. For example, being able to concentrate on the peaceful scene viewed from a mountain top reduces the attention a patient can pay to his discomfort. If, in addition, he can feel the mountain breeze on his face and be totally absorbed by the fragrance and vividly experienced surroundings, he will pay even less attention to the discomfort of his symptom;
3. so alter his sense of time that a lengthy period of pain will be perceived as brief, and a short spell of relief as prolonged comfort;
4. end the feeling of discomfort entirely; or
5. substitute a mild localized disability for a more serious and incapacitating symptom.

## Adjunct to Psychotherapy

The increased capacity for memory recall that occurs in hypnosis provides a useful means of facilitating the explorative aspects of psychotherapy.[39] This is especially useful when psychosomatic symptoms originate in the unresolved problems of the past. Perhaps the intensely trusting relationship in hypnosis is responsible for aiding the uncovering process, particularly in instances where resistance impedes free association, blocks dreaming, or prevents a lessing of the defenses. On the other hand, the mental event itself might provide access to memory. We do not yet understand the relative importance of these two factors.

Now we can examine the principles in some detail.

## Relaxation and the Placebo Effect

The clinical literature is replete with assumptions that a patient is hypnotized once his physician or therapist has administered a hypnotic induction procedure to him. Most patients who submit willingly to the repetitive, calming, and reassuring tones of an induction procedure will feel relaxed and calm, but they are not necessarily hypnotized; we have already discussed the criteria of hypnosis above. Patients can appear to be very relaxed, and they might even truthfully declare that their symptoms are relieved, whether or not they have experienced hypnosis. Such improvement associated with relaxation in the absence of hypnosis is in most instances also related to the faith the patient has in the hypnotist and in the procedure; it is usually very difficult if not impossible to separate the effects of the relaxation per se from those that follow the firm belief and expectation that the intervention will be helpful, namely, the placebo effects.

In the individual clinical case, it matters little whether hypnosis, relaxation, or placebo is responsible for the shift; this is applicable where there is no attempt to generalize from a particular event or to develop additional strategies to help the patient further. Where claims are made, however, for therapeutic effectiveness, it becomes important that there exists a greater understanding of the other potentially therapeutic factors in the case.

The therapeutic value of faith has consistently complicated the understanding of treatment methods; Osler directed the attention of doctors to the frequency with which they are ignorant of their own faith cures when prescribing medication, and their sensitivity to those that are performed outside of their ranks.[40] The importance of the placebo effect has been increasingly acknowledged in recent decades.[41-44]

It is readily seen that a successful therapeutic interaction in hypnosis depends on just those criteria that encourage the placebo response. A trusting relationship, positive expectations, and faith in the procedure and the person administering it contribute to one of the three dimensions already mentioned.[27] Physicians who use hypnosis effectively are usually highly sensitive to the importance of encouraging the positive aspects of the transference, fostering trust, and enhancing the patient's anticipation of success. Many modern physicians, however, particularly those trained during the years of the burgeoning technology since World War II, have had little opportunity during their training to develop much regard for this exercise. For them, the good doctor has been he who possesses technological skills and knowledge. Devoting time and attention to inspiring faith has been reminiscent of the charlatan of necessity compensating for his ignorance. Even the bedside manner, much a part of the traditional doctor of the past, has rarely been actively encouraged in most schools.

On serious reflection, it is soon apparent that, in life and death situations, the advantage of skills and knowledge far outweigh the relevance of any other qualities in the physician. In the less critical illnesses that will probably improve regardless of the medical attention, however, an environment that fosters relaxation and a sense of confidence is probably equally, and at times even more important.

Judicious use of the hypnotic induction procedure, applied with a minimum of fanfare, provides a helpful vehicle for the achievement of relaxation and the placebo effect. These can be attained without theatrical embellishments, by making use of the transference and the trust that are embedded in the induction procedure. After a discussion with the patient about the potential benefit, the procedure is introduced as a vehicle for the suggestions that will lead to greater comfort. The patient's readiness to accept the physician's suggestions provides the context for the kind of communication that might otherwise be interpreted as patronizing or paternalistic.

The following clinical example illustrates some of what has been stated here, and also demonstrates the complexity of the clinical situation with its overlap of relaxation, placebo, and hypnosis:

Hypnosis was requested for a 22-year-old unmarried man on the surgical service who had been bothered by continuous hiccoughs for eight days. They had begun shortly after a cholecystectomy and, apart from subsiding during sleep, had continued uninterrupted since their onset. The patient felt exhausted.

The clinical encounter was complicated by the ceaseless and obtrusive heaving of his abdomen as he lay almost flat on his back, and the fact that he had become partially deaf as a result of an antibiotic that he had taken in the past. His left arm was connected to a continuous intravenous drip.

His unfortunate history revealed that he had been healthy until the age of seventeen when an infection of his kidneys suddenly made its appearance, leading to surgical removal and a subsequent kidney transplant. A few months prior to our meeting he had been admitted to hospital with pneumonia attributed to the necessary use of immunosuppressive drugs. As the pneumonia improved, cholecystitis supervened; this led to a cholecystectomy followed two days later by the complication of a faulty drainage tube. Within hours after this had been adequately attended to in the operating room, the hiccoughs commenced. That was eight days before our first meeting.

Despite his hearing loss, and the disruptive nature of the hiccoughs, every effort was made to establish some relationship with him by discussing his complaint, his medical problems, and his past history. He was the only child of a working-class family, involved since his first illness at seventeen in an undemanding supervisor's job. In answer to direct questioning, he talked of his enjoyment, when well enough, of hiking on mountain trails. When given an opportunity to discuss his concern and anxiety about the gall bladder disease that appeared for the first time while he was recovering in the hospital from the pneumonia, he went to some length to explain that he had become used to disappointments in recent years, and that he was more enthusiastic about having the surgery than his physicians had been because he was keen to have the problem behind him. He denied any sense of anxiety or concern.

He had never been exposed to hypnosis, but was hopeful that it would help end the hiccoughs. Because of his hearing difficulty, the induction procedure had to be delivered in a loud voice. He was encouraged to relax by closing his eyes and thinking about being on a mountain top surveying the surrounding valleys and hills. He was then asked to allow his right arm to relax completely and to float into an upright position. He was then encouraged to permit it to float over to the upper part of his abdomen and rest there; the relaxed feeling would then spread to the abdominal musculature. He was told this would relax the muscles so that the hiccoughs would become gentler and less frequent. He was encouraged to continue to imagine himself in the mountain setting, described to him in elaborate detail.

About 20 minutes after the commencement of the induction procedure, the hiccoughs gradually decreased in intensity and frequency. He was instructed in how to induce hypnosis on his own, and advised to practice the procedure after waking as often as he wished. He was told that when he opened his eyes and wakened from the hypnosis he would continue to be relaxed and comfortable, that he would have a feeling of well-being, and that the condition of the hiccoughs would continue to improve. After a period of about 45 minutes from the commencement of the induction, he was asked to waken, and as he did so the hiccoughs ceased.

On a return visit about four hours later, he was found lying with his eyes closed, his hand resting on his upper abdomen, and with no evidence of the hiccoughs. In answer to questions, he recounted that he had been symptom-free for almost an hour after the first session, but that the self-induced exercises had then been difficult to do because of constant but necessary nursing interruptions. He had finally succeeded, however, about half an hour prior to my return visit. He rapidly agreed to the idea of another induction procedure to reinforce his own abilities, and chose to remain in that completely relaxed and hiccough-free state at the end of that procedure, prepared to lie with his eyes closed and his hand on his abdooen, totally relaxed, until the time of his evening meal.

Next day, when visited, he was walking about the ward, cheerful and bright, having rid himself of both his symptom and the intravenous apparatus. He was extremely grateful and very surprised at the ease with which he had been able to respond. He left the hospital a few days later.

His hypnotizability was not measured at any point, and in discussing the event he referred only to the remarkably relaxed feeling he had had. A review of the event does not clarify what the active therapeutic principle had been. The whole procedure had been carried out in a very solicitous setting. My hand had often rested gently on his forearm during our initial discussion, and my manner and comments were purposefully reassuring. He had been reminded during the history-taking that most patients would have been deeply disappointed had they been exposed to the repeated major illnesses that he had had to endure. He had indicated that he had not discussed his concerns with any of his physicians, and prior to the request for hypnosis had not been interviewed by a psychiatrist. Given the strenuous nature of engaging in conversation with him because of his deafness, it was entirely plausible that at no time prior to our interview had his feelings about his illness been adequately discussed with anyone.

It is pertinent that we ask what the role of hypnosis was in this case. Would a psychiatric interview repeated once or twice, with no hypnosis, but demonstrating an understanding for his concern about his health, have been sufficient to alleviate the symptoms? What role did his motivation for hypnosis and his faith in it play? How effective on its own could the relaxed state have been?

In the clinical context, where controlled studies are rarely possible, the answers to these questions remain elusive. In this case the hypnotic technique played an important role, but not necessairly hypnosis per se. A more systematic study of relaxation, placebo, and related states will, we hope, lead to a greater understanding of the variables, and a refinement of the concepts.[45]

The clinical literature carries innumerable reports of similar cases.[10, 46, 47] Those interested in case histories rich in clinical details should refer to them.

## Focused Attention

No induction procedure is likely to succeed without the active cooperation of the patient. This involves his redistributing his attention and focusing it on an idea, an object, an image, or a part of the body recommended by the physician. He may be asked to alter the feelings in a part of his body; if he succeeds in experiencing this, he probably achieves hypnosis, but the success of the treatment is not dependent on it.

This principle of concentrating attention uninterruptedly on a series of ideas without necessarily altering one's perceptions or experiencing hypnosis is captured in an effective one-session treatment designed by Spiegel to help patients quit smoking.[48]

Once the induction procedure has been administered, the physician presents a well thought out statement regarding bodily health, smoking, and motivation. It is, in essence, a 15-minute monologue which is offered to the patient after he has been told that, in this state of intense concentration, his mind will be especially receptive to the ideas and wishes that are of importance to him. He is then instructed to practice, on his own, brief but frequent self-induced hypnotic procedures in which key motivating phrases are repeated.

The substance of the physician's statement might have been mentioned many times in previous conversation with other physicians, but by presenting it to a patient programmed to listen to a formal statement delivered this way, the physician emphasizes and adds importance to the phraseology which, under ordinary circumstances, might seem like a sermon. The circumstances here are structured for the patient to give his undivided attention to the matter at hand. He might sit motionless, his eyes closed, his arm in the levitated position, engrossed for 15 minutes or more. The procedure of hypnosis conveys explicitly to him that this is what he is expected to do. The effect can rarely be equalled without it.

It is readily apparent that this therapeutic principle is particularly suited to treatments aimed at the control of other habits such as nailbiting and overeating. Conditioning procedures are often included.[49, 50] Patients are told, while concentrating intently on the problem, of the unpleasant feelings, tastes, or smells that will occur should they fail to follow their resolve.

Strong suggestions to reinforce self-esteem make good use of the patient's ability to focus attention on what is being told him. It can be assumed that the more deeply hypnotized he is, the less distracted will the patient be, and the more effective the suggestions. From the widespread response to the method of Coué[51] and the clinically useful ego-strengthening techniques of Hartland,[11] however, there is reason to believe that positive response to suggestions of general well-being is not necessarily dependent on the degree of hypnotizability. A close study of the correlation is needed.

## Perceptual Alteration

This large category makes use of an essential aspect of hypnosis, namely the capacity of the person to alter the way in which his internal and external reality are experienced by him. People vary in their ability to accomplish this, which they can do in different ways:

*They can replace an uncomfortable or unwanted feeling with one that is more comfortable.* They can obscure a painful throb by developing a tingling sensation in and around the painful area, to "screen out the hurt from the pain." This suggestion can be offered directly to the hypnotized patient in pain. He is usually advised, first, to concentrate on a tingling feeling in his fingers and hand. Because mild tingling not infrequently occurs spontaneously in the levitated hand, suggestions directed to intensifying that experience are likely to succeed. The patient is then directed to "permit the hand to move to the affected area," thereby strengthening the dissociated feeling in the limb and reinforcing the experience of hypnosis. When applied to the affected part, the patient is advised to "permit the tingling (or numb) feeling to drain from the fingers to surround (or replace) the painful sensations or screen out the hurt." Contrary to popular belief this method can be especially useful in the relief of bodily aches and pains that arise from physical illness.

In the same vein, other undesirable feelings can be replaced by imagining pleasant ones. For example, the cold, numb, or tingling sensations in the finger tips due to Raynaud's disease can be displaced by thinking of the warm and comfortable feelings that are present during the summer months. Images that are familiar to the patient are more easily experienced. In many instances, the patients become aware of an increased warmth in the fingers, and at times the rise in skin temperature can be measured. This leads to improvement in the clinical picture.[10]

I have referred earlier in this chapter to a case of psoriasis that improved after the introduction of suggestions in hypnosis.[9] This patient, a man in his mid-30s, had suffered from psoriasis for 20 years. The condition had improved somewhat in the summers, but never completely. He was able to recapture in hypnosis the warm feeling of the sun beating down on his shoulders as he sunbathed, and encourage its spread to adjacent areas of the skin on his body. He felt the warmth in his skin, the temperature of which, on one occasion, was found to have risen over 2°F. Although it did not disappear entirely, the psoriasis improved to a great extent, and much more than it ever had in 20 years.

Encouraging a smooth feeling in the skin of fingers affected by warts, or a cool feeling in the head of a patient experiencing the prodromal features of an attack of migraine, appear to influence not only the discomfort associated with the illness, but the illness itself. It is this impact of hypnosis on the pathophysiology and pathological structure itself that attracts the interest of clinicians, even though laboratory confirmation of these effects has been difficult to achieve. Until the mental mechanisms involved in this impressive psychosomatic interaction are understood, the event of hypnosis will continue to invite, in some quarters, explanations of magic and mystery.

*They can redirect their attention.*   This is accomplished by shifting attention from the discomfort to an imagined and pleasurable or otherwise captivating situation that becomes more demanding. This can be applied to circumstances in which organic pathology might or might not be present.

An attractive situation can be one alluded to above, namely, a view of the surroundings from the top of a high mountain. The peaceful scene can then be described in detail, and the patient, when able, will be encouraged to experience the event vividly. The mountain breeze, the fragrance, the sounds, and the colors can all become a part of his reality, as will the succession of surrounding valleys and moutanins, and the prevailing calm.

This is but one example of the kinds of images that can be created by patients to distract their attention from a site of pain or discomfort. Left to their own devices, patients have reported exhilarating flights of fantasy, identifying closely with a seagull, an eagle, or a ship at sea. Imagining they sense the touch and the temperature of their environment strengthens the therapeutic value of the experience.

The value of relating the nature of the fantasied image to a characteristic of the illness, and then, by altering the former influencing the latter, is well demonstrated by the following method.[10] The young patient with asthma, having been induced into hypnosis, is advised to watch a television movie in his mind's eye depicting cowboys riding on horses. The horses are running very fast and they are breathing hard and fast, like his breathing. When he repeats that he can see and feel this, he is told that the horses are beginning to run more slowly. Their breathing is becoming slower and easier, and his breathing is slowing down too.

Erickson, in a viedeotaped interview, captures an essential element in the value of these alternative realities by recounting how he had explained the role of hypnosis to a woman with intractable pain.[52] She had wanted to know how, in his view, words would help her when all the methods of modern medicine had failed to offer her relief. He answered by asking her, encouragingly, what would happen to her pain if a tiger were to enter through the door. She conceded that the arrival of the tiger would dominate the situation.

*They can alter their sense of time.*   This is done in order that a period of pain can be perceived as brief, and a spell of relief perceived as prolonged. This ability to alter the perception of time is a part of the hypnotic experience. It can be accomplished by patients who are hypnotizable, and is unlikely to occur in those who are not. Clearly, its value will be most apparent in conditions of prolonged, recurring pain.

*They can remove the sense of discomfort, or substitute a mild localized disability in place of a more serious and incapacitating symptom.*   These two principles can be considered together because of their similarity, and because the circumstances in which they are used are generally alike. They work most effectively in the relief of symptoms of psychogenic origin, in the absence of detectable physical disease.

Because the psychodynamic forces behind such symptoms continue to exert an influence, any attempt to modify the clinical picture should take them into account. To this end, before proceeding with any therapeutic intent, it is essential that an adequate psychiatric evaluation be carried out to determine the patient's motivation, preparedness to give up the symptom, secondary gain from the symptom, strengths and weaknesses, and general level of adjustment. It is necessary to rule out evidence of psychosis, or to ensure that if there is a major personality disturbance, it will not be adversely affected by the use of hypnosis. Adequate studies to rule out organic disease must be completed.

In the general psychiatric evaluation, pains should be taken to determine the degree of emotional support that will be needed if the symptoms are, in fact, sacrificed. Continuous psychotherapy might be advisable, or several hours of the physician's time within the first few days might be essential.

Discomfort, pain, or paralysis can be coaxed to improve by degrees; patients can be taught how to induce hypnosis on their own and practice altering the sensation in a part of the body or improving the function in a "paralyzed" limb; they can be taught how to concentrate on the increasing sensations of "life" in the paralyzed muscles until they can feel and then actually see the muscular fibrillations becoming stronger and spreading to involve other groups of muscles; or they can be encouraged, because the pain in a limb has become so embedded in their existence, to retain one small area of pain in a little finger or toe—this will then allow the remainder of the body to function without the more disabling symptom.

## Adjunct to Psychotherapy in Psychosomatic Problems

The treatment of illnesses generally described as psychosomatic in nature is likely to be helped by the inclusion of supportive psychotherapy in the treatment plan. Hypnosis can be useful if the patients are hypnotizable. I refer now not merely to the alleviation of symptoms by means of relaxation and suggestion (which has been reviewed above), but to the other traditional role of hypnosis in therapy, namely, that of aiding in the explorative and uncovering aspects, when this is possible.

Manipulation of memories is a recognized aspect of hypnosis. These can be hidden, or recalled with surprising accuracy in hypnosis; resistance is lessened and defenses seem weakened. The process of therapy is facilitated and accelerated.[39, 53]

## COMMENT

I have presented the use of hypnosis in the treatment of medical disorders by emphasizing four general principles of therapeutic practice, namely: (1) for relaxation and the placebo effect; (2) to refocus attention; (3) to alter perception; and (4) as an adjunct to psychotherapy. Close examination reveals that these principles are not infrequently used together, and that they often overlap. An even closer inspection might produce a few more. The importance of this approach, however, I believe to be the bridging of the gap between laboratory research and clinical practice. The former demonstrates that not all people are hypnotizable, and that their level of response tends to be stable. Clinical descriptions indicate that far more patients respond to hypnotic techniques than can be anticipated from the numbers that do so in laboratory research.

By acknowledging other factors to account for the successful response to hypnotic techniques, we recognize that the findings of the clinician and the laboratory investigator are not incompatible. A therapeutic response to a hypnotic induction procedure is possible without hypnosis occuring, largely because of the beneficial effects of relaxation and placebo which are by-products of the technique.

I have not attempted a comprehensive survey of the areas in which hypnosis can be used. These are adequately dealt with in some of the publications already referred to.[8, 10, 11, 44, 46, 47] It should be remembered that, with initiative and some ingenuity, illness in almost all systems of the body can be relieved by the judicious application of hypnotic techniques. The effectiveness of disciplines as widely different as anesthesiology, oncology, nutrition, and rehabilitation can be greatly improved by the inclusion of aspects of hypnosis. Preoperative calm, postoperative comfort, a sense of well-being with an interest in food in the presence of terminal illness, and increased motivation to move a paralyzed limb, are all possibilities.

Techniques are numerous and provide a number of different ways to achieve either a sense of calm and well-being, or a more dramatic altered perception.[34] As with all efficient treatments, the technique of hypnosis is likely to be most effective when the diagnosis has been clearly defined; the presence or absence of physical disease should be established, because either influences treatment strategy. The treatment should be in the hands of those who are not only familiar with the practice of hypnosis, but are trained also either in the principles and practice of psychotherapy or in the management of medical disorders.

## References

1. Chong TM: The Truth About Hypnosis. Singapore, T.M. Chong, 1975
2. Mesmer FA: Mémoire sur la découverte du magnetisme animal. Geneva, 1774. With the Précis historique écrite par M. Paradise en mars 1777. Paris, Didot, 1779. English version: V.R. Myers (Trans.), Mesmerism by Doctor Mesmer: Dissertation on the discovery of animal magnetism, 1779. Published with Frankau G, Introductory Monograph. London, Macdonald, 1948
3. Bailly JS, et al.: Rapport secret sur le mesmérisme, ou magnétisme animal. (Secret report on mesmerism or animal magnetism.) Paris, 11 August 1784 (not published). Signed: Franklin (Chairman), Debory, Lavoisier, Bailly (Reporter), Majault, Sallin, d'Arcet, Guillotin, Le Roy. Reproduced in Bertrand A: Du magnétisme animal. (On animal magnetism.) Paris, J.B. Baillière, 1826, pp. 511–516. Reproduced in Binet A, Féré C: Animal Magnetism. French original, 1887. English translation, New York, D. Appleton and Co., 1888, pp 18–25
4. Braid J: Neurypnology: The rationale of nervous sleep considered in relation with animal magnetism, illustrated by numerous cases of its successful application in the relief and cure of disease. London, John Churchill, 1843. Edited version: Waite AE (Ed.), Braid on Hypnotism: Neurypnology. A new edition edited with an introduction, biographical and bibliographical, embodying the author's later views and further evidence on the subject. London, George Redway, 1889. Reprinted as: Braid on Hypnotism: The beginnings of modern hypnosis. New York, Julian Press, 1960
5. Bramwell JM: Hypnotism: Its History, Practice and Theory. London, Rider and Co., 1903, reprinted 1930
6. Charcot JM: Oeuvres Complète. (Complete Works.) Paris, Aux Bureaux de Progrès Médical, 1886, 9 vols.
7. Janet P: The Major Symptoms of Hysteria: Fifteen Lectures Given in the Medical School of Harvard University. New York, Macmillan, 1907
8. Bernheim HM: Hypnosis and Suggestion in Psychotherapy: A Treatise on the Nature and Uses of Hypnotism. French original of first part, 1884; second part, 1886; with a new preface, 1887. English version: Herter CA (Trans.), 1888. Reissued with an introduction by E.R. Hilgard, New Hyde Park, New York, University Books, 1964
9. Frankel FH, Misch RC: Hypnosis in a case of long-standing psoriasis in a person with character problems. Int J Clin Exp Hypn 21:121–130, 1973
10. Crasilneck HB, Hall JA: Clinical Hypnosis: Principles and Applications. New York, Grune and Stratton, 1975
11. Hartland J: Medical and Dental Hypnosis and its Clinical Applications. Baltimore, The Williams and Wilkins Co., 1966
12. Weitzenhoffer AM, Hilgard ER: Stanford Hypnotic Susceptibility Scale, Forms A and B. Palo Alto, California, Consulting Psychologists Press, 1959
13. Shor RE, Orne EC: The Harvard Group Scale of Hypnotic Susceptibility, Form A. Palo Alto, California, Consulting Psychologists Press, 1962
14. Orne MT: The nature of hypnosis: artifact and essence. J Abnorm Soc Psychol 58:277–299, 1959
15. McGlashan TH, Evans FJ, Orne MT: The nature of hypnotic analgesia and placebo response to experimental pain. Psychosom Med 31:227–246, 1969
16. Diamond MJ: Modification of hypnotizability: a review. Psychol Bull 81:180–198, 1974
17. Hilgard ER: Hypnotic Susceptibility. New York, Harcourt, Brace and World, Inc., 1965
18. Evans FJ: Suggestibility in the normal waking state. Psychol Bull 67:114–129, 1967
19. Morgan AH, Hilgard ER: Age differences in susceptibility to hypnosis. Int J Clin Exp Hypn 21:78–85, 1973
20. Hilgard JR: Imaginative involvement: some characteristics of the highly hypnotizable and the non-hypnotizable. Int J Clin Exp Hypn 22:138–156, 1974
21. Barber TX, Calverley DS: "Hypnotic behavior" as a function of task motivation. J Psychol 54:363–389, 1962
22. Orne MT: Hypnosis, motivation and compliance. Am J Psychiatry 122:721–726, 1966

23. Zamansky HS, Scharf B, Brightbill R: The effect of expectancy for hypnosis on prehypnotic performance. J Pers 32:236–248, 1964

24. Orne MT, Evans FJ: Social control in the psychological experiment: antisocial behavior and hypnosis. J Pers Soc Psychol 1:189–200, 1965

25. Evans FJ: Hypnosis and sleep: techniques for exploring cognitive activity during sleep. In Fromm E, Shor E (Eds.), Hypnosis: Research Development and Perspectives. Chicago, Aldine Atherton, 1972, pp 43–83

26. Shor RE: Hypnosis and the concept of the generalized reality-orientation. Am J Psychotherapy 13:582–602, 1959

27. Shor RE: Three dimensions of hypnotic depth. Int J Clin Exp Hypn 10:23–38, 1962

28. Tart CT (Ed.): Altered States of Consciousness: A Book of Readings. New York, John Wiley and Sons, 1969

29. Ludwig AM: Altered states of consciousness. Arch Gen Psychiatry 15:225–234, 1969

30. Hilgard ER: Dissociation revisited. In Henle M, Jaynes J, Sullivan JJ (Eds.): Historical Conceptions of Psychology. New York, Springer Publishing Company, Inc. 1973

31. Sarbin TR: Contributions to role-taking theory, I. Hypnotic behavior. Psychol Rev 57:255–270, 1950

32. Sarbin TR, Coe WC: Hypnosis: A Social Psychological Analysis of Influence Communication. New York, Holt Rinehart and Winston, Inc., 1972

33. Barber TX, Spanos NP, Chaves JF: Hypnotism: Imagination, and Human Potentialities. New York, Pergamon Press, Inc., 1974

34. Weitzenhoffer AM: General Techniques of Hypnotism. New York, Grune and Stratton, 1957

35. Benson H: The Relaxation Response. New York, William Morrow and Co., 1975

36. Benson H, Beary JF, Carol MP: The relaxation response. Psychiatry 37:37–46, 1974

37. Glueck BC: Psychophysiological correlates of relaxation. In Sugarman AA, Tarter RE (Eds.): Expanding Dimensions of Consciousness. New York, Springer Publishing Co., (in press)

38. Luthe W, Schultz JH: Medical Applications, 2. In Luthe W (Ed.), Autogenic Therapy. New York, Grune and Stratton, 1969

39. Wolberg LR: Hypnoanalysis. New York, Grune and Stratton, 1945

40. Osler W: Medicine in the nineteenth century. In Aequanimitas A (Ed.), Volume of Essays. Philadelphia, Blakiston, 1904

41. Beecher AK: The powerful placebo. JAMA 159:1602, 1955

42. Shapiro AK: A contribution to a history of the placebo effect. Behav Sci 5:109–135, 1959

43. Evans FJ: The placebo response in pain reduction. In Bonica JJ (Ed.), Pain, 4, in Advances in Neurology. New York, Raven Press, 1974

44. Kroger WS: Clinical and Experimental Hypnosis. Philadelphia, J.B. Lippincott Co., 1963, ch. 26

45. Position statement on meditation. Official Actions, Am J Psychiatry 134:720, 1977

46. Meares A: A System of Medical Hypnosis. New York, The Julian Press, Inc., 1960

47. Haley J (Ed.): Advanced Techniques of Hypnosis and Therapy: Selected papers of Milton H. Erickson MD. New York, Grune and Stratton, 1967

48. Spiegel H: A single treatment method to stop smoking using ancillary self-hypnosis. Int J Clin Exp Hypn 18:235–250, 1970

49. Cautela JR: The use of covert conditioning in hypnotherapy. Int J Clin Exp Hypn 23:15–27, 1975

50. Dengrove E (Ed.): Hypnosis and Behavior Therapy. Springfield, Illinois, Charles C Thomas, 1976

51. Coué E (1857-1926) French Psychotherapist: devised system of autosuggestion. Encyclopedia Britannica, 6. Chicago, William Benton, 1963

52. Erickson M: The Artistry of Milton Erickson MD, 2 (Videotape). Haverford, Pennsylvania, Herbert S. Lustig MD Ltd., 1975

53. Schneck JM: Principles and Practice of Hypnoanalysis. Springfield, Illinois, Charles C. Thomas, 1965

Ian Alger

# 10
# Family Therapeutic Approaches to the Medically Ill Patient

In the past 10 years there has been a parallel development in the fields of family medicine and family therapy. Family medicine approaches the patient as a member of a family, and is concerned not only with the total medical condition of each individual in the family, but also with the relationships within the total family. It is more than a return to the general practitioner, and it is an approach which has the increasing acceptance of the medical profession.

Family therapy represents a change in the way mental illness and psychiatric problems are viewed. Attention is not just on the individual, but rather on the individual in context, especially in the context of family. Although this viewpoint challenges more traditional concepts, family therapy has also been increasingly accepted by professional groups.

From a broader perspective, one could conclude that our society is now more ready to accept the idea that cause and effect are not so simply related to one another as linear explanations would have had us believe, and that behavioral phenomena, including illness and the way it is dealt with, can best be understood by examining those behaviors in their social contexts. In brief, circular explanations which include multicausal effects and feedback loops are now found to be more acceptable than linear cause-and-effect explanations.

It is readily apparent why there should be a close relationship of understanding between family physicians and family therapists, and why the insights and work of each should be valuable to the other. This chapter will explore some of the approaches in family therapy which can be useful in helping families to deal with medical illness.

## FAMILY THERAPY APPROACHES

In an excellent review of the literature surveying the relationship of families to the development of psychosomatic illnesses, Grolnick notes that illness can be seen on a spectrum from perceived discomforts, hypochondriasis, through psychologically related physiological dysfunctions, to clearly organic entities.[1] No matter where it may lie on this spectrum, any illness in a member of a family creates a current problem for both the patient and for the other family members, and may have profound effects on the transactions among members, on the very quality of life experienced, and indeed, on the actual survival of some members. In other words, once an illness appears in a family member, it affects the operation of the family system and may create chronic and severe problems. Because all members of a family are affected, it can be seen why a family therapy approach may be effective, whereas an approach which deals only with the prime patient may prove frustratingly inadequate. Common experience has shown that a headache which serves to provide an excuse not to participate as a partner, whether for the night at the theater, or for a sexual encounter, is often intractable when only the aching head, and not the aching relationship, is considered.

A medical illness always has a profound effect on the individual who is sick. Depression is perhaps the most frequent accompaniment, and has been related to the feelings of helplessness, vulnerability, and dependency that often are the consequences of illness. The actual physiological changes also play an important role in this type of depression. Reactions to the enforced dependency and diminished competence will be dealt with in unique ways depending on the personal characteristics of each patient, and in turn will have an effect on the other family members, and on the functioning of the family unit.

When illness occurs in the family, the family is required to assume a nursing function, involving actual care and a rearrangement of its usual routine. Families that are rigid and not flexible will find such demands disruptive, and the family system may resist such demands. This, in turn, may create feelings of rejection and further depression in the patient. His responses, in turn, may foster guilt feelings and additional rejection from the family. In a more functional family, the nursing role will assume not only the necessary physical responses, but also a compassionate response which induces feelings of comfort. This type of regression to a dependency state, and the consequent gratification, is functional in a loving and cooperative family, and when the interval of sickness is over, such a family can return to its former state of equilibrium, and the family members can once again assume their usual roles and patterns of interaction.

Chronic illness poses a different problem because, although the disruption of ordinary functioning in the family occurs, the necessity for a long-term adaptation by the family, with possible continuing nursing functions, means permanent alteration in the usual family operations. A healthy family may possess the flexibility and the inventiveness to make such an adaptation, while at the same time considering the needs of other family members, and giving them adequate priority.

In a sense, a measure of the healthiness of a family may be the extent to which adversities, whether illness or other stresses, succeed in evoking adaptational responses in individual family members, as well as the family as a group, which allow for the crisis, but which also permit a new alignment so all members are considered and cared for.

Even in healthy families, some stresses exceed the limits of that group's adaptability, and help from extended family, from networks of friends and co-workers, and from agencies, as well as professional helpers and caretakers, is needed. The healthy family can assess such a situation and seek help, while the less adaptive family may retreat in its social isolation and, only when the symptoms are quite marked, seek help from a family therapist or a family physician or both.

There are two features of illness which are important to identify, since they play such an important part in the dynamics of the family, and on the overall effect that the illness will have on both individuals and on the total family system. The first issue is the degree of disability. Neither naming a specific disease entity, such as the "flu" or "arthritis," nor defining its severity in the usual sense, such as acute or chronic, or mild or severe, gives an accurate measure of the actual disability which the illness will create for the afflicted individual, nor the degree of dysfunction which may be created for the family as a totality. The factors which determine the degree of disability are numerous, complex, and open to a degree of deception which makes the issue of disability a most crucial one in terms of the manipulative value of an illness. Sometimes the individual patient wishes to exaggerate his degree of disability for reasons of simple malice or, perhaps, for reasons of complex transactional factors. This raises the second feature of illnesses which is so important to consider when one is assessing family dynamics. This second feature is the responsibility factor. For the most part, illness can be seen by both the afflicted and his friends and relatives as something over which he has little control, either in the getting of it or in the getting rid of it. True, a favorite style in some families is to tell the sick one that he was asking for illness when he went without a hat or when he overdid it on the tennis court; and in one sense these insights may be true to an extent. However, as yet we have little evidence on how to assess the deliberate generation of a heart attack. Biofeedback has convinced us that we are able to affect our physiology, but the linkage is not yet very clear. It is also true that sick persons are frequently accused of not wanting to get better and of using their afflictions in the games they play with others. These truths notwithstanding, the ill person usually holds a very powerful card in the dynamics of family manipulations precisely for the reason that he can assume the posture that the illness is happening to him. In this sense, the illness takes on many of the characteristics of neurotic symptomatology, with all the strategic advantages so neatly outlined by Haley in his explication of double-bind maneuvers.[2] The consequences of this double set of factors, the degree of disability and the nonresponsibility for the illness, may be the development of intense suppressed rage on the part of the caring members of the family, with the installation of a progressively more destructive feedback cycle of extremely damaging proportions.

In these introductory comments, I have tried to touch some of the factors which will be detailed in clinical examples to follow. I described the way illness can be incorporated into the family interactions in a manner which may be either temporary, or which may in less healthy families convert into a chronic dysfunctional homeostasis. I also mentioned that, whether the illness is psychosomatic or organic in nature, it can serve the same function in this dynamic balance. The whole issue of the effects of family dynamics and functioning on the development of psychosomatic conditions is another much more complicated issue. This subject has been reviewed, as mentioned, by Grolnick, and also is examined in a provocative paper by Weakland,[3] who calls for exploring the neglected edge of family somatics. Meissner too has written a most valuable contribution on family dynamics and psychosomatic processes.[4] Finally, extremely provocative studies and concepts have been developed by Minuchin et al. in their work on psychosomatic illnesses in children.[5] In concert with family therapy approaches, they write that they have begun to look beyond the individual per se to the individual in his social contexts, and to the feedback processes that exist between the individual and his context. Their hypotheses involving the nature of family dynamics which may predispose to the development of psychosomatic conditions are challenging. Aside from the etiologic significance of their work, they describe their therapeutic efforts as directed towards making interventions in the individual, in the family, and in the interactions and feedback loops existing among family members. This work confirms that, regardless of the origins of the illness itself, the intervention which is most effective is one which includes the family, the context of the patient as well as the patient, and not just the patient himself. It is in this perspective that the following clinical material will be presented. The material comes from cases in my own practice, or patients whom I have treated in hospital settings where I have worked. Often the issue of a medical illness arose as a crisis in the course of treatment of a family I was already seeing around other issues. Sometimes the cases were referred specifically because of the stress being produced by the presence of a medical illness. In the material I will attempt to focus on some of my understanding of the family dynamics involved, and on my therapeutic interventions and my rationale for them.

## FATAL ILLNESS

Death, the final transition of our lives, always hovers; but in the vitality and rush of everyday living, denial pushes death's inevitability out of focus. Illness brings the awareness of its possibility closer; but one expects to recover from acute sickness and learns to endure the chronic ailments. At times, however, an illness is clearly life-threatening, and the somber truth at some level seeps through the patient's denial and flows into the consciousness of relatives and friends. Everyone involved is challenged to cope, and the course of such a fatal illness can transcend the tragic. It can be the experience through which family members have a chance to meet more intimately than they ever have before. In some instances, the family therapist may have the opportunity to be a part of that experience.

*Case 1.* A brief family therapy intervention was made at the time of a crisis. The goal was to provide a new perspective for the family in the face of the impending death of the wife's father. Such situations represent a "normal" crisis in life, but can be the nucleus around which continuing problems and suffering can become organized. Judicious intervention is aimed at preventing such an unfortunate outcome.

The consultation interview took place with the husband and wife, who were accompanied by another couple who were friends and who were supportive during this period of stress. A week earlier, the wife's father had suffered a severe heart attack and since that time had been in a coma in a hospital, given no chance for recovery. The mother had died three years earlier, and the father had lived alone in retirement about 100 miles away in a quiet coastal town. The daughter, Anna, was married to Dick and had two children. Dick worked as a truck driver, away from home about two weeks in every month, and Anna worked to provide extra support for the family. It was at work that she made friends with Bill and Nancy, who accompanied the couple to the family session.

Anna was the younger of two girls, and her married sister lived in another state but had been notified of father's heart attack. Anna related how she had always tried to be quiet and stay out of trouble at home. She had always looked for approval from her father but found him difficult to be close to. During the interview she fought back tears as she told how she had always wanted his love, but how, even recently, she had been unable to communicate with him. "I saw other girls with their fathers and wanted it to be close like that," she said. Her way of adapting was to become quiet and self-sufficient. She looked after not only herself, but others as well. Her husband, Dick, was himself an outsider who had been bullied and belittled by his father, and who depended very much on Anna.

When Anna began to feel the stress of her father's illness and could no longer continue in her usual role of caretaker, Dick was unable to move from his usual role of dependency and take charge. Instead, he became more dependent and was involved in an accident with his truck. In many families a complementarity of roles is a stabilizing factor, and flexibility in such systems permits an alternation of responsibility, so the caring functions can be reversed. When this is not possible, as in the situation with Anna and Dick, the stress on one member creates further stress on the other, and the family's function decompensates.

This family sought consultation because of Anna's stress. A therapist could approach the problem as one of facilitating Anna's grief reaction, but this would have the shortcoming of dealing with her as an individual outside the context of her actual life. A family therapy approach would be to also consider her networks of support, both in her family and in her friendship and work networks. This broadened assessment can then clarify where some intervention in the system may be effective and can assist in avoiding the focus being placed on the isolated individual and her grief.

In Anna's case the distant sister and some other relatives to whom she felt little closeness offered limited support. Her friends, Bill and Nancy, were much more involved and were offering support both in practical ways as well as emotionally. Finally, her husband Dick, although in considerable stress himself, was available as a possible source of strength, and a therapeutic decision was made to enhance his position as the provider of support for Anna. In the consultation, the focus on individuals was lessened by delineating the two couples present. As a model, Bill and Nancy were asked how they were experiencing the crisis, and they responded and went on to elaborate feelings about their own parents and the relationships they had with them. In the course of this, Bill held Nancy's hand, and this was seen by Dick when part of the session was replayed on videotape. The use of video-replay in therapy can be a useful adjunct and has been described by the author elsewhere.[6] In the session, I spent considerable time talking to Dick and emphasizing the competence he showed in taking care of the damaged truck after his accident with it. Dick said that his boss had a lot of confidence in him, and Anna confirmed how organized Dick was in emergencies. Dick also talked about low blood sugar that both he and Anna had, and used this as an explanation of his own difficulty at times in coping. I suggested after a time that this might be a way to avoid experiencing painful feeling and observed that the topic of blood sugar came up when painful feelings were emerging. Following that discussion, I asked Anna if there was anyone now who really did look after, and as she struggled for an answer, Dick took off his coat and shortly was holding her hand, as Bill had held Nancy's. Dick then talked about his own search for strength and his struggle to learn more about his own feelings. He said that he had attended a counseling group to try and become more aware of himself. I supported him again with my expression of genuine respect for his efforts at growth.

In essence, then, the consultation session served to allow me to give something to Dick, and to thereby help him give something to Anna. The focus was not on her having to go through an inner process of grieving alone, but rather on helping her see that she could look for support from her husband when she was no longer able to handle the caretaking job for the whole family. Although she had given up hope of ever obtaining the love and response she had wanted from her father, and although his impending death made such a hope even more impossible, she now could begin to take support from her husband as he was supported by the therapy to risk a more nurturing role. Without intervention from outside helpers, like the friends and a family therapist, Anna might have continued in her stress and could have developed increasing bitterness and depression. The case illustrates how one consultation may be extremely useful in shifting a family's method of adapting.

Case 2 describes a brief intervention, but the context is different from the former example in that the patient, who was the son, had been seen by me previously in therapy for a lengthy period. Thus, the family therapist is often maintained as a peripheral part of the family's network, to be called into more intensive involvement at the time of medical and other crises.

*Case 2.* Michael called to tell me his mother was terminally ill with cancer and had been in hospitals and nursing homes for months. Recently, she had returned home with round-the-clock nursing and was slowly dying in great pain. When we saw each other the main issue on his mind was whether or not he should arrange in some way to give her an overdose of her pain medication to end her suffering. He was extremely anxious and agitated about the situation and his sense of desperation was extreme. The distress was amplified by a series of other losses in his life. His career as a successful free-lance writer had in recent years been declining, and he reported that many of his old contacts and friends seemed to have drifted away and deserted him. This was producing financial pressure. Furthermore, a woman with whom he had lived for several years had recently broken with him, and before that his marriage had ended when he left his wife over a disagreement as to whether they should have another child.

His isolation was more complete. His sister had been repeatedly hospitalized over the years with schizophrenia and was now travelling alone, with almost no money, and had been a constant source of worry to the mother. Michael's father had died many years earlier, and his mother had taken over the family business and had run it successfully, continuing to provide support for the daughter, but finding her a constant source of anxiety and irritation. Michael had been a disappointment to his parents, both of whom had wanted him to enter a profession. The mother was an especially controlling woman who had always downgraded Michael's achievements in writing, and he felt that his talents had never been recognized by either parent. At home he had adapted as a youngster by an independence expressed in rebellion and withdrawal, and recalls the complaints of others throughout his life that he was late or argumentative or stubborn and uncooperative. It seemed that he repeatedly duplicated this early system of relationships in his life and found himself alone, embittered, and often depressed.

As the mother's illness had progressed, she did not mellow, but increased her usual method of coping by controlling everything. She insisted on running her own treatment program, thereby alienating several doctors and, although she manipulated her way into other hospitals, she eventually was transferred from all of them into nursing homes, where she was a source of difficulty to the staff. During this time, more and more responsibility fell to Michael, who was the only relative available to help. He began to administer her finances, and become increasingly involved in day-to-day decisions. With the other stresses of his own life, and with this enforced closeness to his mother, his ambivalence was heightened. In our sessions he talked of his compassion for her suffering and of his frustration with his own helplessness to do anything about it. He also became increasingly aware of his hostility to her and resented her self-centeredness and her intense drive to control.

At this stage, the therapy had several goals. The first was to provide the reconstitution of the relationship with me after a period when therapy had been discontinued. The reconnection was easy, and this immediately provided one branch of a support system. The second thrust was to encourage communication and cooperation with the medical and hospital care-providers. This strengthened an auxilliary support system for Michael, and also relieved his feelings of guilt as he learned over and over how much difficulty others were experiencing with his mother. The third therapeutic aim was to encourage a different stance with his mother. The old adaptation of withdrawal and resistance could not work now since he was actually the only responsible person. Although he was not getting support or appreciation from his mother for his effective efforts in this new role, he was able to appreciate his own adult performance and to continue making the necessary arrangements, even to the point of obtaining excellent nursing care at home when nursing homes no longer were available. It was at this point, during the final weeks, that he became preoccupied with a feeling that it was his responsibility to end her suffering. In a home visit I was able to experience the pressure he felt and to appreciate how alone he felt with his dilemma. The ambivalence had become more sharply defined in the last weeks, but he was able to recognize that his own needs to control, developed in the workshop of his controlling home, now led him to feel an exaggerated urgency to solve everything for his mother. He also saw that the emergence of his hostile feelings threatened him and fueled the anxiety-ridden conflict. The approach encouraged was an attempt on his part to spend time with his mother acknowledging with her the pain they both felt in the suffering and unhappiness. With an acceptance of the inevitability of her death, and by turning more of the responsibility for the relief of her pain over to the doctors and nurses, Michael was able to find relief from the obsession that he must solve it by himself. Some resolution was accomplished, and his mother's death subsequently left him with little guilt, less bitterness, and an experience in which he felt that he had responded instead of withdrawing into his own isolation.

The family therapy approach attempted to consider Michael in the context of his current life where he had experienced multiple stresses and a loss of many of his supports; in the context of his past family life, where he had adapted by withdrawing and isolating himself; and in the context of his present dilemma, which had heightened as he was drawn back into the nexus of his intense ambivalence and, as the only responsible adult, could not easily avoid direct confrontation with his mother and their relationship. By helping him find more understanding of his own duplication of the original family system within the actual current relationship with his mother, I was able to encourage his finding a different resolution to his conflict about ending her life, and he was able to experience his own capacity to relate in a new way to his mother and now possibly to others.

The situation of Case 3 resembled the former case in that a crisis developed as the patient's father became terminally ill with cancer, and the daughter, Marge, who had been in individual therapy with me, asked that I consult with her family. The point to be emphasized is the flexibility necessary for successful work with families. This capacity has at times been lost by therapists who have worked with an individual model. In that model, the focus is on privacy and confidentiality in the relationship and primarily on the intrapsychic conflicts. Family therapy has a dual approach. From a theoretical base it holds that the intrapsychic functions (concepts and adaptational patterns) can be understood only in the context of human interactions and social sets, both historical and current. In addition, family therapy also utilizes as a therapeutic method the conduct of therapy in family groups, where many members of the family in addition to the identified patient assemble for a therapy session. The necessary flexibility is, therefore, both in the theoretical as well as in the practical realm.

*Case 3*. Marge was one of six sisters, and two still lived with their parents although Marge was 21 and her sister two years younger. Both parents worked, but the father had been operated for a bowel cancer three years before and was intermittently being treated with chemotherapy. He had been effective in providing for the family and had maintained an outgoing and cheerful attitude about life, using denial to obscure his own dissatisfactions. His wife was an anxious person who had always taken a dependent position in relationship to her husband. Marital problems had always been hidden behind concern for the six daughters. One sister had made an adequate adjustment but was a continuing source of worry. Marge was intelligent but socially inept, and had gained acceptance as well as rejection by continually bouncing back and forth in relationships as the resource person and the "fixit maven." In the crisis of her father's illness, however, this capacity had been useful, and she constantly acted as consultant to his illness because she worked in a clinical lab and was able to get the latest information from doctors on cancer treatments and on the nuances of chemotherapeutic agents.

As the seriousness of the illness became more apparent, denial was escalated, and the underlying hostilities buried more deeply. Tension increased in the family, and one day Marge asked if I could visit her family. I agreed, and it was arranged that I should come to dinner. Everyone knew I was Marge's therapist, but the family meeting was not structured as therapy. Rather, I said I welcomed the chance to know her family better and continued that we might be able to talk together about how the family was managing. My goal in that meeting was to make entry into the family, and I succeeded in establishing a comfortable relationship with the father and the mother. Janet, the sister, was not hostile but stayed rather aloof.

This earlier meeting laid the groundwork for a second and much more stressful session. Joseph, the father, had been hospitalized for further treatment as his condition worsened. The illness seemed clearly terminal, but he had agreed to a special procedure with direct perfusion of the liver with a new experimental chemical. I visited him in the hospital and met with the whole family in his room. Everyone was under tremendous stress, and the women in the family were taking turns keeping a 24-hour vigil. Joseph seemed pleased to see me, and we held each other's hands throughout the meeting. He was calm, and everyone was able to speak easily about the sadness and difficulty of his dying. He then asked if he could talk alone with me for a while, and when the others left, he cried and told me he never would have agreed to the procedure had he known the pain and discomfort he would have to endure. He asked me to talk with his family, and then he became peaceful and, in fatigue, drifted to sleep.

In a room in the hospital I met with the mother and daughters, and we talked about their feelings of helplessness, fear, and sadness. They were able to support one another and to plan a better schedule so they would not be so tired in their attempts to stay beside him. All of them cried and then seemed to accept the inevitability of his death.

Two days later he died, and the following week I visited their home. A normal grieving process seemed to be going on. Relatives had been very loving and supportive, and when the four of us talked, feelings of regret, but not guilt, were expressed. Since then the mother has continued to work, has expanded her friendships, and both girls have moved to their own apartments.

The value of the family approach was that it was easy to move into the family at a time of crisis and to intervene in a way to provide relief at the time, and to help prevent the development of disabling guilt.

*Case 4.* A woman psychotherapist in her late forties came to see me, asking to join one of my groups. She told me that a few years earlier she had been operated on for breast cancer and since that time was on long-term chemotherapy. Although she knew the grave prognosis, and although there had been metastases to the bone, she maintained a positive interest in life and said she was anxious to belong to a group so she could continue to improve the quality of her human relationships. She also told me sadly that several other therapists had been reluctant to have her join a group when they learned of her illness. I welcomed her into a group, and for the two years until her death she was actively involved in the life of the group.

There is no need to dwell on the fact that family structure in our society is undergoing rapid and extensive change. Divorces multiply, and geographic distance and the mobility of the society have made the extended family truly extended to the point frequently of invisible diffusion. With such changes, the traditional support systems and family networks have been weakened and often lost, and individuals are more isolated and helpless in their aloneness. Pat was in some ways typically caught in this dilemma, and yet in other ways she had uniquely struggled to maintain networks of support. Several years earlier she had decided to leave a marriage of over two decades in which she had been very unhappy. This was a courageous act, because her husband gave very little financial assistance, and she had to return to school to complete her professional training so she could better earn her own living.

The two daughters in the family were already old enough to be on their own, so Pat ventured into a new world.

Over the years she had succeeded admirably in her field, but her children had moved to distant states, and she lived alone. She had established a close relationship with a man, and they loved one another, but although they considered moving together at times, this plan never was completed, and they maintained separate apartments and considerable separateness in their lives. As Pat's illness developed, she grew more and more anxious to find a place with her man, and put pressure on him to move. This served mainly to cause his withdrawal, and when she joined the group, this reciprocal dance was one of the important dynamics she wanted to work on.

The group functioned basically as a foster family for her and, in this sense, played a role which it frequently plays, since the families of many people are so dispersed, leaving them lonely and disconnected. Pat was accepted into the group almost from the beginning, and there was complete frankness about her cancer and about the questionable prognosis. The "family" therapy in the group consisted of the building of this expanded network within the group. Pat was given great support by the group and by me to pursue her career. She continued to take postgraduate courses and was very open to studying and applying new techniques of therapy. She herself took many courses in family therapy and also taught the method to others.

Her role in the group was frequently that of nurturer, and she freely offered help, compassion, and understanding to others. I supported this role for her, and allowed her to function as a co-therapist at times. In this sense, she and I frequently modeled mother and father for the group. Then the role would flip, and she would be very needy and burdened, and the group would take over the nurturing role and give her great support. Just as in a family a healthy capacity for members to alternate and shift roles is a sign of the family's viability and adaptability, so too in the group this possibility provided everyone with the acceptance and nurturing they needed as life created problems and presented its flow of crises.

The group also encouraged Pat to explore her relationships with her own family and, although there was distance between her daughters and herself, and, although she felt continuing problems with her mother (now living in retirement in the south), Pat did move to change these relationships. On trips to the west to visit her daughters, she established a new understanding with them, and was very proud of their increasing ability to accept their rights to their own lives. She became less sensitive to rejection, and was able to step back and let them move in their own directions without experiencing every such move as a direct personal rebuff. She also developed a better interaction with her own mother, and she was able on one notable occasion to say "no" to an excessive demand from her mother without feeling guilty or resentful.

Finally, as her illness became more severe and when eventually the spread of the disease disabled her further, the group took on the nursing role of family. Members reached out to Pat, socialized with her, visited her, and gave her their love and friendship. When she no longer could attend sessions, they called and visited her until the time of her death, which at the end was swift.

The group went through a period of mourning. Her dying was personally felt by us all, and her example of courage and her constant striving for life was deeply felt by everyone. The therapy in the family of her group had brought growth to each one involved, and her therapy with her own family brought Pat a new freedom and human equality with her mother and a new sense of connectedness with her daughters. At the time of her dying, her children returned to be with her, and all the work Pat had done found a closure at her funeral where friends, colleagues, group members, and family came together to mourn her loss and to celebrate her life.

## FAMILIES AND INSTITUTIONS

In the last section I wrote of the changes in family life in this society and showed how a therapy group functioned as an extended family for Pat. Other institutions in the society frequently function in the place of families, and their effect can be either supportive or destructive. Institutions are often brought into the family life to provide a kind of barrier between struggling partners, much in the way that a child and his problems can be triangulated into a marriage so the partners don't have to deal directly with their own struggles. In this way too, the legitimate functions of institutions such as hospitals can be sabotaged, and the resulting backlash from the institution can develop a runaway reaction which can overwhelm the family system and effectively destroy the primary patient in the process. The next two cases are relevant to this issue; in one instance, the institution was triangulated in a destructive way, while in the other, the institution functioned to support the family in the determination of its own destiny.

*Case 5.* This family is one which over three generations has earned the label of a "multiproblem family." In this instance many of the problems were medical in nature and, although the etiology of the various illnesses is varied, they all have been used in the family dynamics to help people avoid closeness and to allow manipulation of other members. The point of this vignette is to show how a member of the family, the wife of one son, was identified by the family as having an "individual" drinking problem. The fact that her drinking was not dealt with as a family problem and that this approach was supported by physicians and hospitals perpetuated the maintenance of a very maladaptive family homeostasis.

The husband had been dominated throughout his life by his father, toward whom he had great ambivalence. He constantly strove to gain the father's acceptance, and was hurt and furious that his younger brother seemed to be the one toward whom the father turned. The mother was a strongly manipulative woman who developed an alliance with the older son, Phil, and the parent couple kept their own relationship at a distance by this triangulation. Whenever this maneuver didn't work, illness was brought in as a barrier and manipulative lever, and the mother suffered from weakness and fainting, and drank excessively but intermittently. Phil's father developed heart and prostate problems, and after his wife's death his illnesses became the center around which his own life and those close to him were controlled.

When Phil married Shirley the equilibrium in the family of origin was disturbed. Phil began to organize his own family life, and two girls were born. But the new family was threatened by Phil's parents' attempt to drawn him back into his old position between them. When Shirley began to drink, this was both a medical and a family problem, but it was labeled "Shirley's problem;" and Phil and his parents and the medical and mental health systems colluded (without conscious deliberateness) to have her admitted to a mental hospital for treatment. This focus on her became a permanent and habitual way for the three generations of this family to deal with important emotional issues. Stresses in the family exacerbated Shirley's drinking, and she became a scapegoat and was either rehospitalized or threatened with readmission.

As noted, when the mother died after a prolonged illness with malignancy, the father continued to suffer from chronic heart problems, and Phil developed joint symptoms diagnosed as posttraumatic, phobias related to heart disease, and attacks of dizziness. Shirley found lumps in her breast which were removed and benign, but her anxiety over breast cancer remains. The younger daughter has chronic skin problems, and the older one has severe behavior problems at school. The "multimedical problem family" uses all the ailments at times to maintain a homeostasis which allows a continuity but which prevents the members from freely developing their individual potentials as human beings and which perpetuates a family system which is constrictive and rigid. The scapegoating of Shirley and her alcoholism became the final common path which was used whenever the other illnesses and symptoms no longer maintained control in the system.

I do not mean to simplify the problem of alcoholism, which at this point seems to be a combined medical and family disturbance. The course of treatment in this family was disappointing. Family sessions were held with Phil and Shirley after both had had many years of individual therapy with other psychotherapists. The children were seen with the parents in some family sessions, but the family dynamics already described would usually promote further drinking, which then was very destructive and resulted in a new scapegoating of Shirley and a return to the same family impasse. With the death of the father imminent, Phil has begun to develop new strengths. In therapy he has understood the dynamics, but each attempt by any member to change the structure releases a responsive onslaught of symptoms in the family system.

During family therapy, Phil's parents could not be induced to join sessions, and they continued, with Phil's collusion, to view the problem as primarily Shirley's.

This example reveals that when alcoholism was not dealt with as a family problem but was isolated as a problem in an individual, institutions of medicine and the mental health system taught the family to deal with their family problems by institutionalizing the individual. The result is a dysfunctional family which is extremely resistant to change.

The following illustration demonstrates the positive effect a non-rigid institution can have on the lives of family members faced with a crucial life decision.

*Case 6.* The patient was a man who had just reached 40 when stricken with bulbar polio, leaving him a quadriplegic who could not be sustained without respirator breathing support for more than a few minutes. He was married, with two children, and after two years the patient, Ben, and his family had accepted the fact that he would spend the remainder of his life in an intensive respiratory care center.

The center in which he was a patient had a full rehabilitation program which included a group of mental health professionals who tried not only to work with the "staff family" at the center, but also to include the total family of each patient in the rehabilitation and counseling program. Ben was a lawyer and showed an amazing capacity to assess and accept his situation. He coped with the kidney problems which developed, as they ordinarily do in patients who are so immobilized. And he coped with the necessity of being so physically dependent on others for his smallest needs, whether it was scratching his nose or adjusting an electric page-turner so he could read through an arrangement of mirrors from his respirator.

He and his wife, Marion, were very devoted to each other and very concerned with each other's welfare and future. Ben decided that, because he loved Marion and because he was so unable to participate in most of life's activities, he wanted to offer her the option of divorcing him and remarrying so she could establish a new family life for herself and the children. I deliberately report that he offered her the option, because their relationship was one which fostered a mutually respectful interaction. Marion could have chosen to remain married and to establish a life as essentially a single parent; but for her own reasons she decided that a fuller life was possible for everyone if she went ahead with the divorce. The couple discussed their decision with the staff, but the staff made no attempt to influence this decision. I believe this was the remarkable thing about the institution. A more rigid and closed system might have exerted pressure on the family to maintain a more traditional format. Marion might have then left the marriage with feelings of doubt and guilt, and there would have been an alienating experience with the center and the nursing staff who would continue to care for Ben each day. Marion might also have decided to stay in the marriage, but if she really had wanted to establish a different life, she might have stayed with bitterness and consequent depression. It is important to note again that the family made its own decision and to realize that I am not saying that their decision has any universal validity. Rather, I am saying that it had validity for them, and the institutional system within which they were operating at the rehabilitation center provided an open understanding and acceptance of their decision which made it possible for the entire family and staff to continue to live in an integrated, cooperative, and loving way.

Marion visited Ben every week, and his children remained close to him. The new husband became a friend and openly discussed issues which affected the children, so Ben continued to feel himself as an important part of that life. Because of his own personal strength, Ben arranged to obtain grant money and undertook the direction of an important legal research project from his respirator, with the assistance of law students who were hired under the grant.

The case illustrates the important point that it is not the illness, but rather the degree of disability which determines how dysfunctional a family will become. The disability is clearly not related just to the medical and organic factors, but rather to the degree of functional impairment of the total human being. In this instance, Ben demonstrated his determination, his maturity of judgment, his own self-confidence and ability to care for others, and his intense motivation to use his mind and intellect when most of his muscular system was permanently lost. These resources defined the extent of his disability, and he and his family in the context of a caring and open institutional system created a unique and very functional life style for themselves.

## CHILDHOOD ILLNESS AND THE FAMILY

If it is true that the presence of a new child in a family greatly changes the structure and function of that family, it is especially true that the occurrence of illness in an infant or child can be catastrophic in consequence and, unless dealt with effectively, can become a chronic and destructive organizing force in the family. In the introduction of this chapter, I noted that there is considerable lack of clarity as to the nature of the relationships between family dynamics and the occurrence of certain psychosomatic illnesses. But I also wrote that regardless of the etiology, once an illness does occur in the child, the way the illness is dealt with by the family system will determine how powerful that illness will be in the future of that family and in the future of the separate members of the family.

Two cases will be described briefly. One demonstrates a chronic situation which might have had an earlier and more felicitous resolution had a family therapeutic approach been attempted when the child was young. The work of Liebman et al in similar cases has demonstrated a follow-up improvement result of astonishing success.[3a] The second case is one in which early family therapy intervention was effective, and a possibly chronic and disabling family problem averted.

*Case 7.* Vera consulted me when she was 35, complaining that she felt isolated. Although she had been in therapy for the past seven years, she still wanted to feel more comfortable with people and decided to join a therapy group. She lived alone, had completed college, and was earning a good living in work she enjoyed as a director of her own management company. She soon related that her 32-year-old sister, Laura, had been a tremendous problem for her most of her life. As 12, Laura had developed asthma, and since then had spent about half her life in hospitals. Vera had been designated as the caretaker in her family, and since the age of fifteen she had taken major responsibility for Laura. After college she had moved with Laura to a southern state which was recommended for the asthma. But when that didn't help, the sisters moved back to New York and took apartments in the same building. Vera described being frequently awakened at night by a phone call from her sister, who would gasp her distress and then hang up. The hectic ride to the hospital in the ambulance followed. Laura became increasingly dependent and demanding and wanted to accompany Vera on all her social dates.

When Vera began to work, she gave support to Laura, and the dependency continued until the time she consulted me. The father had died four years earlier, and at that time both girls had gone into treatment together. This therapy was reported to have eased the dependency situation to some extent, but a very constrictive bond still remained. The mother, with whom Vera had always had a distant and strained relationship, lived alone in another part of the city, and had always claimed that her own illnesses prevented her from being able to care for Laura.

The history demonstrates how a whole family system can be organized around one person's chronic illness, and how Vera had become the prime caretaker in the family so that others' needs always were given more priority than her own. In the extended family history it was striking to note that in every generation, one sister in the family had taken such a role, and that one of the mother's sisters had continued to supply financial support to the patient's mother through her entire life. This pattern of one sibling taking over a parenting role and continuing in that overresponsible position is a common family dynamic in dysfunctional systems. In the present case, Vera had been unable to shift the family structure even during conjoint therapy with the sister. The treatment decision was to have Vera enter a heterogeneous psychotherapy group with the plan that this group would become a new extended family for her, a new family in which she would not be allowed to take the usual overresponsible position. The strategy was effective, and Vera found that this new group was interested in *her* needs. This was a very different experience for her, and she began to make a new network of friends outside the group. During the second year of therapy, she met a man whom she married several months later. This change in her life of establishing her own family created a new crisis in the life of the original family. The mother began to experience increased symptoms and complained to Vera that Vera was no longer showing care for her sick sister, who was now complaining to the mother in an old pattern which formerly had resulted in Vera's rushing back into the caretaking role.

This time new factors created the necessary impetus for Vera to hold her own course, and she confronted Laura with the importance of her getting work herself so she could become more self-sufficient. This move was encouraged by Vera's husband, who wanted to keep their money for a better future for Vera and himself. This move created another crisis, and the mother sought help from a therapist who suggested a family consultation. The result was that both Vera and Laura began sessions again with this family therapist to negotiate a new relationship among themselves and the mother. In the meantime, Vera continued to work in her own therapy group and continued to find reinforcement for the idea that in any system the needs of every member must be met, even the needs of the caretaker.

Changing an established system after over twenty years of habitual functioning is extremely difficult and often impossible. In this case the daughter who was designated to live in the parent role with her sister managed to shift the system through the help of a new "family" in her therapy group and through the subsequent development of her own nuclear family unit. Had family therapy been available when Laura first developed her asthmatic symptoms at age 12, the dysfunctional family organization might have been changed in a relatively short time, and much pain might have been avoided.

Case 8 is another illustration of a family returning for brief therapy in a crisis when a therapeutic relationship had been established earlier.

*Case 8.* Jill and Len had been married a year, and before the marriage, I had treated Jill for several years in individual therapy and then had seen them as a couple while they decided whether or not they would marry. They met when Jill was 30 and Len was 50. He had been married previously, had divorced, and was just beginning a new career in academic life after a successful business career. Jill too was starting a new career in social work after having worked for many years as a teacher. Both were in a transitional stage of their lives and, in their marriage, found a common solution to their different needs.

The question of a child was unsettled because a baby was important to Jill for what she would gain in terms of being fulfilled as a mother, while it was important to Len because of what he might lose in beginning a second cycle as a father. Both had fears. She feared she might lose a chance to be a mother; he feared he might lose a chance to be successful in a new career because of the burdens of a family.

The dilemma was solved by pregnancy; and when the baby arrived, I received an excited call and the message that it was the happiest day in Jill's life. I must add that Len seemed very happy too. Two weeks later I received another call, this time frantic. The baby had developed jaundice, and examination by the pediatrician and then by a pediatric hematologist produced a tentative diagnosis of blood dyscrasia. The following day I learned the baby had been hospitalized and there was the possibility of a grave prognosis. The couple had been told that in any case the child would need periodic blood transfusions until her teens, and then a splenectomy could be performed. I saw them in an emergency consultation and found Len to be somewhat distraught and Jill to be overcome with anxiety and panic. The family therapy approach was to provide a place where the couple could express their anxiety together. Because of the earlier dynamics expressed in the father's ambivalence about having a child, a very close bond had occurred immediately between Jill and the baby, and Len had become excluded. I saw the couple frequently during this crisis period, making myself available on the phone and providing information about specialists who might be consulted. At home during the immediate phase there was considerable blaming of Len by Jill, and she talked of leaving him because he showed so little interest in caring for her and the child and instead seemed only interested (to her) in the obligations he had at work. He was under considerable stress himself because he was in the final stages of preparing for his doctoral orals.

The baby was released from the hospital after a transfusion, and Jill continued to stay home full-time to care for the baby, extending her leave-of-absence at her job. She became more and more depressed and found no comfort from anything Len could do. At this time a focus on her as an individual would have been a possibility because she was now clearly suffering a clinical depression. By continuing to keep the focus on the family system, however, and by supporting both parents in the sessions, they began to be able to give and receive support from one another. As I continued to support their closeness as spouses, the danger that mother and child might develop too close a symbiosis faded.

Many stresses had come together at the same time in their lives. Their new marriage, the difference in their ages, the beginning of new careers, and then the baby followed by the illness; all had concentrated to produce a major time of crisis. The fact that there was no support system of relatives for either of them added to the stress, and my being able to provide a source of support at this crucial time sustained them for a period during which they made a transition and were able to begin to care for one another instead of blaming one another.

The importance of being able to mobilize family strengths at the time of crisis cannot be overemphasized. The family approach facilitated the restructuring of the family and encouraged a new dynamic of mutual support. An individual approach towards Jill's depression might have focused the problem on her, and in this way might have been the beginning of a chronic pattern of dysfunction in that family. The fact that the diagnosis later turned out to be too pessimistic, and the baby needed no further transfusions and seems to have had only a transient problem, is happy news, but does not have relevance to the points made in regard to the value of the family therapeutic approach.

## CARDIAC ILLNESS

Affairs of the heart have always had a central place in human life, and in medical illnesses it is no different. Sudden death from a heart attack causes fear and anguish among relatives and friends. Anxiety in a wife over her husband's possibly impending heart attack may only mask her underlying hostility toward him. On the other side, a man's fear of such an attack may result in phobic anxiety, or may give him the excuse to withdraw and avoid all the annoying responsibilities that accrue at middle age.

Survivors of attacks may experience a totally new perspective on life and develop a different sense of values about the priorities in their lives, while others may use denial in order to continue their predetermined course, while their wives and children may become fearful and overconcerned. As with other illnesses, the degree of disability is related to the total life adjustment that is made and not alone to the actual pathology of the particular condition.

The cases to be described here involve ways in which a family therapy approach was useful in not supporting the development of cardiac invalids and in not promoting the development of cardiac neuroses.

Case 9 is reported to illustrate an approach to someone who has suffered coronary occlusion, has recovered, but is using his fear of the illness to avoid crucial problems in life which are very disabling.

*Case 9.* Norm was in his early forties when he consulted me. He was a business manager, married, with two children, and had suffered two heart attacks, the last one over a year previously. He was obviously overweight and spoke in a mild, somewhat deferential manner. He reported that he had worked over seven years in individual and group therapy, but he was now seeking help because he was very unhappy in his marriage and extremely dissatisfied with the progress of his own career. He felt that he continually made moves to sabotage his progress just at times when he was about to achieve success.

He described his family life as a tortured morass of quiet provocativeness and bitter frustration. Both children had learning problems at school, and both had difficulty in relating to peers and tended to be reclusive and morose. His wife was described as anxious and demanding, and he said that she was continually critical of him. She complained that he was not active enough in pursuing his career, in creating interesting social friendships, and in participating in physical activities. Her anger at his passivity was only made worse as he tried not to exert or excite himself because of his heart "problems." This reaction in turn caused his wife to become more angry, and if we turn to cybernetics for a description of this process, we would say that a positive feedback loop had been established which was promoting a runaway reaction with increasing tension and the attendant dangers.

At the beginning of therapy I told him that his life did indeed seem very bleak and stressful and that I could only promise that I would try to help him create some better way of living. I went on to say that such a project carried with it a risk, and we should clearly understand the risk together before we began. I told him that I would move in therapy with no regard for his fear about his heart. I said that any attempt to avoid stressful material in the therapy would likely render our task hopeless, and that unless he were willing to personally take the risk that he might face a fatal heart attack during the therapy, I would rather not work with him. I continued that in his search for a better life style he obviously wanted to have a more dynamic interpersonal life and that this would involve his engaging more directly and forcefully in his human interrelationships. He felt it was a blunt approach, but he also said that he was willing to take the risk and that he felt relieved that I had spoken in the way I had because he now felt that he was really talking to someone who was taking him seriously. He felt there was hope that his life could be different.

When we began, I asked to have his wife come in for sessions; and we concentrated on taking the two children out of the center of the field, where they had become a major distraction for the couple and prevented a clear definition of the underlying serious problems in the marriage. A detailed account of the therapy is not necessary here, but within a year Norm had decided he wanted to separate from his wife and build a different life for himself. With this decision, his own anger became more accessible, and, as this happened, his wife became quite violent. Through the storm and violence his decision remained firm, however, and there was fortunately no further heart attack, and the divorce was completed.

The brief follow-up is that after 10 years, he has had no further attack. After the decision for divorce, he continued for a period in individual therapy, and his wife consulted a therapist she had previously worked with for some further help. She has made a successful new life for herself, as has Norm.

The somewhat happier ending is less to the point than is the therapeutic strategy which was employed; namely, that the family therapist encountered the system and clearly defined a contract which called for risk-taking on the part of the patient and for his participation in therapy in the total context of his family.

Case 10 illustrates how illness in one family member, whether it be a psychiatric illness or a cardiac illness, can be used in some families to obscure serious dysfunction in the marital pair.

*Case 10.* Barbara was the middle of three daughters in a family where the mother assumed a very protective and controlling position and the father retired into relative obscurity. The youngest daughter had married and moved out of the state, but although Barbara was also married she continued to be periodically drawn into an overresponsible role vis-a-vis her older sister Helen, who had stayed in a dependent relationship following an earlier psychotic break.

In the original family Barbara and her mother had actually played the parental roles. This pattern was evident over the previous two generations, and consisted of the mother and second daughter in each generation playing these parts of the parental pair, while the fathers of necessity were placed in, and accepted, a more passive and isolated position in the family.

Barbara had originally sought family therapy with her husband, partly because of her dissatisfaction with his passivity, and in the course of treatment she had moved out of her overresponsible role with him and had learned to lean on him for support. His advice about the political strategies she might use in her work situation were valued by her, and a mutuality of respect was growing between them as they related with one another in a more equal adult way.

The crisis occurred when Barbara's grandmother (her mother's mother) began to decompensate with age. The mother and grandmother had functioned as a parental pair in that generation, just as Barbara and the mother had functioned as a parental pair in the next. When the grandmother slipped into a more helpless child role, the mother turned to Barbara for help with sister Helen, whose psychiatric condition was called upon by the mother as a cause for concern. Because of the changes she had made in therapy, Barbara was no longer comfortable in this old role, and suggested a three-way session with her mother and sister. This actually carried forward the scenario of Barbara and mother (the parents) coming to therapy for the sick child (Helen). Realizing this, Barbara suggested her father be asked to join the session, and I concurred. When she heard of this plan, the mother objected by saying that the father would talk too much and take up too much time. As if on cue, four days before the scheduled session, the father suffered a "heart attack" and was hospitalized in an ICU with changes in his EKG. Dynamically he had upped the ante when Barbara tried not to be a co-parent. Now there were two "children" to worry about; Helen, the psychiatrically ill one, and father, the medically ill one.

Barbara rushed to the hospital where she was met by her mother, who warned that the father likely had become sick because of the pending family session. This attempt by the mother to keep the system from changing was abetted by the father when, through his tears, he told Barbara that he had named her executor of his will, and wanted her to promise to care for her mother and her sister when he was gone.

In an amazing tribute to Barbara's determination to maintain her therapeutic gains, the portentous family therapy session was held, with Barbara, Helen, mother, and father. The session began with Barbara slipping easily into the overresponsible co-therapy role. I immediately stopped her from this, so the mother introduced the concern about Helen's potential for another psychiatric break. The old pattern of placing Helen in the sick-child position was being attempted, but I ignored it and focused on the "mother-father" spouse relationship. The father had been quiet so far, and looked rather depressed, so I asked him what he did for fun. I learned that he loved tennis, but hadn't played for 30 years. I asked his wife if she played, and she said no, and added that she would be terribly worried about his heart if he tried to play. I was not so worried about his heart, because his discharge diagnosis had been hiatus hernia, which apparently had accounted for some insignificant aberration in the EKG. Barbara said she liked tennis, but wasn't too good at it. I then had the opportunity to encourage the two of them to play, and by this means was able to cast the father in role of expert with his daughter. This took her out of her usual responsible position, and also reversed her role with the mother, because now she was going to be doing something which caused the mother to have anxiety, rather than her usual activity of doing things to relieve the mother's anxiety.

I finally told the father that if he wanted to play tennis, he'd have to tolerate his wife's anxiety, and wondered aloud if he could manage that. He said he thought he could. And he turned out to be better than his word. He applied for a city tennis permit, played three times with Barbara, and then continued to go several times a week for games. Follow-up showed that he continued to play during the next three years, and Barbara reported that this once isolated man mentioned recently that he now knew by their first names, over 60 people with whom he had played tennis doubles. There have been no further "heart attacks," and the father has trimmed down by 20 pounds and is a vigorous 60-year-old.

## CONCLUSION

Family therapy basically represents a philosophy which holds that no individual can be understood or related to in isolation. Just as the function of no cell in the body can be understood in isolation, so the behavior of any human being can only be understood in relation to his family, his friends, and his social and cultural context. Medical illness can give the illusion of discreteness, but causation is complex and manifold, and the symptoms and actual disability resulting from the illness are influenced by physiology and psychology, by hormones and emotion, and by learned behavior patterns and attitudes, as well as social context and human interactions.

The team of medical helpers is also made up of individual professionals and paraprofessionals whose impact is not an addition of the input of each, but is rather a larger integration of their individual contributions. It is not just the whole man who needs to be considered in treatment, but rather the whole man in the context of human systems. And it is not just an individual physician, be he generalist or specialist, who can always best render the help, but rather the whole system of helpers who feel able to call on one another's knowledge and skill. Family therapeutic appraoches can be usefully applied by anyone on the medical team. As a member of that team, the family therapist, with his knowledge of more specialized techniques of intervening in human systems especially resistant to change, can at times be particularly useful in helping with the management of patients suffering from medical illness.

## References

1. Grolnick L: A family perspective of psychosomatic factors in illness: a review of the literature. Family Process 11:457–486, 1972

2. Haley J: Strategies of Psychotherapy. New York, Grune & Stratton, 1963

3. Weakland J: Family somatics: a neglected edge. Family Process 16:263–272, 1977

3a. Liebman R, Minuchin S, Baker L: The use of structural family therapy in the treatment of intractable asthma. Am J Psychiatry 131: 535–540, 1974

4. Meissner WW: Family dynamics and psychosomatic processes. Family Process 5: 142–161, 1966

5. Minuchin S, Baker L, Rosman BL, et al: A conceptual model for psychosomatic illness in children: family organization and family therapy. Arch Gen Psychiatry 32:1031–1038, 1975

6. Alger I: Integrating immediate videoplayback in family therapy. In Guerin P (Ed.): Family Therapy. New York, Gardner Press, 1976

Aaron Stein
Stephen Wiener

# 11
# Group Therapy with Medically Ill Patients

The title of this book is an excellent one. It does not use the term "psychosomatic," which invariably brings to mind the idea of a difference or separation between psyche and soma—the mind and the body. Instead, it calls attention to the "physical illness" which is the explicit means of expression of the conflict or tension or stress or maladaptation which the particular person in a given environment and situation is experiencing. It also implicitly points out that treatment of the physical illness is an essential part of the treatment of the whole person's illness or disability or dysfunction.

In a previous report, the statement was made " . . . for most patients with psychosomatic illness, group psychotherapy is a specific and usually (quite) effective form of treatment, and for many it is the treatment of choice."[1] A fairly complete survey of the clinical and experimental work with the psychological aspects of physical illness and disability has not produced any evidence to make it necessary to change the above statement. All findings seem to point to the fact that these patients show the same patterns of dealing with tensions in an immature, if not primitive fashion, leading to the expression of the affects of these tensions through somatic channels, and that these are related to disturbed early relationships.

It will be pointed out below, and this was also mentioned in the previous report,[1] that developmental and psychological factors lead to the establishment in these patients of characteristic reaction patterns culminating in the typical physical illness and dysfunction. The nature of these immature reactions and the way in which they are developed can be specifically and usefully treated by the relationships and interaction that occur in group psychotherapy. Hence, the statement that was made above. An attempt will be made to again demonstrate that

223

the relationships and interactions occurring in group psychotherapy make it more specifically useful in the overall treatment of these patients than other forms of psychotherapy, including some of the more recently utilized active forms of treatment, such as behavior conditioning therapy, biofeedback, etc.

The literature covering the use of group psychotherapy in medically ill patients was surveyed fairly completely through the year 1970.[1] The literature since then, 1970 through 1976, dealing with the use of group psychotherapy in patients with psychosomatic illness, has been reviewed only incompletely, and is briefly summarized here. No attempt was made to review the effectiveness in the various types of conditions—from asthma to ulcerative colitis—in which physical illness is associated with definite psychological factors. The results obtained with group psychotherapy in these conditions was covered in the previous article,[2] and the current literature since then indicates the same findings.

Some excellent reviews of present day concepts of psychological factors in physical illness are worthy of mention. Lipowski has edited a very extensive review of this type which appeared in the International Journal of Psychiatry in Medicine in 1974 and 1975.[2] His review consists of an extensive collection of articles dealing with "Current Trends in Psychosomatic Medicine."

Shontz,[3] in an excellent and very clearly written book, reviews "The Psychological Aspects of Physical Illness and Disability."[3] He discusses the mind-body problem from the concept of holism, the "body experience" in health and illness, including its sensory functions as a "tool for action," as a "locus of the self," and as a "subjective" symbol. He also describes anxiety and fear in relation to disruption of self-integrity, and the effect of these on the patient and the therapist in the treatment situation. He points out how the patient's adaptation to stress and crisis affects him physically and psychologically and, finally, he indicates two types of treatment approaches utilized at the present time: (1) the naturalistic approach which attempts to enhance existing systems of adapting to physical illness and the psychological factors involved, and (2) the synthetic approach which sets up specific conditions to change behavior—the behavioral conditioning approach.

Karush and his associates, in a short but excellent monograph, describe their findings in the psychotherapeutic treatment of over 200 patients with chronic ulcerative colitis.[4] They review the literature, describe the kind of personality and characteristic type of reactions occurring in these patients, and relate these to faulty development of the early mother-child relationship. They indicate that a unified approach involving an internist, surgeon, and psychiatrist is absolutely necessary in the treatment of chronic ulcerative colitis. They point out that, in utilizing psychotherapy, the kind of patient and his needs should determine the type of psychotherapy used. For the sicker patient, a special supportive type of relationship and identification with the therapist is most useful. For the more integrated patients, a more interpretive type of treatment is helpful. This review covers only individual psychotherapy, and Karush acknowledges that other forms of psychotherapy, including group therapy, were not included in the review.

Fisher and Laufer surveyed the literature on the response of heart attack patients in group psychotherapy and found it useful.[5] They confirmed the findings of several other writers who use group psychotherapy in the treatment of patients with heart conditions, namely Ibrahim, et al.,[6] Rahe, et al.,[7] Reckless and Fauntleroy,[8] and Bilodeau and Hackett.[9] All of them found that group psychotherapy lessened the stress that the physical illness imposed on these patients, helped them become aware of the underlying factors involved, and was useful in helping them develop more mature and effective ways of expressing feeling with a concomitant lessening of the symptoms of their physical illness and a greater freedom from relapse and rehospitalization.

Ammon reviewed analytic group psychotherapy as an instrument for the treatment and research of psychosomatic disorders.[10] He found that the relationships and the interactions in group psychotherapy permitted patients to express their aggressive tendencies and conflicts much more freely, something they were not able to do in individual therapy. He thought that this was especially useful for patients with psychosomatic illness and physical illness whose guilt over aggressive tendencies usually prevented them from becoming aware of and acknowledging these and who directed the expression of these through somatic channels. He also found the group supportive toward these patients' emotional reactions and in dealing with their physical illness; in this fashion, the group members acted like a good family.

In a series of reviews of the group psychotherapy literature by various writers, which appeared in the *International Journal of Group Psychotherapy, Volumes 21–26,* summaries of the group psychotherapy literature dealing with the use of group psychotherapy in patients with psychosomatic and physical illness are given.[12] In most instances, the summaries indicate that the use of group psychotherapy with patients with these conditions was helpful. Again, group psychotherapy helped these patients become aware of the emotional factors involved, and the relationships and interactions in the groups helped them express their feelings directly and effectively, instead of through somatic channels. Also, it helped the patients acknowledge and deal more effectively with their psychosomatic and physical illnesses and, therefore, to lessen the amount of symptoms and illness that occurred with a general improvement in their physical health and emotional attitudes.

## THEORETICAL CONSIDERATIONS FOR THE USE OF GROUP PSYCHOTHERAPY IN PATIENTS WITH PHYSICAL ILLNESS

The factors in the developmental history and the characteristic emotional reactions of patients with psychosomatic and physical illness were described in detail in an article previously cited.[1] It is of great interest that Karush, et al. also found essentially the same factors related to disturbed development and abnormal psychological reactions.[4] These findings will be summarized here, because they indicate the difficulties in individual psychotherapy with these patients, and they also indicate the theoretical—and actual—basis for the use of group psychotherapy in the treatment of these patients.

The pathological, psychological susceptibility to ulcerative colitis in these patients begins with the disruption and distortion of the relationship to the parents and other significant persons early in the patient's life. This psychological predisposition leads to mental reactions of a specific kind and play a significant part in all ulcerative colitis patients—and, we may add, in all patients with psychosomatic and certain kinds of physical illness—and a primary role in some. "These predisposing forces are released when symbiotic-like attachments to figures of dependency in the patient's past and present life persist."[4] It is the mother or her surrogate who is the original object of the symbiotic attachment during the patient's first year of life, and this interferes with and permanently alters the child's inherent drive for mastery over each body function as it successively matures. Pathogenic effects upon a young child of the mother's emotional reaction depend on their timing, intensity, and the persistent quality of the mother's invasiveness. In the case of ulcerative colitis, the mother's primary interest in the child is centered on his gastrointestinal functions, both oral and anal; accordingly, the mother's fears, wishes, or demands are unconsciously taken over by her dependent child.

When such patients become adults, the reenactment of the infantile symbiotic needs is expressed in body language. Accordingly, the colitis symptoms represent the symbiotic phase in which intense urges and feelings are truly expressed symbolically by lower bowel activity. These symptoms proclaim the patient's helplessness in an effort to win the mother's attention and concern. At the same time, excessive emotion may also signify rage at the mother figure for allowing the precipitating crisis to overwhelm the patient. When guilt or aggressive impulses cannot be neutralized, the continuing symptoms become a form of self-punishment to which the patient clings as a desperate means of reestablishing the symbiotic tie between himself and the object of his dependency.

The patient's symbiotic needs for dependency are doomed to frustration, resulting in an angry helplessness which may become extremely intense. Acts of aggression by the patient no longer are effective in obtaining comfort and safety through dependency. As a result, the patient may become withdrawn and depressed. Direct emotional expression becomes extremely difficult and is replaced by a nonverbal discharge with the activation of an internal organ system. This bodily reaction may be compared with that of the infant, but it cannot express its specific emotional state and may signify rage, anxious helplessness, a need to suffer, or even a suicidal wish to die. Many of these patients show strong reaction formation primarily directed against sexual drive, against aggression, and against rage and, particularly, envy. The sexual aspect of the lives of such patients is empty with inhibition and avoidance of sexual activity. Other defenses include denial and hostility to objects. Projection, frequent episodes of depression with defensive apathy, and withdrawal, that often result in profound regression and paranoid projection, are also present in many of these patients.

The central internal conflicts are concerned with the unresolved struggle between the wish to be dependent upon a parent or a parental substitute and a grandiose wish to control absolutely the feelings and attitudes of the object of dependency. The majority of such patients also suffer identity disorders with distortion of their masculine/feminine self-image. Karush also feels that dread of a life-saving colectomy is greater than the fear of death and disease. Losing one's body-integrity represents to these patients a castration fear more dreaded than death.

This confirms the findings in the previous study, that the patients' fear and guilt about their disturbed body-image represented a symbolic punitive castration for their aggressive and sexual impulses.[1] In this article, the difficulties and limitations involved in the psychotherapeutic treatment of patients with psychosomatic and certain types of physical illness related to the faulty psychological development and the resultant disturbed reactions and personality characteristics of these patients was described. These disturbances were listed as follows: disturbed early relationships with the persistence of an intense symbiotic relationship to the mother; separation anxiety and depression with, at times, overwhelming reacions to object loss; and intense emotional needs and conflicts related particularly to oral cravings and oral and anal regressive tendencies. Tensions of any kind are poorly tolerated, and at times overwhelmingly result in the mobilization of destructive drives necessitating specific defense reactions to an extreme degree. Weakness of the ego occurs in most of these patients and leads to an inability to deal with emotional reactions or to express them in mature and effective fashion. There are also poorly developed object relationships of the primitive and narcissistic type, especially the passive-symbiotic type. These patients have a punitive, archaic superego resulting in excessive unconscious guilt and ambivalence with a fear of retaliation and punishment. There is a defective body-image and self-image so that the patients do not know their own identity, sexually or as a person, and see themselves in an incomplete or distorted fashion. Defensive reactions in which many of these patients develop reaction formations such as submissiveness, obedience, and pseudo-self-sufficiency, lead to rigid characteriological and social roles in relationships. Finally, many of these patients have extremely little knowledge or awareness of their emotional reactions; they are "emotional illiterates," to use Freedman and Sweet's term.[12] The primitive defense mechanisms of isolation and denial are involved here.

All writers including Karush agree that the individual treatment with psychotherapy of such patients is very difficult. Ludwig pointed out difficulty in treating patients with such complicated and profound disturbances, and stated that the first task of therapy would be an attempt to restore a balance by establishing a contact with the patient.[13] This is the greatest difficulty in treating these patients. They are often reluctant and unable to establish contact with psychotherapy, especially in individual psychotherapy. One of the main reasons for the difficulty in establishing effective therapeutic contact with these patients in individual treatment stems from the nature of the transference they develop to the therapist. As noted above, they tend to develop primitive regressive types of relationships to others, and this shows itself in the individual treatment they receive in terms of a primitive and regressive type of transference to the therapist. The need to establish a symbiotic fusion, the need to attempt to control the object of their dependency (in treatment, this is the therapist), the excessive emotional reactions to any sexual or aggressive impulse, the fear of retaliation and punishment, all combine to make individual psychotherapy very difficult with this type of patient.

The same factors that make difficult the establishment of a relationship for effective individual psychotherapy are specific indications for the use of group psychotherapy with these patients. On theoretical grounds, and as proven by clinical experience, group psychotherapy is especially useful in the treatment of this type of patient.

Most important of all, group psychotherapy is useful in helping these patients enter into a psychotherapeutic relationship. This results from the nature of relationships of the members to the therapist and among the members themselves, which are different in group therapy than in individual therapy, and which facilitate establishment of the psychotherapeutic relationship and interactions. The basic nature of the relationship to the therapist in group psychotherapy differs from the one-to-one relationship because it is lessened in intensity and also because the leader or therapist is shared by all members of the group. Emotional ties among the members of the group consist largely of a number of identifications, the most important of which is their sharing of a common object—the therapist.[14] This is another reason why the transference of the therapist is much less intense and threatening, and is felt on a much more realistic level. The therapist becomes to each member an idolized figure and thus an object for their narcissistic libido.

In the development of a group—any group and particularly a therapy group—certain developmental phases occur. These have been described by many writers; the relationship of these phases to a regressive type of reaction that occurs at the beginning of a group are discussed by Freud[14] and Scheidlinger.[15] Essentially, the phases are as follows. First there is the initial phase of dependency on the therapist in the group, in which each member tries to establish a special relationship with the group leader so as to satisfy dependency needs. In other words, they seek gratification of their dependency needs and, in the sicker type of patients, may even seek some type of symbiotic-like fusion with the leader.

In certain groups of very severely ill patients, as noted by many authors including Karush and Stein, and as will be described in the clinical material given in this report, the group does not develop past this first initial stage. The therapist then has to assume certain roles and to handle the therapeutic relationship in certain fashions which will be described later.

In groups of less severely ill patients who have some ability to establish their own identity and maintain some independence in dealing with their life situations and their illness, the group goes on to certain other phases. As the frustration of the dependency needs expected from the therapist increases, a rebellious anger toward the therapist becomes clear and is manifested by interaction among the patients. They turn away from the therapist toward each other, and they use roles based on unconscious fantasies to interact with each other and try to get the other patients to act out these transference roles. The availability of multiple transference objects which are realistically present in the group and which actually respond, results in a group member "here and now" interaction that constitutes the therapeutic interaction in the group session, and makes it readily available for therapeutic work. Pathological character traits and attitudes become apparent quickly, as do pathological defensive attitudes, and they also are readily available for therapeutic scrutiny. The rigid patient with psychosomatic illness or physical illness of certain kinds who is not aware of the nature and significance of this characteristic style of emotional raction and interaction is helped in this way to become aware of these things and to understand their nature.

Returning now to the transference to the therapist, in phase one—the dependency phase—of the group, this has the same primitive intense, symbiotic-like need for attachment and dependency previously described. The presence of a number of other patients in the group and the need to share the therapist tends to lessen the intensity of this type of transference to the therapist, however, a factor which is extremely helpful in the treatment. In addition, the transference needs are directed toward the other members of the group and are shared by them, so that the intense transference dependency needs are directed towards many individuals instead of just one. This also provides the opportunity to enter into psychotherapeutic relationships and to examine the nature of these relationships, and also gives the patients an opportunity to develop new relationships. The presence of several factors including the sharing of the guilt, the identification with the therapist, and the use of various kinds of spokesmen, enables certain rigid punitive superego attitudes to be dealt with much more readily in the group than in individual psychotherapy.

The presence of other patients provides stimuli for participation, and helps the patient become aware, through their identification, of their emotional reactions and attitudes in a much more realistic and effective fashion than in individual therapy. Projection, denial, and isolation can readily be pointed out by other members of the group, an insight that is of special value to these emotionally illiterate patients. The emotional reactions acknowledged by the other members and the realization that they also have intense forbidden feelings, the understanding and accepting attitude of the therapist and the other members, all help the patients become aware of and express feelings in an effective and realistic way instead of expressing them through somatic channels. The nature of the ties in the group helps the members to supply each other with a great deal of emotional support, particularly in the areas of ego functioning and the strengthening of defenses. These are most useful features for the weak egos and the overpowering reactions of the patients with psychological disturbances associated with psychosomatic and certain types of physical illness.

Most writers agree on the fact that the outcome of any type of psychotherapy depends upon how well the therapeutic interventions match the degree of development and the type of emotional reaction the patient shows. Thus, Karush states,

> Insight therapy is most likely to succeed in patients who have a clear sense of separate identity and have proven some capability for realistic independence . . . Patients with the least differentiate identities, those with symbiotic attachments to others, have difficulty utilizing interpretation and need the therapy in which they can identify with the therapist as an apparently omnipotent parental figure. When such patients identify themselves with this idealized therapist, his strengths and his admired traits become assimilated by them and enable them to add to their ego strength and character armor, so as to alter their vulnerability and excessive sensitivity to disappointments. The therapist offers himself and is seen as a good and consistent parent surrogate, unlike the original object for dependency who was seen as punitive and hurtful. The symbiotic dependency is thus replaced with new insight and new identifications, leading to more independence and more ability to see onself as a separate individual. At the same time, the pathogenic somatic activity becomes less important as a maladaptive emotional discharge, and emotions are recognized in a realistic fashion and dealt with in a much more mature and realistic fashion.[4]

In the clinical material that follows, both types of patients are described. In the group led by one of us (S.W.), the very sick patients involved could not go beyond the phase one of dependency on the therapist. Accordingly the group therapist assumed the role needed to provide the realistic support and gratification of dependent needs and displayed an attitude that helped the patients identify with him as a "good and consistent parent surrogate." In the examples given of individual patients in regular therapy groups, these more independent patients were able to go on to the other phases of the group, and, with the group's help, interactions and confrontations occurred which helped them become aware of the underlying emotional reactions connected with their physical symptoms.

## CLINICAL EXAMPLES

The first example will deal with experiences of a small group of patients with severe physical illness treated with group therapy in the Psychiatric Out-Patient Department of a large general hospital.* In the examples of sessions with this group, there are from 4–6 patients present. There had been others in the group, but one died and the others dropped out. The six patients who comprised the group were diagnostically severe character disorders with anxiety and depressive symptoms, alcoholism, masochistic tendencies, etc.

The present group therapist (S.W.) began his work with this group under difficult circumstances. There had been a long delay from the time their former group therapist left until the present group therapist began to work with the group because of the early departure of the former therapist, and also because a strike at the hospital had forced closing of the clinic so that the group was unable to meet.

*The Mount Sinai Hospital, New York, N.Y.

There had also been considerable fearful and depressed reactions of the group members to the death of one of the group members—a woman who had a mastectomy because of breast cancer. In addition, from the beginning of the time that the group met with their present therapist, many medical emergencies and illnesses on the part of various group members had occurred. This led to increased anxiety, fear, and the expectance of some medical catastrophe on the part of the group members. This characterized the attitude of the group members when the present therapist first began working with them. It was due in part to a feeling they had that their former therapist had not been available for them, in terms of helping them during these periods of crisis.

All of these factors, from the beginning of the present therapist's work with this group, posed problems as to how the therapist should function in the group and what role he should assume in leading the group discussion. It was obvious that this very sick, both psychologically and physically, group of patients had many complex needs, including medical and social service, as well as psychological. Although the stated purpose of the group was to have them discuss the reactions related to these problems and needs, the constant threat of becoming severely ill physically and the many emergencies in their family and social situations inevitably focused the group discussions on these factors, rather than on emotional reactions to these.

One of the difficulties with their former therapist had been his attmpt to take the role of a confronting therapist who tried to get them to discuss their emotional reactions to these situations. It was obvious to the present therapist that, while this would be most desirable, it would not be possible with this very severely ill group of patients and their many urgent realities, complications, and emergencies. It was felt that they needed a different kind of relationship to the group therapist; one that would help them with their urgent medical and social needs, as well as with their psychological difficulties. The attitude of the patients when they began the group discussion with this present therapist brought this out very clearly, and the first session to be summarized below clearly indicates how they turned to the therapist for help with their severe distress in many areas.

Brief descriptions of the patients comprising the group follow.

Mrs. C. B. is a 49-year-old married Hispanic woman and the mother of four grown children. She has a three year history of progressive exacerbation of deep vein phlebitis with the complications of pulmonary embolism and angina. A year ago, she was admitted to the psychiatric service of the hospital because of a severe depression, the treatment of which was complicated because of persistent tachycardia with antidepressants and her refusal to continue with ECT. Her depression appears to have developed from a severe sense of guilt over feelings that she has been a bad mother, a bad wife, and a bad Catholic, for having had several abortions and a tubal ligation to avoid earlier problems with thrombophlebitis during her second pregnancy. She also tends to blame herself for all the problems that occurred in her family. She has, during her frequent periods of depression, a severe loss of self-esteem together with a sense of impending doom. She feels that her depression and her physical difficulties are her penance for her past bad behavior. In the group, she is supportive to other members, but has difficulty in accepting the support and concern of other members for her own difficulties. Despite some tendency to projection, the diagnosis is probably severe character disorder associated with episodes of severe depression.

Mr. A. T. is a 32-year-old married white male with a history of congenital bicuspid aortic valve dysfunction. Two years ago, he had the aortic valve replaced following development of severe aortic insufficiency. He had been in individual therapy for a year prior to coming into the group when his doctor left the hospital. He is a tall, grossly obese man, who enjoys being the center of attention and often interrupts in the group to take over the spotlight. Recently, he developed hypertension; despite this, he continues to be obese and to smoke. In the group, Mr. T. slowly has been able to give up his demands for attention and to discuss to some small extent his anxiety about his health and himself. Recently, his wife had a miscarriage due to probably congenital aortic stenosis in the infant, which was very depressing to Mr. T. He spoke of his feelings freely in the individual sessions, but was not able to speak of them very freely in the group. He is a comparatively new member of the group. The diagnosis is an inadequate character with anxiety and depression.

Mrs. G. S. is a 56-year-old widow with a history of chronic spinal arthritis, apparently secondary to trauma following an automobile accident. This led to her retirement from a career as a fairly responsible administrator; since then, she has been unable to assume the responsibility of a job. Early in her adolescence, her mother died, and this was followed by the death of her father and brother as the result of accidents and unexpected illnesses. Also, her husband died suddenly shortly after their marriage. Widowed at an early age, Mrs. S. has been left with a sense of catastrophic expectancies for herself which seemed to be fulfilled following her own accident. She is obsessively anxious about her own health, and her anxiety is so extreme that she is frequently unable to evaluate realistically the various illnesses she has. She is very self-preoccupied, and frequently is very jealous of the younger members of the group. She often leads the group into discussing trivial details about illness and will avoid discussing the restrictions of her own very limited life style. At the beginning of the group, she was troubled by the loss of her individual therapist. Her diagnosis is a severe obsessive character with rather prominent schizoid features.

Mr. K. J. is a 42-year-old unmarried, unemployed chronic alcoholic with a 20-year drinking history. He wears a thick moustache to hide the results of a cleft palate repair. He is sexually impotent; at present, this seems related to psychogenic factors. He also has healed bilateral hip fractures, one of which was suffered last year following an infrequent but severe drinking spree after a violent quarrel with his father and the death of another group member, to whom Mr. J. was deeply attached. Mr. J. lives with his aging parents in an atmosphere of great friction and tension. His father has also been a chronic alcoholic. Mr. J. refuses to consider his own role in his present problems, externalizing them on to his family and outsiders. He constantly states that he is about to get married or about to get a job, obviously unrealistic statements in view of his rather deteriorated condition. He is openly tense and anxious, with slow speech and a circumstantial manner of speaking, possibly related to organic factors connected with his chronic alcoholism. He has been unable to maintain any relationships outside the group, nor has he been able to obtain a job. In the group, Mr. J. developed his only real relationship, a friendship with a woman who had been in the group prior to her death from metastatic cancer. She had helped him to begin to recognize he had personal emotional needs which he was not satisfying. Her sudden death left Mr. J. with a deep sense of loss and depression, from which he has not yet recovered. His diagnosis is an inadequate character disorder with alcoholism and depression.

Mrs. H. M. is a 57-year-old widowed woman with two divorced daughters. Two years ago, she had a left mastectomy for breast cancer with positive lymph nodes. Four years ago, she had an attack of viral meningitis, which apparently left her with some residual memory impairment and led to her early retirement as a rather successful executive secretary. During the group session, she was frequently preoccupied with and upset by the physical complaints of the other group members. She stated that she feared she might develop their symptoms. At times, she upset other group members with her persistent efforts to ward off the other members speaking of their depression, just as she attempted to ward off speaking of her own depression and fears of her illness. By complaining about the others, she displaced on to them her own anger, fear, and guilt, just as she would displace on to her discussion of her two daughters' difficulties, her own feelings of frustration, anger, fear, and guilt. Prior to her meningitis, she had helped a male friend live through his own wife's death—something that must have touched her own awareness of the probable course of her illness. She was troubled by the limitations that her disease imposed on her physical appearance and the loss of use of her arm, as well as the symptoms induced by chemotherapy. Despite this, in the group, she tried to help the others face their situations more optimistically and tried to make efforts to change their lives. The unwillingness of the others in the group to go along with her efforts plus a growing fear that her cancer was returning ultimately caused Mrs. M. to stop attending the group. Follow-up has indicated that she has benefited from the group therapy, has reached more acceptance of her illness and its consequences, is helping her daughters with their difficulties and their children, and is doing some volunteer work. Her diagnosis is character disorder with anxiety and depressive reactions.

Mrs. C. M., a 32-year-old divorced Hispanic woman, mother of three sons, has a history dating back 11 years with peptic ulcer disease, which occurred at the time of her first pregnancy. Her ulcer condition has always been exacerbated at times of separation and stress. Past treatment has included several surgical procedures including a Billroth II, and later a surgical correction of this procedure. Medical treatment has not given significant relief to this woman. She is an attractive, somewhat overweight person who gives an outward impression of being self-assured, but also gives evidence of being very troubled by her responsibilities, particularly that of being a mother. She presently has considerable difficulty with her three children, all of whom seem to be overly dependent on her. The present situation is complicated because she is introducing a new boy friend into the home. Because of these tensions, the patient was recently hospitalized again for ulcer symptoms. She is an anxious, depressed, somewhat unrealistic person who tends to deny the significance of her illness and the difficulties in her family life. Diagnostic impression was of a mixed character disorder with prominent depressive features.

## Summary of a Group Session

Mr. T., a new patient with a heart condition, joined the group at this session, one of the early sessions. Following the introduction of Mr. T., there developed an interaction in which Mr. T. expressed an appeal for group approval and support, yet at the same time tried to deny the significance of having heart trouble. During the same session, the other male in the group, Mr. J., had also returned to the group following recovery from a hip fracture during a drinking spree resulting from an argument with his own alcoholic father. These two men bid for the attention of the group. The women in the group reacted by making unrelated comments over the limitations on their own physical health, and this led the group to discuss their respective disabilities. This regressive return and recounting of symptoms avoided any discussion of the competitiveness for attention in the group.

The group then proceeded to consider the effect that Mrs. C. B.'s phlebitis had on her being unable to continue work at a time just following her husband having been laid off for three months. During this time, Mrs. B. had felt intensely guilty about not being able to contribute to the family welfare. She is constantly struggling with her need for attention, her anger at her rejecting husband, and her deep guilt over demands on her family, as well as her need for punishment for her earlier abortions and tubal ligation. While Mrs. B. could only speak of these events in a very unconnected fashion, the group responded sympathetically and supportively to her overwhelming sense of guilt. Mrs. B. became very self-conscious and ashamed and could not accept the support of the group or reduce her sense of guilt about her illness.

At this point, Mr. T. again assumed control of the group discussion and stated that he felt that, if people have to suffer, it ought to be more worthwhile. He catalogued a group of difficulties, both physical and financial, in which he implicitly asked the group how much their therapist could be depended on to help them with the multiple demands that his and their medical condition necessitated. While expressing great anger at his inability to work, he also indicated a strong, passive demand for gratification of many unresolved dependency needs.

Mr. T., in his first group meeting, echoed many of the themes which were evoked by the group at the beginning of their work with the present therapist. They had been depressed, fearful, and angry due to a recent loss of a group member from metastatic cancer and the long delay between the transition from their old therapist to their new group leader. Furthermore, the addition of Mr. T. and Mrs. B. following the death of the group member, and their feeling of a lack of a sense of the availability of their new therapist, brought out considerable group support for Mr. T.'s questions. It was quite obvious that despite the avowed purpose of this group—to discuss these emotional reactions—the members felt that the former therapist had been too inactive in helping them resolve the complex and urgent psychological, social service, and medical needs of their severe illness.

While asking about the availability of their new therapist to help them, the group began to discuss the sense of devaluation they felt as a result of their illnesses and disabilities and the imposed restrictions and limitations. This devaluation was ascribed to others in their lives, but also immediately followed remarks to the effect that the group members felt their former therapist didn't understand them. It appeared from the group's comments that the prior therapist had acted more as a catalyst to confront the group members with their emotional reactions, something with which most of the members were unprepared to deal. While the group was clearly stating that they needed someone to depend on to help them to manage their illnesses and their emotional problems, their significant associated self-devaluation and the sense of devaluation of them by their former therapist clearly helped to crystalize the less apparent negative group transference to their former therapist. This, and the addition of the new member who demanded attention, led them to react so that he served as a spokesman for their unresolved feelings of loss, anger, helplessness, and dependency. The group continued to discuss various derivative issues of self-devaluation such as birth defects in three of the group members or their children, the sense of being avoided by friends who were afraid of "catching something," and the associated sense of a taint that each group member felt due to their illness.

The discussion of these feelings of being defective brought the group to further consider the effect of their illness on spouses, family members, and others; an issue which was so sensitive that it had never fully been approached by the group. Whenever such sensitive issues occurred, the group diverted the discussion back to the characteristics of the illness. While the members themselves severely criticized others for devaluing themselves and for avoiding people due to their illness, the members themselves could not discuss their own feelings openly about the effects of their illness on their relationships.

This focus of the group discussion on physical illness has actually been a strong form of group resistance. The group members approach this topic, but only when there are no present medical crises in any of the group members. This session stood out as one of those sessions. It further clearly indicates the necessity of having a somewhat more psychologically minded group member or members to point out such avoidances in the group, to help the group leader in confronting the tendency of the group to avoid their emotional reactions to their life situations. Although they resent others seeing them as ill, they see this way themselves.

Another factor demonstrated by this group is that there is a need that these groups provide significant support to deal with their illnesses which is not presently available to them from a spouse or family or friend. A few of the patients who are severely ill or dying, at times have the emotional resources sufficient to meet the stresses and limitations of their illness. For most of the patients, it is very necessary to have the group offering support, real assistance in managing the course of a debilitating illness, and the opportunity to gain information about their illness, as well as having available someone, the therapist and the other members, to monitor their physical health between visits to the clinic. Previous studies with cardiac patients suggest that this last function of the group is perhaps most vital, as indicated by the reduction of mortality in the more severely ill patients who attend group therapy.[16] Additionally, the reduction in stress by always having available someone who knows their case seems very important in helping the group members deal with and lessen the strains, medical and psychological, associated with their illnesses.

Nevertheless, the more independent and self-directed patients may attend several group sessions while readjusting their lives and activity levels to their illnesses, but then find that the group's continual focus on somatic problems and complaints interferes with their ability to discuss their own emotional reactions. These patients briefly use the therapist and the group situation as a transition back into their own environment. This emphasizes the importance of careful selection of patients for this group, something that is not always possible realistically.

### Summary of a Group Session

Another group session followed the hospitalization and return of Mrs. M. to the group after an episode of phlebitis and leukopenia. Mrs. M. had become increasingly depressed when she fractured a rib (metastatic?) following a fall. With the return of her phlebitis and a coincident episode of leukopenia, Mrs. M. was convinced that her breast cancer was returning. This fear was related to the attitude of her own physician, and also occurred on the anniversary of her mastectomy the preceding year. The rigors of chemotherapy had produced severe weight gain, edema, and baldness in a woman whose physical appearance had been very important. Her release from the hospital had only slightly diminished her fears about her dying, and Mrs. M. had assumed the role of the group member who had died the previous year following a series of hospitalizations.

Mrs. M. had also previously been very jealous of a new group member who recently had a mastectomy but without any metastatic indications. During this woman's brief stay in the group, Mrs. M. began to express some of her own depression and anger over her illnesses, and it appeared that her recent hospitalization had presented her with an acute crisis, since it seemed to her that everyone believed her case was hopeless. In the face of extreme weakness and increasing anxiety, Mrs. M. began to approach her own feelings about death. While obviously incompletely facing many of her own feelings about her own possible approach to death, Mrs. M. gave a very moving account of the sense of loss of meaning in her life following her encephalitis, her retirement, the death of her husband, and her mastectomy.

Mrs. M. had preceded this discussion of her feelings by describing a dream she had several weeks before her hospitalization in which she was standing on an ice-covered lake while two small boys called for help. Although she wanted to go to their aid, she realized that the ice was very thin and she could not reach them by herself. She became very anxious about the boys, although they were in no immediate danger. While looking around, Mrs. M. had noted two men nearby who seemed not to heed the cries of the small children. Mrs. M. now called to these men also, but they ignored her. Following some rather concrete interpretations involving the present season and difficult weather, the group and the therapist suggested the possibility of the sense of the helplessness and isolation in the dream which Mrs. M. seemed to feel. It suggested her own sense of helplessness in the face of her illness while her psychiatrist and medical doctor (and her husband and present lover) standing nearby seemed unable to allay her fears or stem her cancer. While some of these meanings were suggested to the patient, the complex interrelationships were mainly focused on the sense of helplessness and her fear of being in danger of death from her disease.

These patients found themselves much more able to confront their affects and deal with these specific feelings than to deal with the associated dynamics. The genetic origins of these feelings were too anxiety provoking, as well as too distant, for patients whose consciousness was preoccupied with their illness, the fear of death and the struggle for survival in the present moment.

## Discussion

In summary, these two sessions present a sample of the more psychologically oriented sessions which occurred over the course of a year of weekly ninety-minute group therapy meetings. These patients with severe medical illness in acute, chronic, and terminal stages, present a series of reactions of dependency, fear, anger, rage, guilt, envy, isolation, loss, depression, pain, and unhappiness. While these patients present many of the same features as usual psychiatric patients, the presence of a significant and frequently life-threatening intercurrent illness requires several modifications of usual psychiatric techniques in order for the therapist and the group to be readily useful and consistently available to such patients.

In a group composed of members such as these, the patients seldom move beyond the authority-seeking, dependency-gratifying phase of usual group formation, the first phase of group development. Due to the threat from their illness, and the associated loss of self-esteem, loss of job and financial security, and the general uncertainty that severe illness imposes, such patients frequently are able to give up their dependency-seeking positions only when they and the other group members are not threatened by present physical deterioration or medical emergencies. Both of the reported sessions occurred during such times in the course of the present group. Of interest also is the fact that both of these reported sessions occurred when a new member entered the group. The entry of the new member seemed to help the older group members lose some of their own self-preoccupations as they attempted to welcome the new member and to inform them about how the group worked, as well as giving them an opportunity to express the negative aspects of the transference.

Another interesting aspect of resistance is represented by the general tendency of the patients to mainly use denial as their chief form of defense. Although Hackett et al. have shown that denial seems to lead to some increased survival in cardiac patients, there is not much other evidence presently available.[16] Yet, such a hypothesis seems to support data which would suggest that if such denial reduces stress and consequent catecholamine output, there may be a lessening of the inhibition of body response systems which are responsible for repair of damaged tissue in cardiac patients. Such research in cardiac patients and cancer patients has been carried out, but often without the milieu of simultaneous group therapy or group counseling. The experience with group therapy reported here definitely supports Hackett's work in showing that it was often necessary for the patients to deny present threats of their health which they were later able to deal with when the acute crisis had been medically managed. A final note is that the individual dynamics and the current state of the physical and psychological health in such patients made it necessary for the therapist to constantly reevaluate what had been going on in the group sessions so he could judge the degree of interpretive comments that such patients could tolerate without further stress to their already imperiled physical and psychic systems.

Another aspect of importance in terms of managing this type of group was the need for helping these people be alert to warning signs that their illness was reoccurring either in an acute or more deteriorative state, such as Mr. T. with difficulties with his heart valve and intermittent chest pain and Mrs. B. with her recurrent phlebitis. Often the content of the group would focus on particular medical difficulties that these patients were having, but suggestions by the therapist frequently resulted in medical interventions which prevented subsequent hospitalizations or further exacerbations of their illness. In doing this, the therapist was going along with the need of the group members for an authority figure who would gratify their dependent needs, but this increased their receptiveness to the suggestions for health-sustaining behavior. This further consolidated a cohesiveness among the group members which did not seem to previously exist under the former therapist.

Another important result of the therapist gratifying patients' needs for an authority figure who would be helpful in satisfying to some extent their dependent needs, was the degree to which the hopelessness of many of these patients in regard to their present physical illnesses was reduced or influenced by the opportunity to see that certain steps that they could take themselves would diminish the pervasiveness of their present physical symptoms. A simple example of this is that one woman rearranged her refrigerator so that the most used items were on the top shelf since, due to weakness, she frequently had trouble stooping to pick things off the bottom shelves. Encouraging these types of simple behavioral management reduced the sense of hopelessness and helplessness in such patients and allowed them to further increase their own efforts toward managing and controlling the degree to which their present symptoms interfered with their daily activities.

Related to the earlier discussion of the relationship of patient improvement and subjective feelings of greater self-worth, was the relationship between their decreased sense of isolation due to their illness and their decreased sense of hopelessness over improvement. This relationship seemed most significant in those patients in whom there was some sense of a need for being punished for any past behavior, such as what occurred in Mrs. M. with her mastectomy and Mrs. B. with her phlebitis. Both these women very closely identified with the therapist and adopted a more introspective method in terms of approaching their own behavior, although their underlying extreme sense of guilt made it very difficult for them to recognize the underlying conflicts. It was during such times in the group process that these women's emotional problems were the focus of the group discussions that their overall symptoms diminished most significantly. When the problems of other patients who had medical emergencies involving themselves or other patients recurred, the loss of this focus of the group on their feelings and their reactions seemed to result in subsequent reexacerbation of their symptomatic tendencies.

Another example of how the group helped these patients is shown by the situation of Mrs. B., who showed a tremendous intolerance to antidepressants. Intermittently, however, she was able to tolerate sufficient doses of antidepressants to show a diminution in her depressive symptoms. When such situations occurred in conjunction with periods of closer identification with the therapist and a diminution of the sense of guilt about her family, the patient began to improve.

## Some Additional Clinical Examples

The above summary of a couple of sessions of a group composed of patients with severe physical illness illustrates the difficulty in dealing with such patients. As was indicated in the discussion, however, physically ill patients who are able to be more independent and manage their life situation better can tolerate a more interpretive type of therapy. Accordingly, such patients can be placed—and it is now the usual practice with these patients—in a regular group therapy group. The type of group, a regular therapy group, assumes the task of self-investigation and discussion of the emotional difficulties.

A couple of examples of patients with physical illness who were helped in a regular therapy group will now be given.

Mrs. T. K., a 50-year-old married health professional with one son, had had tachycardia, angina, and a persistent mitral murmur following an attack of rheumatic fever some 20 years previously. She also had severe bleeding with her periods, which at times had led to a need for hospitalization and a D and C. There was much guilt over the death of her parents and the death of her defective first-born son. She had been in individual therapy with another therapist for many years with considerable improvement. She still, however, had a great deal of anxiety, guilt, and fear connected with her somatic symptoms, periods of anxiety and depression and some speech difficulty. She sought therapy for this. Because of her great sense of guilt and the self-consciousness related to a speech difficulty, she was placed in a regular therapy group.

From the first, she was an articulate and participating member of the therapy group, and her speech difficulty rapidly cleared up. She persisted in bringing her somatic fears and complaints about her heart and her period to the group. The group members were initially sympathetic and supportive, but as she persisted in monopolizing the group sessions with her fears and complaints about these, the group members, led by the therapist, began to confront her with the fact that these somatic complaints were evidence of her resistance to dealing with less conscious and very strong feelings of competitiveness, jealousy, and aggression.

There were heated group discussions as the patient resisted this confrontation. Also, her seemingly submissive, but manipulative attitude directed toward the group members and the therapist in trying to get them to go along with her needs for physical examinations and various kinds of physical treatment began to subside. Finally, she was able to bring out the aggression, anger, and the fear and guilt connected with these and her competitiveness with her family and her husband. The result was a marked improvement in her feelings of anxiety and depression and a marked diminution in her preoccupation with her physical complaints.

It was obvious that this improvement stemmed from the relationship and interaction in the group. With the new relationships in the group (identification with the self-investigative tendencies with the other members of the group and the therapeutic approach of the therapist) she was able to give up the strong resistance that was focused on her preoccupation with her physical complaints. She was also able to realize that she had the same aggressive, competitive, angry, guilty, and fearful feelings that the others did and was, with the group members support and confrontation, able to discuss this. The most important thing was that her preoccupation with her physical complaints, which had led her to make frequent visits to the doctors and to seek various kinds of medication and treatment to deal with them, lessened markedly since she was able to handle the rather simple task of managing her not too severe physical illnesses.

Mr. C. T. is a 50-year-old executive who has been married twice and has two children, one by his first marriage and one by his second. During the past several years, he has developed moderately severe diverticulitis, high blood pressure and frequent anginal pains. He is overweight and a heavy smoker. Physical examination has indicated high cholesterol levels and an occasional cardiac arrhythmia. Mr. T. is a very intelligent and capable person, extremely articulate, who presents himself with an air of great independence, self-sufficiency, and a need to help and direct others. All of these mask underlying strong passive-dependent needs, and great guilt and fear about his anger about these.

Mr. T. had been in individual analytic therapy for several years with another therapist. He found the closeness in individual therapy and the interpretive comments of the individual therapist extremely difficult for him to cope with, feeling them as censure directed toward him which made him feel guilty and angry. He, therefore, sought group treatment and was placed in a regular group. He also immediately became an articulate and active participant in the group discussions. While he was eager and willing to discuss all types of emotional tensions and difficulties and problems in an intellectual, analytic way, he was unable to articulate any of his own dependent needs or his fear and associated guilt over his physical condition. When the group, with the aid of the therapist, confronted him with his avoidance of discussing his own physical complaints and needs and his own emotional needs, he attempted his usual resistive tactics of intellectual analysis of the underlying emotional factors. Aided by the therapist, the group persisted in trying to get him to express directly his own feelings of anxiety, depression, helplessness, dependency, and, most important of all, his great fear that his physical complaints might lead to serious, if not, fatal physical illness.

Getting this patient to talk about his dependent needs and physical symptoms came only after heated interactions and discussions in the group. They repeatedly pointed out to him his counterphobic disregard for his own physical health and his avoidance of discussing these, as well as his impatience with any one else in the group discussing dependent needs or physical complaints. Finally, he was able to begin to discuss these things and undertook a series of physical examinations which clarified for him the rather moderate extent of his physical illness. He was able to discuss this in the group and with their help, like the previous patient, was able to assume a more realistic attitude in taking care of himself and dealing with these things. He was able to stop smoking, go on a diet, begin to take regular periods of exercise and rest, with resultant marked improvement in his physical complaints.

Here again, the relationship and reactions in the group helped this patient face the anxiety, fear, rage, and guilt connected with his resistance, and his characteristic attitude of being self-sufficient and independent when underneath he really did not feel so. By identifying with the other patients and with the attitude of the therapist, he began to look past this resistance to see the nature of the fear, guilt, and anger that were involved in his avoidance of his discussing his dependent needs and his physical complaints.

Both these patients are examples of how patients with physical illness or somatic illness or complaints can be treated in a regular therapy group. As was emphasized above, however, such patients have to be sufficiently independent and able to manage so that they can be confronted with their resistance—excessive physical complaints with one patient and denial of physical complaints with the other. Both these patients had had individual therapy, which was helpful to some extent, but it was not sufficiently able to help them face the emotional factors involved in their dependency needs and physical complaints.

## SUMMARY AND CONCLUSIONS

The clinical material just described underlines the theoretical points made earlier, namely that because of the faulty psychological development and the pathological disturbances found in patients who express emotions through somatic channels, group psychotherapy is a specifically useful form of treatment. It enables these patients to enter into a therapeutic relationship more effectively than in individual treatment, and enables them to become aware of and deal with their pathological, characterological disturbances and overly reactive emotional attitudes.

The characteristic kinds of emotional disturbances occurring in these patients have been previously summarized and stem from the persistence of the disturbed symbiotic relationship with the mother and mother-surrogate. They have developed faulty object relationships, separation, anxiety and depression, intense emotional needs, conflicts over oral and anal cravings and aggressive tendencies, overwhelming tensions that are poorly tolerated and result in primitive defensive reactions with expression of emotions through somatic channels, weakness of the ego, a punitive of archaic superego, defective body image and self-image, a rigid characterological and social role, and emotional illiteracy or lack of awareness of their emotional reactions.

We have tried to indicate in this report how, in group psychotherapy, the relationships that are established, and the interactions that occur, help these patients overcome their pathological aggressive relationships and emotional attitudes and reactions so that emotional expression may find more realistic, mature, and effective channels rather than through somatic illness. The diminution in intensity of the primitive transference directed toward the therapist and its deflection on to other members of the group enable these patients to overcome their regressive fixation at the passive symbiotic level, and thus to enter into a useful psychotherapeutic relationship. The establishment of relationships with the therapist and each other through a series of identification enables these patients to enter into the relationship necessary for the therapy, and their sharing of the idealized figure of the leader or the therapist also helps them become aware of and discuss their feelings, as well as helping them lessen the guilt and fear of punishment stemming from their excessively harsh primitive superego. The more severely ill patients, psychiatrically by means of the idealized identification with the therapist, are able to develop more realistic and helpful attitudes in dealing with their illness. The less ill, somewhat more independent patients, who have been able to manage to establish a separate identity and realistically handle certain difficulties, can go on to the next phase of the group in which the transference manifestations related to their dependent needs are focused on the other members of the group and the interactions that occur make available for therapeutic scrutiny the pathological nature of their character traits and their emotional reactions. They are able to become aware and express emotions in the accepting atmosphere of the group, and express these feelings realistically and directly instead of through somatic and autonomic nonverbal channels. The presence of the other group members provides support and helps the patient work out new relationships and new ways of dealing with emotional tensions. The group psychotherapy thus enables the patient with psychosomatic illness and certain types of physical illness to enter into a psychotherapeutic relationship more quickly and more effectively and to deal with his psychopathology in such a way that there is a more useful realignment of intrapsychic forces, resulting in the fact that the psychophysiological regression is no longer expressed through psychosomatic symptoms. As stated in the beginning of this paper, it is because of these findings that we consider group psychotherapy as a "specific and usually quite effective form of treatment for patients with psychosomatic and certain types of physical illness, and for many it is the treatment of choice."

## References

1. Stein A: Group therapy with psychosomatically ill patients, In Kaplan HI, Saddock BJ (Eds.), Group Treatment of Mental Illness. New York, E.P. Dutton, 1972
2. Lipowski ZJ (Ed.): Current trends in psychosomatic medicine, I and II, Int J Psychiatry Med 5:303–612, 1974, and 5:3–336, 1975
3. Shontz FC: The Psychological Aspects of Physical Illness and Disability. New York, Macmillan Publishing Co., Inc., 1975
4. Karush A, Daniels GE, Flood C, O'Connor JF: Chronic Ulcerative Colitis. Philadelphia, W. B. Saunders, 1977
5. Fisher B, Laufer LG: A survey of the literature on psychological factors in heart attacks, the response of heart attack patients to group psychotherapy and recommendations for further investigation. In Wolberg LR, Aronson ML, Wolberg, AR (Eds.), Group Therapy, An Overview, New York: Stratton Intercontinental Medical Book Corp., 1977
6. Ibrahim M, Feldman J, Sultz H, et al.: Management after myocardial infarction: a controlled trial of the effect of group psychotherapy, Int J Psychiatry Med 5:253–268, 1974
7. Rahe R, et al.: Group therapy in the outpatient management of postmyocardial infarction patients. Psychiatry Med 4:77, 1973
8. Reckless J, Fauntleroy A: Groups, spouses and hospitalization as a trial of treatment in psychosomatic illness. Psychosomatics 13:353–357, 1972
9. Bilodeau C, Hackett T: Issues raised in a group setting by patients recovering from myocardial infarction. Am J Psychiatry 128:73–78, 1971
10. Ammon G: Analytic group psychotherapy as an instrument for the treatment and research of psychosomatic disorders, In Wolberg LR, Aronson ML (Eds.), Group Therapy: An Overview, New York: Stratton Intercontinental Medical Book Corp, 1975
11. Group Psychotherapy Literature (1970–1975), summarized by various writers. Int J Group Psychother Vols. 21–26, 1971–1976
12. Freedman B, Sweet BS: Some specific features of group psychotherapy and their implications for selection of patients. Int J Group Psychother 4:355, 1954
13. Ludwig A: Psychotherapy of rheumatoid arthritis, Bull Am Psychoanal Assoc 8:177, 1952
14. Freud S: Group Psychology and the Analysis of the Ego (Standard Edition, 18:67–143). London, Hagarth Press, 1955
15. Scheidlinger S: The concept of regression in group psychotherapy, Int J Group Psychother 18:3–20, 1965
16. Hackett TP, Froese, AP, Vasquez E: Psychological management of the CCU patient. Psychiatry Med 4:89–105, 1973

Pietro Castelnuovo-Tedesco

# 12
# Psychotherapy for the Nonpsychiatric Physician: Theoretical and Practical Aspects of the Twenty-Minute Hour

Everyone knows that a large proportion of the patients seen in the context of the practice of medicine have some kind of emotional disturbance. The estimates usually given vary from 25 to 50 percent;[1, 2] some even say 80 percent.[3, 4] Although it is difficult to establish a "true" figure, it is clearly very high. Moreover, patients with definite organic disease also may have significant emotional difficulties which openly or subtly complicate both the primary illness and its treatment.

This experience inevitably has compelled attention to the role of the nonpsychiatric physician in caring for the emotionally troubled. There is a consensus, at least among those who write on these topics, that the psychiatrist, alone, cannot deal with this large number, and that the nonpsychiatrist should share in this effort. This seems important not only for plain and practical reasons, having to do with the many patients who want help, but also because responsiveness to their emotional distress is essential to keep medical care "human" and prevent its becoming mechanized and impersonal.

For obvious reasons, psychiatry has been seen as the discipline that would provide physicians with the understanding and the means to deal with their patients' emotional difficulties. It also has become apparent that, somehow, psychiatry as taught in medical schools, even during the last 20 years, has not equipped practitioners to give the help sought by patients. It has been customary to assume that this lack of familiarity with basic psychotherapeutic skills was true primarily of the older physicians, who had not had the benefit of expanded psychiatric teaching in medical school.[5, 6] Yet in a 1967 study of recent U.S. medical graduates, 49 percent felt that they had not learned as much psychiatry as they would need to practice medicine in their specialty.[7] In a 1975 study of New Zealand general practitioners, 64 percent agreed that training to deal with neurotic illness is one of the most urgent needs in medicine; 65 percent thought they would like to undergo further training in the management of neurotic disorders.[8] Such feelings are not limited to one country, but are broadly common among physicians, certainly in western countries where such surveys have been made.[9-11] At any rate, awareness of these common deficiencies has led to special programs designed to enhance the competence of physicians in the area of psychological medicine.

Because these courses are a relatively new development, they have not followed a set format. In fact, there have been many questions about their goals, content, duration, and methods of presentation.

## HISTORICAL REVIEW

During the past 25 years, many postgraduate programs aimed at teaching psychiatry to nonpsychiatrists have sprung up in this country, in Great Britain and the British Commonwealth, and, to a lesser extent, in Western Europe. In the United States they were especially numerous during the early and mid-1960s, when the National Institute of Mental Health subsidized them on a large scale. For example, in 1963, psychiatric training programs for general practitioners were awarded $7,000,000;[12] this figure includes funds both for residency training and short-term programs.

Programs have varied all the way from the traveling workshop[13] to the dinner seminar[14] or to long-term courses which provide the practitioner some grounding in psychopathology, psychodynamics, and personality development.[15-17] Some courses have been organized around the personality of their leader, who has provided impetus and guidance as well as the bulk of the instruction;[18-19] sessions consist of case presentations by the practitioner, largely from his own case-file, followed by discussion.

Often, descriptions of programs do not convey accurately what was actually taught.[17] Generally, in the more successful ones, the personal relationship between instructor and trainees is the fulcrum of the course, perhaps more significant than its stated content. Parenthetically, this personal relationship is akin to a positive transference that sustains motivation and effort, and promotes learning through identification with the instructor. Most programs strive to be practical and to give help with everyday clinical problems. They depend on a combination of didactic techniques and group discussions, especially the latter. The lecture, as the only or principal vehicle for teaching, typically meets with a cool response,[4, 20] whereas an informal give-and-take atmosphere is best received.[21, 22] Recent efforts also have included newer technics, such as the actor-patient, instant playback video tapes, patients serving as "teachers," physicians role-playing their own patients, and emphasis on group dynamics.[20, 23]

A most difficult question has been how to promote clinical skills and which skills to emphasize. Some programs have tried mainly to "sensitize" the practitioner, by increasing his awareness of emotional states and encouraging him to listen to patients and speak with them informally about matters of personal concern. Other programs have stressed "interviewing," again as a means of helping doctors "talk" with patients. Still others have included "psychotherapy," but there has been a considerable range to what has been meant by this label. "Psychotherapy" might be simply a matter of promoting communication with patients or an approach with a specific and structured format. In the latter case, instruction in psychotherapy often has taken place late in the program, after more basic kinds of information have been transmitted.[16] Another issue has been whether to teach psychotherapy or just patient management and how much emphasis to give to drug treatment. During the 1950s and early 1960s, "talking" skills (interviewing, psychotherapy, etc.) were stressed, whereas recently the orientation has been more toward psychopharmacology and the management of symptoms by means of drugs.[5, 11, 24] Implicit in this choice has been some feeling that this would come easier to physicians, and would be less likely to evoke resistance.

Over the years, the programs that have featured psychotherapy in some form have been sufficiently numerous that it is difficult to give even an approximate list of the principal ones. As early as 1939, Maurice Levine conducted seminars for nonpsychiatrists in Cincinnati, and from this experience came *Psychotherapy in Medical Practice,* by now a classic.[25] This book is noteworthy also because, together with Binger's *The Doctor's Job*[26] and Bird's *Talking With Patients,*[27] it is one of the first attempts to apply psychoanalytic insights to the practical work of the nonpsychiatrist.

Other pioneering efforts were those at the University of Minnesota, led by Thomas A. C. Rennie and John M. Murray*,[28] and those by T. A. Watters in New Orleans.[29] A major early contributor was Michael Balint. In the late 1950s at the Tavistock Clinic in London, Balint developed the now well-known "Balint groups." From his work came many publications, most prominently *The Doctor, His Patient and the Illness*[18] and *Psychotherapeutic Techniques in Medicine.*[19] Balint groups became quite popular during the 1960s, and were introduced also in the United States,[30] Canada,[31] and Europe.[32-35] In essence, a Balint group consists of about 10 doctors who meet once a week with a psychiatrist to discuss their patients; the group may go on for years. Emphasis is placed on the doctor-patient relationship, on understanding the patient's conflicts, and on promoting self-awareness in the physician.

Other key programs with emphasis on psychotherapy have been that of M. R. Kaufman at the Mount Sinai Hospital in New York,[15, 36] that of the Zabarenkos at the Staunton Clinic in Pittsburgh,[37] that of A. Enelow at the University of Southern California in Los Angeles,[5, 16, 17] and that of P. Castelnuovo-Tedesco at the Harbor General Hospital, also in Los Angeles.[38-42] There have also been programs with outstanding leadership that have aimed at teaching psychosomatic medicine, rather

---

*The distinguished faculty included also Walter Bauer, Douglas D. Bond, Henry W. Brosin, Donald Hastings, M. Ralph Kaufman, John Romano, and Harold G. Wolff.

than psychotherapy and basic psychiatry, to the nonpsychiatrist.[43-45] Because these, although related, have had a different orientation, their contribution is recognized but will not be considered in detail.

It is worth noting that over the years this area has generated great interest, that the pertinent literature is a large one, and that its tone typically is optimistic. In reviewing over 100 contributions of the past 20 years on psychiatry for nonpsychiatrists, I was impressed by their authors' apparent desire to accent the positive. Although difficulties are acknowledged, often they seem understated, and the headlines usually are assigned to their programs' achievements. Overall, I found only two articles that spoke quite candidly of their efforts as failures and tried to account for these results.[46, 47] Both are most informative. They show the importance of collaborating from the earliest phases of planning with the medical group for whom the program is being organized. It is essential also that the leadership of the medical group be involved and support the program. Attendance by physicians may be poor, even though initially they may have requested the program, if various sources of resistance go unrecognized. Finally, a program is likely to have trouble if it promotes an approach which the practitioner finds at variance with his accustomed style of working with patients.

The next section will be devoted to a description of the Twenty-Minute Hour, as an example of a structured approach to psychotherapy for the nonpsychiatrist. The concluding section of this paper will consider some issues about teaching psychotherapy to nonpsychiatrists that are central to planning a training program.

## THE TWENTY-MINUTE HOUR

### What It Is and How It Came About

The Twenty-Minute Hour is an approach to brief supportive psychotherapy that was developed specifically for the nonpsychiatric physician. Its chief characteristics are that it is simple, time-limited, and specific enough to be easily learned. It is safe and effective, even when the opportunities for personal supervision are limited. Moreover, although it is a true, integrated psychotherapeutic experience, it does not require that the practitioner learn a new theoretical system, special skills, or change his orientation toward his work. He simply needs to extend his usual way of working with patients. The approach was designed to fit well with the practitioner's individual style and with traditional medical practices. It has grown out of direct experience with the needs, capacities, and limitations of nonpsychiatrists in dealing with the emotional difficulties of their patients.

The Twenty-Minute Hour originated at the Harbor General Hospital in Los Angeles, when, in 1960, the author began a program for medical residents which centered on their learning a limited kind of psychotherapy. Since that time, the program has grown and diversified by including residents from other clinical departments in addition to those from the department of medicine; it has continued, with support from the National Institute of Mental Health, to the present. This work has been reported in a number of publications,[38-42] including a book, *The Twenty Minute Hour: A Guide to Brief Psychotherapy for the Physician,* which appeared in 1965.[39] The reader is referred to these writings for a more complete description than will be possible here.

The Twenty-Minute Hour was designed to deal with the common resistances that nonpsychiatrists typically show in response to the task of involving themselves in psychotherapy. These will be examined later. For the moment I want to say simply that attention to these is essential to establish a successful program.

Time is the fundamental parameter of the Twenty-Minute Hour. Time was seen, from the beginning, as the central variable which influences the practitioner's capacity to do psychotherapy. The reason routinely given by physicians for excluding psychotherapy from their practice was not that they did not "believe" in it, but that it required too much *time*. This, in turn, was based on the premise, accepted as fact, that the magic unit of 50 minutes is necessary for psychotherapy. Obviously, a busy practitioner cannot set aside so much time for each of his emotionally upset patients. Although this claim contains much reality, however, it is also commonly used as a rationalization for avoiding psychotherapy altogether. A period of twenty minutes was chosen because it represents a unit of time which a practitioner could be expected to spend with a patient and which can be fitted without too much strain into a busy office practice. Other benefits accrue from a short session: it limits the patient's resistance and the inexperienced psychotherapist's fear that he may "run out of steam" before the end of an hour or that he may get involved beyond his capacities. It also helps to insure that the work will be focused and not waste itself on trifles. Yet those who try twenty-minute periods for the first time often are surprised by how much can be accomplished during the session.

The basic format of the Twenty-Minute Hour is a maximum of ten treatment sessions, each of 20-minutes' duration. The initial contact with the patient (which may last 1–2 hours) aims at an assessment of the problem, and includes a medical history and a physical examination. The history exphasizes the chief complaint, the present illness, and, in particular, the *social context* in which the patient's difficulty has developed. The remaining sessions, of 20-minutes' duration at weekly intervals, are devoted to psychotherapy.

The doctor's first task is to use his initial basic history to identify the sources of friction and dissatisfaction currently at work in the patient's life. He needs to know not only the patient's complaints and how they evolved, but also how they relate to his characteristic mode of living, bearing in mind that any life pattern—no matter how successful—has built-in stresses and sources of conflict, and that, inevitably, these reflect themselves in the illness. The doctor, therefore, must inform himself about the patient's work, his current family relationships, his customary daily activities, and also learn something about his background. Moreover, there are three questions which he must answer in each case. Every patient with emotional difficulties—so the doctor is advised—has trouble primarily with *one key person in the present*. Often, however, the patient is unaware that his distress has developed in the context of that relationship. The doctor's task is to help the patient discover, by talking, (1) who that person is, (2) what the trouble is about, and (3) what alternatives are open to the patient to make that relationship more satisfactory. Reaching an answer to the first two questions is akin to achieving a "diagnosis." It spells out the problems to be solved or, at least, ameliorated. Pursuit of the third question in a series of consecutive conversations with the patient is the "psychotherapy" portion of the work, which aims at change or, at least, at a rethinking of the problem. Admittedly this approach involves oversimplifications, yet it makes the task specific and realistic and provides the student with guidelines that greatly increase his comfort and sense of direction. This, in turn, often makes the difference between early abandonment of the task and pursuing it to successful completion.

The whole treatment effort rests on the formulation of a plan in terms that are simple and basic enough to be readily shared and accepted by both doctor and patient. In keeping with his training and usual practice, the doctor employs the initial workup to reach some understanding of the presenting problem. If he decides that the patient's difficulty is primarily emotional in origin, he needs to say this to him—tactfully, but directly and without equivocation. The patient usually does not resent this because it is offered as the conclusion to a painstaking workup and not as a casual opinion. The doctor also should identify for the patient the person with whom he appears to have trouble and clarify what this trouble is about. Finally, he needs to advise the patient that to help him with his emotional problem, he would like to see him each week for 20 minutes. To this end, he should set up several consecutive appointments. He also must explain that the purpose of the visits will be to discuss in more detail the particular relationship which, jointly, they have defined as central to the current difficulty. Coexisting "organic" problems can be treated concurrently by the appropriate means.

As this program is carried out, in most instances the patient improves and feels better. The pressure of symptoms diminishes and, even when they do not disappear altogether, they are no longer so strange or frightening, and are better understood and tolerated. Although improvement may be modest, it is nonetheless evident, and the patient usually appears much more comfortable. After approximately 8 to 10 such consecutive interviews, enough resolution has taken place that treatment can be concluded. One must keep in mind, however, that symptoms may recur, and that the patient may need to return perhaps months later for further psychotherapy.

How should the doctor conduct himself as a psychotherapist? We emphasize that the doctor should not simply be a listener and sit sphinx-like while the patient painfully brings up his worries. He needs to interact with the patient and converse with him about his problems in a spontaneous and friendly way. To be effective, the doctor must feel comfortable. It helps if he can be himself and follow naturally the bent of his own personality rather than some stereotyped notion of how a psychotherapist acts. It is important to acknowledge that personal styles differ, and that some doctors are naturally more talkative or directive, while others are quieter and more restrained.

Inasmuch as the nonpsychiatrist lacks a theoretical orientation in psychiatry, in what terms, then, is he to understand the patient's problems? This predicament is not easily solved. Some have given the practitioner an accelerated indoctrination in psychodynamic principles, while others have offered a prolonged apprenticeship. The Twenty-Minute Hour program emphasizes that much can be accomplished with the ordinary, untutored psychological understanding that everyone relies on in daily life. For reasons too lengthy to be pursued here, physicians often do not employ in their work with patients the interpersonal skills by which they manage the more personal aspects of their own lives. The physician, in other words, really knows more about people and their motivations than he typically gives himself credit for. Rather than theoretical training, which is necessarily lengthy and complex, the physician needs encouragement to trust the interpersonal skills that he already possesses so that he may allow himself to apply them in behalf of his patients.

To make this issue more specific, we give the practitioner the following example. We ask him what he would do if a close friend sought his help because he was having trouble with his wife or his boss. Probably, we say, you would begin by listening to him and then you might ask questions to clarify your picture of the problem. Above all, you would give your friend an opportunity to unburden himself of feelings. Also, you would express concern and sympathy. Then, very likely, you would point out some aspects of the situation that your friend had overlooked and that would help place matters in a different, more positive light. You might even suggest steps that he might take to help resolve the difficulty, and, finally, you would ask your friend to let you know how things turned out and invite him to keep in touch with you. The second time you saw your friend, you would listen to the further developments of the story, repeating the same procedure, and so on. More details could be spelled out, but the general approach, so simple really, is clear enough. The doctor is urged to treat his patients in much the same way, to help them to express themselves freely, and to convey to them interest, friendliness, encouragement, and also a measure of good sense.

Two other points that are basic to the Twenty-Minute Hour program pertain to the prescription of drugs and the giving of advice. Often, as his first therapeutic gesture, the practitioner is inclined to prescribe a tranquilizer or an antidepressant. We recommend that the doctor try, if possible, to restrain this impulse, which is dictated more often by his own discomfort and his urge to "do something" right away than by the patient's clinical condition. At times, psychotropic drugs are helpful, but it is best if they are given later, in the context of a growing relationship, and with a clear idea of how they fit into the overall plan. The doctor needs to grasp that, while drugs can *assist* the psychotherapeutic program, they do not *replace* it.

About advice, the attitude of practitioners tends to be ambivalent. On the one hand, they would be inclined to dispense it freely, because advice (like drugs) is easy to give and does not require much effort. At the same time, they often feel guilty about giving it at all, because they have heard during their training that advice is bad and should be avoided, especially on major decisions (e.g., about marriage, vocation, etc.). We explain to practitioners that advice-giving is not only permissible, but at times quite useful. The advice, however, should make sense to the patient and represent a course of action that he can reasonably be expected to follow. It should not be what the doctor would do if he were in the patient's shoes. The best advice is that which evolves naturally from an attempt to weigh, jointly with the patient, his conflicting wishes and fears and the available alternatives.

Most patients clearly profit from treatment by the Twenty-Minute Hour, if they are appropriately chosen for it in the first place. Occasionally, however, if nothing has happened by the 10th session, the patient will need to be referred to a psychiatrist. Instruction is given in the program about how to refer a patient; it is important to explain that a referral is more acceptable to the patient at this point because the practitioner already has made an effort to deal with the problem himself.

The effectiveness of the Twenty-Minute Hour (and, incidentally, of similar short-term psychotherapies) depends largely on careful patient selection. The Twenty-Minute Hour is not a cure-all. To the extent that it is applied randomly, patients will be included who really are unsuited for it and who will show a disappointing response. The Twenty-Minute Hour is best restricted to the *milder* emotional disturbances that are seen so commonly in the everyday practice of medicine. Basically, these are of recent onset, of no more than moderate severity, and related to fairly clear-cut situational difficulties and interpersonal stresses. The chief symptoms are anxiety-depression or preoccupation with multiple physical complaints. Although troubled and upset, the typical Twenty-Minute Hour patient shows no major regression. This can be determined by his continued capacity to function in his accustomed social role. In particular, work effectiveness, a dependable and easily ascertained index of ego integrity, has not been undermined. By these criteria, the patients who should be excluded are those whose disturbances are severe and/or chronic and who show substantial ego impairment. Specifically, these are the obviously psychotic (including depressives with suicidal risk), the obviously psychopathic (including drug addicts, alcoholics, and emotionally unstable characters), those with complex neuroses (e.g., phobic patients), and those with the more serious psychosomatic disorders (e.g., ulcerative colitis).

At this point I wish to underline that the Twenty-Minute Hour, while stressing patient selection, does not require that the practitioner know how to make a *formal* psychiatric diagnosis, a difficult skill that inevitably presumes much training and experience. Rather, we convey the importance of arriving at a *functional* assessment of the patient, based on his performance. More important than deciding which of a dozen textbook labels best fits the patient, is the capacity to pick out, by the criteria outlined above, those with mild disturbances who are likely to respond to brief psychotherapy. Other patients should be referred to the psychiatrist for more prolonged treatment.

A positive feature of the Twenty-Minute Hour, mentioned earlier but deserving emphasis, is its safety and essential freedom from complications. Because it is time-limited, it has both a clear beginning and an end. The practitioner learns how to start and where to stop, two aspects of psychotherapy that otherwise he commonly finds difficult. Practitioners also worry that, if they treat a patient with psychotherapy, they may inadvertently trigger a serious emotional storm or somehow cause the patient to get worse. With the Twenty-Minute Hour, this, in fact, is extremely unlikely, because the doctor confines himself to the patient's current, consciously perceived, realistic problems; maintains a consistently supportive attitude; and avoids dealing with buried conflicts. Our experience has been that nonpsychiatrists are uniformly overcautious in approaching their patients' emotional struggles. They need, if anything, encouragement and reassurance that their psychotherapeutic efforts are fundamentally safe and, if consistently pursued, will be rewarded by success.

## PSYCHOTHERAPY BY NONPSYCHIATRISTS—
## PROBLEMS AND SOLUTIONS

This section will be devoted to some of the central issues which, in our experience, influence the attitude of practitioners toward psychotherapy and their willingness to learn it and practice it. I wish to point out at the outset that, while some physicians may recognize the value of psychotherapy in the abstract and even the merit of referring a patient to a psychiatrist, most find it difficult to regard psychotherapy as a *medical* technique which *any* physician (themselves included) might apply in the course of his daily practice. Although unfamiliarity with psychiatric techniques may be widespread among physicians, it is only a well-selected group that chooses to take part in psychiatric courses for nonpsychiatrists. In fact, those with long experience in organizing such programs have noticed that often there is a small core that returns to take the same course year after year.[5, 36]

In other words, the number of physicians for whom these remarks ultimately may turn out to have relevance is unfortunately quite restricted.[12, 46] Yet, no matter how small the number of potential "customers," it seems important to try to identify the conditions under which learning best takes place. Among physicians there is considerable resistance to psychiatry, and attempts to teach psychotherapy or anything else that is psychiatric generally meet with an uphill struggle. Therefore, it is valuable to recognize explicitly these attitudes and common forms of resistance so that they may be taken into account and dealt with as much as possible. The success of any training program depends on its capacity to come to terms with the following issues.

### Active Mastery as a Basis for Learning

The practitioner needs to put what he learns into active use. He can learn only if he has the opportunity from the very beginning to *be* a psychotherapist and apply himself to the actual treatment of one or more patients. Also, he learns as he goes along. Too much time spent listening to experts and watching *them* interview patients (as takes place in some programs) is not helpful. In the Twenty-Minute Hour program, the emphasis throughout has been on *doing,* on what is done and why, and the student finds few occasions to take a back seat. From the beginning, he is involved in treating a patient and comes to grapple with his anxiety about being a psychotherapist. Plentiful support and encouragement during supervision help him to get started.

## Problems of Professional Identity

For the physician, attempting psychotherapy often means running the risk of stepping outside his professional role, as he perceives it—in short, of not being a doctor anymore. This view equates the practice of medicine with the management of "organic" problems; "mental" and "organic" aspects of behavior are seen as far apart. It is helpful to clarify for the practitioner that in truth they belong together and, more importantly, that he need not replace or unlearn his accustomed ways of dealing with patients, but only to broaden and extend them. The wish to help a patient with his psychological troubles in no way requires that the physician give up his hard-won knowledge of "organic" disease nor his interest in it. He can use the stethoscope or the listening ear, as needed.

The issue, however, is not simply that physicians prefer to deal with "organic" problems. Throughout its breadth, medicine is becoming ever more specialized, and physicians are increasingly uncomfortable and wary of stepping outside the narrow perimeter of their usual practices. Events of the last few years, such as extravagant malpractice claims, the new emphasis on peer review, and the assignment of various tasks to paraprofessionals, certainly have not stimulated among physicians a desire to broaden the scope of their work or their area of responsibility. The tendency, rather, has been to restrict and compartmentalize one's practice to make it, as much as possible, safely predictable. These factors, unfortunately, are difficult to change, yet recognizing them openly may help to mitigate their effects.

## Attitudes Toward Psychotherapy

Most physicians have great difficulty coming to a clear conclusion about psychotherapy, and their attitude typically is ambivalent. On the one hand, they see it as mysterious, magical and arcane. On the other, they suspect that there is nothing to it, that it is all "just talk." This, in turn, derives from the view that to do something *for* a patient, one must do something *to* him (i.e., perform a test or a physical examination, give him a medicine, or subject him to surgery). Because in psychotherapy nothing *visible* is done to the patient, the thought emerges that perhaps the whole thing is a sham.

Other problems with psychotherapy, as far as the average physician is concerned, have to do with its very name. The "psych" root evokes thoughts of things that are "mental" and vague, far removed from what is "organic" and comfortably concrete. Years ago, while making arrangements to teach The Twenty-Minute Hour to members of a clinical department, I quickly discovered that these physicians had no interest in the program when it was presented as a form of brief psychotherapy, but were enthusiastic when I agreed to teach them how to "do counseling." They never knew that the label was changed, but that the program otherwise remained the same. On the other hand, even such simple strategems are not always successful. One resident complained that, when he attempted to deal with his patients about their personal problems, he felt more like a marriage counselor than like a doctor. Again, the problem of identity kept cropping up.

These negative attitudes toward psychotherapy are reflected in a reluctance of the physician to charge for any psychotherapy he may offer his patients. The nonpsychiatrist is inclined to look on his therapeutic efforts as forms of personal benevolence rather than as a medical treatment which warrants a fee. Obviously, this view is not conducive to the acceptance of psychotherapy in the therapeutic armamentarium or to its frequent use.

These are difficult problems for which no fully satisfactory solution exists. The Twenty-Minute Hour tries to deal with them by providing the practitioner with an approach that has an identifiable format. Its step-by-step procedure, which approximates that of other medical interventions, seeks to counteract the fear that it is something totally amorphous, "just talk." During the training program, attitudes toward fees for psychotherapy need to be approached directly and considered in detail; an appropriate fee schedule should be recommended.

### Time

As noted earlier, time is a very real issue for the physician who would employ psychotherapy in his practice. Because he is called upon to see dozens of patients in the course of a day's work, the period that he can spend with any one patient is sharply limited. Even though the issue of time typically serves to rationalize the doctor's failure to use psychotherapy, one must recognize that the traditional 50-minute hour is not applicable to the pace of a general medical practice. It is pointless, therefore, to teach the nonpsychiatrist forms of psychotherapy based on a time frame that does not fit the structure of an average practice. When this is attempted, the message is given that the training is purely academic and not intended to have practical application. On the other hand, twenty-minute periods are perceived as feasible for at least a portion of the patients; they approximate the time limits the physician is accustomed to.

### Language and Communication

Any program that seeks to teach psychological medicine must consider very carefully the language it speaks and whether it is adequately shared and understood by the physician. Experience has shown that the practitioner typically finds psychiatric jargon irritating and confusing. Unfailingly, it has a negative effect on communication. By contrast, using plain English to describe basic emotions and common situations of conflict helps to convey that we are not dealing with abstract or esoteric issues, but with the stuff of daily life. For this reason, the Twenty-Minute Hour avoids almost entirely formal psychiatric diagnosis, and emphasizes instead the importance of understanding the patient in simple, everyday, common sense terms. In short, the language of a program is at the core of its effort, and determines to a large extent how much acceptance a program achieves.

## Knowledge and Skill

The practitioner usually is the first to admit that he knows very little about psychiatry. One alternative is to give the practitioner a concentrated course in psychopathology and psychodynamics, but such an approach may simply serve to impress him with how much he still needs to learn. The Twenty-Minute Hour instead emphasizes the practical understanding of people the practitioner already possesses, and advises him that with this knowledge there is much he can do to help his patient. The problem is not so much one of teaching the physician new material that he needs to know, but of helping him to recognize what he already knows so that he can apply it in the clinical setting. For this reason, we make no special attempt to teach psychiatric diagnosis or techniques of interviewing, although pointers in these areas may be given from time to time as they fit a specific case. Mainly, we do not wish to detract from the practitioner's reliance on his own skills and capacities and try, instead, to encourage these as much as possible. The issue of psychiatric interviewing provides a good example. Although we try to clarify what sort of historical ifnormation (e.g., the current social context) will help the physician to understand his patient, the method by which this information is to be obtained is left largely up to him. We take for granted that he will not be as adroit as an experienced psychotherapist. We want him to develop his own style and, therefore, do not wish to suggest that there is a "right way" of talking to the patient. More important is whether the physician is able to pursue his goal and act on his own, because in his practice he must function without having to rely on guidance by a psychiatrist.

At the same time as we emphasize the potential of the relatively untrained psychological sense of daily life, it is important to acknowledge that the practitioner's skill as a psychotherapist *is* limited. This has distinct implications for the kind of psychotherapy that he is equipped to carry out. Because he lacks a theoretical grounding, the practitioner should not be expected to involve himself in any psychotherapy that is intensive or prolonged, specifically aimed at interpretive uncovering, or requiring that he manage the complex issues of transference. The alternative, of course, is *really* to train the practitioner in psychotherapy, but this requires much more time and a degree of interest in learning psychotherapy that the physician usually does not possess. Moreover, this approach, if successful, is likely to draw the physician away from his original specialty and turn him into a psychiatrist.

For all these reasons, a form of brief, supportive psychotherapy, like the Twenty-Minute Hour, which aims at symptomatic relief and alleviating interpersonal conflict, has seemed especially suited to the professional needs and capacities of the practitioner. It has clear boundaries that keep the practitioner from drifting and getting lost.

## The Emotional Climate of a Training Program

This discussion would be incomplete without some reference to the emotional climate in which the training takes place. In his work with practitioners, Balint stressed the importance of the drug "doctor"; what the physician gives to the patient through the action of his own personality probably is his most powerful therapeutic agent.[18, 19] To psychiatrists this may seem obvious, yet often it is precisely the obvious that requires emphasis, and Balint, to his credit, chose to make the point strongly. Balint also realized that, if the practitioner is to convey to his patient a sense of contact and relatedness, he, the practitioner, needs to have experienced something similar in the context of the training program. Although the relationship should not become one of therapist and patient, a feeling of personal involvement between teacher and student—akin to a positive transference—is crucial for successful learning. It is not possible to pursue here how the relationship between teacher and student should be managed. Clearly, there is a range of options that depends in part on the personality of the instructor. Some features, however, can be highlighted. A training situation that is overwhelmingly "factual" and aims at imparting the "newest" techniques (as might be done in a refresher course on internal medicine or ophthalmology) is not likely to be effective. At the other extreme, if the "magic" of a charismatic leader largely substitutes for course content, the trainee's involvement in practicing psychotherapy may depend excessively on the maintenance of the relationship between teacher and student, which then is likely to prove quite prolonged.

In turn, this brings up questions about the optimal duration of a training course. There are, again, no clear answers, and I speak with less conviction on this point than about other aspects of this large topic. Our program was 3–4 months long; Balint's groups ran for years. I suspect that *very* short experiences (e.g., weekend refresher courses, two-week "crash" courses, etc.) have a too heavily didactic orientation and, therefore, may not be very helpful. Very long experiences, on the other hand, probably require more than the average physician wishes to invest, and appeal principally to a select number. Also, they are more likely to result in a *coterie* of followers than in a group of students who have successfully accomplished a course of training.

## CONCLUSIONS

I have reviewed the topic of psychotherapy for nonpsychiatrists and have recommended the Twenty-Minute Hour, a form of brief psychotherapy, because its simple and well-defined format makes it readily taught and practical to apply. I have tried also to clarify basic issues that need to be considered in planning a training program for nonpsychiatrists. Because this paper deals with *psychotherapy* (rather than psychiatry) for nonpsychiatrists, some topics deliberately have been omitted that would have been included if the larger subject were being discussed. Obviously, other areas besides psychotherapy are pertinent to the care a nonpsychiatrist can provide to an emotionally upset patient. One can list here such topics as the use of psychotropic drugs, the evaluation of suicidal risk, the psychiatric emergency, the hypochrondriacal and/or "difficult" patient, the management of common sexual problems, the management of alcoholism and drug addiction, the problems of particular age groups (e.g., adolescents, the elderly), etc. These readily find a place in a program that emphasizes the teaching of psychotherapy.

Almost 20 years of experience with the Twenty-Minute Hour have confirmed its usefulness in the hands of the nonpsychiatrist. Its limitations have less to do with the approach itself than with the observation, again, that nonpsychiatrists are not easily drawn to the practice of psychotherapy. It is only fair to add, however, that nonpsychiatrists are not alone in their uncertainty about psychotherapy. In psychiatry, too, the attitude toward psychotherapy is less wholeheartedly positive than it was 20 years ago; some members of the profession even believe that psychiatrists should concentrate on the biological aspects of their field and that psychotherapy should be left largely to the nonphysician and to the paraprofessional.[48] Also, as has been mentioned, the trend toward specialization continues to grow in all fields of medicine, and is proving difficult to reconcile with a holistic approach, in practice even if not in theory.

Yet, other trends also are emerging. A lasting concern that medical care be responsive to individual needs and human complexities is leading gradually to the realization that this goal cannot be achieved solely by emphasizing technology and efficiency and that it is necessary to continue to enhance holistic values and to find application and expression for these, both in training programs and in day-to-day practice. Two recent developments are particularly in keeping with this outlook. The first is a resurgence of interest in psychosomatic medicine under the heading of liaison psychiatry. The latter deals with both administrative and clinical issues and emphasizes the working relationship between psychiatry and the other clinical specialties. The second is the new field of family medicine, which aims at comprehensive care in the context of the family unit. Although, after two decades of effort, the task of teaching psychiatry to nonpsychiatrists remains complex and marked by unsolved problems, it is reasonable to say that the experience gained so far has been noteworthy and that it will find a place in the contributions that now are being prepared.

## References

1. Stepansky PE, Stepansky W: Psychiatry in family medicine: an old role restated. Psychosomatics 13:380–387, 1972
2. Brown JW, Robertson LS, Kosa J, et al: A study of general practice in Massachusetts. JAMA 216:301–306, 1971
3. Lipsitt DR: Some problems in the teaching of psychosomatic medicine. Int J Psychiatry Med 61:317–329, 1975
4. Kaufman MR: The psychiatrist's dilemma. J Mt Sinai Hosp 34:389–395, 1967
5. Naftulin DH, Donnelly FA, Wolkon GH: Psychiatry education programs for nonpsychiatrist physicians: a 10-year perspective. Compr Psychiatry 15:133–139, 1974
6. Fisher JV, Mason RL, Fisher JC: Emotional illness and the family physician. Psychosomatics 16:171–177, 1975
7. Castelnuovo-Tedesco P: How much psychiatry are medical students really learning? Arch Gen Psychiatry 16:668–675, 1967
8. McAllister JJ, Lindsay JSB: Psychiatric illness in general practice: a survey of opinions. NZ Med J 82:155–158, 1975
9. Freeling P: Teaching general practitioners about psychiatry. J R Coll Gen Pract 21:629–633, 1971
10. Walton HG: Medical practitioners seeking post-graduate training in psychiatry. Br J Med Psychol 38:63–73, 1965
11. Owen A, Winkler R: General practitioners and psychosocial problems. An evaluation using pseudopatients. Med J Aust 2: 393–398, 1974
12. Hardin Branch CH: Psychiatric training and the general practitioner. Am J Psychiatry 122:485–489, 1965
13. Meade BT, Fishman JJ: A different project in postgraduate psychiatric education. J Med Educ 38:103–110, 1963
14. Pierce CM: The dinner seminar in a program for general practitioners. South Med J 59:1184–1186, 1966
15. Kleinschmidt HJ, Kaufman MR, Diener H: Experiences in teaching basic psychiatry to medical practitioners at the Mount Sinai Hospital, New York. J Mt Sinai Hosp 30:385–400, 1963
16. Enelow AJ, Adler LM: Psychiatric skills and knowledge for the general practitioner. JAMA 189:91–96, 1964
17. Enelow AJ, Adler LM: Organization of postgraduate courses in psychiatry. Arch Gen Psychiatry 12:433–437, 1965
18. Balint M: The Doctor, His Patient and The Illness. New York, Pitman, 1963
19. Balint M, Balint E: Psychotherapeutic Techniques in Medicine. London, Tavistock, 1961
20. Lurie HJ, Gallagher JM: Innovative techniques for teaching psychiatric principles to general practitioners. JAMA 221: 696–699, 1972
21. Hooper D, Roberts FG: Workshop training in psychotherapy. Br J Med Psychol 49: 177–182, 1976
22. Sheeley WF: Postgraduate education in psychiatry for the practicing physician. Med Clin North Am 51:1363–1374, 1967
23. Harris CM, Long BEL, Byrne PS: A teaching method course in Manchester general practioners teachers. Br J Med Educ 10: 193–197, 1976
24. Rittelmeyer LF, MacKintosh A: Psychiatric education in a family practice residency. Va Med Mon 101:629–631, 1974
25. Levine M: Psychotherapy in Medical Practice. New York, Macmillan, 1942
26. Binger C: The Doctor's Job. New York, Norton, 1945
27. Bird B: Talking With Patients. Philadelphia, Lippincott, 1955
28. Witmer HL (Ed.): Teaching Psychotherapeutic Medicine: Experimental Course for General Physicians. New York, Commonwealth Fund, 1947
29. Watters TA, Atkinson JW: Some interesting experiences in teaching psychiatry to general practitioners. South Med J 50:579–586, 1957
30. Pittenger RA: A method of training physicians in psychotherapy. Paper presented at the American Psychiatric Association Meeting, May 1960
31. Stauble WJ: Courses in psychiatry for family doctors. Can Psychiatr Assoc J 8:104–110, 1963
32. Green A: La formation des practiciens a la psychotherapie. Semaine Therapeutique 39:341–343, 1963

33. Chertok LG, Bourguignon O: The Balint group and preventive industrial medicine. Int J Psychiatry Med 3:395–402, 1972

34. Loch W: The doctor-patient relationship in general practice: implications for diagnosis and treatment. Int J Psychiatry Med 3: 365–370, 1972

35. Alby JM, Sapir M: Le groupe Balint. Rev Practicien 26:1717–1720, 1976

36. Kaufman MR: The teaching of psychiatry to the nonpsychiatrist physician. Am J Psychiatry 128:610–616, 1971

37. Zabarenko RN, Merenstein J, Zabarenko L: Teaching psychological medicine in the family practice office. JAMA 218:392–396, 1971

38. Castelnuovo-Tedesco P: The twenty minute hour: an experiment in medical education. New Engl J Med 266:283–289, 1962

39. Castelnuovo-Tedesco P: The Twenty Minute Hour: A Guide to Brief Psychotherapy for the Physician. Boston, Little, Brown & Co, 1965

40. Castelnuovo-Tedesco P: The twenty minute hour: an approach to the postgraduate teaching of psychiatry. Am J Psychiatry 123: 786–791, 1967

41. Castelnuovo-Tedesco P: The twenty minute hour revisited: a follow-up. Compr Psychiatry 11:108–122, 1970

42. Castelnuovo-Tedesco P: The twenty minute hour: a technic of brief psychotherapy. South Med 64:33–37, 1976

43. Engel GL: Psychological Development in Health and Disease. New York, Saunders, 1962

44. Reichsman F: Teaching psychosomatic medicine to medical students, residents and postgraduate fellows. Int J Psychiatry Med 6:307–316, 1976

45. Reiser MF: Changing theoretical concepts in psychosomatic medicine. In Arieti S (Ed.), American Handbook of Psychiatry, 4. New York, Basic Books, 1975, p. 477–500

46. Enelow AJ, Myers VH: Postgraduate psychiatric education: the ethnography of a failure. Am J Psychiatry 125:79–83, 1968

47. McLean PD, Miles JE: Training family physicians in psychosocial care: an analysis of a program failure. J Med Educ 50: 900–902, 1975

48. Ludwig AM: The psychiatrist as physician. JAMA 234:603–604, 1975

Stuart A. Waltzman

# 13
# Treatment of the Dying Patient and The Family

## INTRODUCTION

For the most part, humans are future-oriented beings. One common way of coping with the disappointments of the past and present is concentrating through fantasy (or behavior) on anticipated future gratifications or accomplishments. For many people, the experience of being alive implies the possession of the freedom to assume that the future will provide numerous possibilities to construct and repair relationships, learn new skills or refine old ones, gratify ambitions, and maintain or enhance self-esteem. The fantasy of repairing what is damaged, replacing what is lost, or constructing something new is especially prevalent during the earlier stages of the life cycle, but is present, to some extent, throughout life as long as the reality of death is at least partially denied. In addition, a sense of continuity as well as a potential for change are components of the feeling of being alive which help to control concerns of annihilation.

When death becomes more than an abstract concept, the loss of the freedom to be future-oriented presents an overwhelming stress which requires significant coping skills. These are further taxed by losses of the sense of body integrity, physical abilities, relationship capacities, and many other activities that contribute to the maintenance of self-esteem. Each individual who is coping with dying manifests adaptive capacities which are expressed uniquely and which confront family, friends, and the health care team which must assume responsibility for the overall direction and implementation of treatment.

Partially in response to the increasing needs of the terminally ill population, as well as other factors not yet adequately defined, there has been a significant growth of interest and a rapidly expanding literature concerning the psychosocial needs and problems of the dying patient, his family, the health care team, and the setting in which the care takes place. Although there have been many valuable theoretical discussions and practical recommendations for the care of the dying patient, the present state of research in the area leaves much to be desired. Most of the literature is anecdotal or suffers from a lack of precise definitions and criteria for comparison of patient groups, standardized instruments possessing clear reliability and validity, and rigorous longitudinal studies. The clinical care of the dying patient has also lagged behind other advances in medicine in spite of the increased publicity and frequent conferences sponsored by those interested in thanatology.

In fact, the discipline of thanatology, in attempting to formulate certain basic principles with which to guide others, has promoted several questionable theses. The first stems from the incontrovertible reality that death is an inevitable part of life. It is then assumed that death must be ultimately dealt with as all unpleasant realities are, namely, with acceptance. This "acceptance" must be accomplished not only by the person dying but by the culture, including those to whom his care is assigned. While it is impossible to argue against the inevitability of death, this point of view also has other more subtle implications. The first is that any other point of view about death, including the view that one's uncontrolled personal annihilation is a tragedy, is then considered an adaptive attitude lower on a hypothetical hierarchical scale. Although it would seem obvious that the acceptance of death as a reality would ease the passage toward it, and in fact many people who are dying appear to experience this attitude, it is still not acceptable to many. In addition, it is difficult to define acceptance and to precisely delineate the constellation of attitudes and behaviors which should accompany it. Whether one views death in these terms or in terms of a desired or undesired hereafter or cosmic union, it appears to be an issue whose resolution should not be placed on the already overburdened shoulders of the dying, the bereaved, and the health care team unless as individuals they actively seek or are consoled by exploring it.

The second questionable thesis stems in part from the first, and immeasurably adds to the burden of those mentioned above. This involves the notion that the dying as well as the bereaved must pass through certain prescribed stages, experience specific feelings, and last, but certainly not least, openly discuss these with others. What follows is frequently a well-intentioned, but misguided effort to help the people involved conform to a theoretical notion rather than allow their unique individual expression of their suffering. This frequently results in a significant feeling of failure by all involved with all its attendant implications.

Nevertheless, the thanatology movement has contributed significantly to the increasing awareness by society of the issues of death and dying and the higher level of humane care now being offered in many facilities and by numerous people in all disciplines. In spite of this improvement, there is much work to be done, because many segments of society have fostered and reinforced a general ignorance about how the individual copes with dying and how families cope with the process of bereavement.

## DEATH: THE CULTURAL MILIEU

The cultural milieu has considerable importance in determining overall attitudes toward death and dying, and our culture has been changing rapidly. The traditional elevated status of the elderly has shifted to youth, and even the middle-aged attempt to incorporate the standards and dress of the young. Modern living arrangements have changed drastically and there has been a shift toward geographic mobility and small family units. The decline of the extended family structure has contributed to feelings of estrangement and lack of support, in addition to a decrease in direct exposure to death.

In rural societies, animals, infants, children, and young adults frequently died, and there was little insulation from direct contact with death. There was little feeling of control over the forces of nature, in contrast to the present day need to view everything, including death, as a potential for mastery. At times, it appears as though anything that reminds us of our lack of mastery tends to be demeaned or excluded. In Western society, there rarely are epidemics or disasters that tend to remind us of our vulnerability, and our achievements in modifying these forces have contributed to our quest for omnipotence. Death has also become visually less evident because of the shift of the dying from private homes to institutions and the relative availability of medical comforts.

In spite of its greater visibility in previous generations, and presumably its greater acceptance, the meaning of death has always presented the human being with one of his most frightening challenges. An endless amount of projections and wish-fulfilling fantasies have always pervaded belief systems concerning the meaning of death. The trauma of death on the survivors has also resulted in a host of rituals, which vary in detail but appear to share the goals of adjusting to or controlling personal annihilation, object loss, guilt, and anticipated potential punishment. Conceptualizations vary from attempts to totally ignore the omnipresence of death to the seductive but highly speculative theoretical formulations which promote the fear of death as the determining factor in human character formation, creativity, and mental illness.[1]

We must, however, be careful to avoid the all-encompassing generalizations which prevent an understanding of certain subcultures as well as individuals. Although it appears to be true that open communication about death and contact with the dying is discouraged in much of our culture, this may be limited to the technologically advanced segments. Garrity and Wyss recently reported the results of an historical survey and questionnaire study of contemporary death practices in Kentucky. They compared Appalachian and non-Appalachian regions and found that, in terms of death visibility, they are tending to become more similar. In addition, the questionnaire survey indicated that "death denial, avoidance, and invisibility are not the norm in Kentucky, contrary to what has been suggested in much of the death literature describing trends in Western society."[2]

## THE SETTING OF DEATH

Unless death is sudden, it is very likely to occur in an institution. More than two-thirds of deaths occur in hospitals, nursing homes, or other similar institutions; and in cities, the amount is even higher.[3] Most of the deaths occur in hospitals, with the vast majority occuring in general hospitals. The occurrence of death in hospitals or nursing homes usually results in the patient's loss of the comfort of dying in familiar surroundings with his family around him. The variable of who has control over their lives at the time of death determines where people die. The more physically or emotionally debilitated people are, the more likely it is that they will die in an institution, because the decision concerning their death will be made by their families, friends, or health professionals. Death in institutions is significantly out of the control of those who are dying. Unfortunately, most institutions and their staffs still invest more energy attempting to deny the impact of the dying patient and bereaved family than encouraging transactions between them. The predominant reasons for this, lie not only with the needs for administrative convenience and emotional distance, but also in the personal characteristics, background, and training of the members of the health care team.

## THE PHYSICIAN

The physician has traditionally been the individual with the most responsibility for the management of dying patients of all ages and, in spite of the fact that this responsibility is increasingly being shared with others, he still remains a key figure. Although the desire to relieve suffering and forestall death is central to the practice of medicine, there have been indications that prior to entering medicine, concerns about death are an important preoccupation of the future physician. Feifel et al. have reported an empirical study which focused on physicians' feelings about and reactions to death. His group conducted in-depth interviews with internists, surgeons, and psychiatrists, and compared their responses with medical students, seriously or terminally ill patients, and apparently healthy "normal" individuals. Feifel felt that the results supported the contention that physicians, as well as medical students, tend to have an above average fear of death and use their profession to attempt to master personal concerns about it. They also found that physicians were more likely to reflect on their own mortality when learning of a death and were more apprehensive about the dying process than either the physically ill or the healthy, "normal" group.[4]

In his training, the physician becomes desensitized not to death, but to the symbols of death. Dysphoric emotions, stimulated by contacts with severely ill and dying patients, provoke a variety of adaptive defenses. While these defenses make it possible for doctors to diagnose and treat illness without being overwhelmed by interfering preoccupations with disease and death, these concerns are usually not far removed from consciousness. In fact, physicians have been noted to postpone medical care for themselves and manifest other evidence of significant denial of illness.

As he becomes more experienced, the physician assimilates large amounts of scientific data and this, combined with the sophisticated use of modern scientific equipment, contributes to increasing his self-esteem. Nevertheless, the increasingly complex information to be learned and machinery to be mastered further isolate the physician from his own feelings and those of others, thereby allowing him to deny threats of pain, disintegration, and death.

Our rapidly expanding scientific era of medicine has contributed to increasing physician specialization, especially in many illnesses that lead directly to death. This results in the shifting of patients from one specialist to another and the avoidance of confronting the personal issues of dying with the patient. It especially protects the physician from directly dealing with the anger, helplessness, and increased dependence of patients who may not be improving. To be impotent in the face of rampant disease strikes at the heart of the physician's narcissism. Under these circumstances, and especially if the patient reminds him of someone in his own personal life, the physician may react with denial, disappointment, disgust, anger, or indifference. "Discontinuous special care giving" is protective for the physician, but tends to isolate the patient and his family.[5]

In spite of these difficulties, there have been changes in physician response to dealing with dying patients and their families. In the late 1950s, Oken did a combination questionnaire and interview study in which attending physicians at a large Chicago hospital were surveyed in regard to informing the cancer patient of his diagnosis and the reasons for their decision to inform or disguise. About 90 percent of the respondents indicated that they did not tell patients their diagnosis. Those that did, employed euphemisms, and only did so if issues of practical importance (e.g., financial responsibility) were involved. It was also clear that, while physicians claimed that "experience" was the determinant of their policy, this did not bear up under critical observation.[6] Recently, however, Rea, Greenspoon, and Spilka reported an exploratory study of the attitudes and behaviors of 151 physicians in 10 medical specialties toward terminally ill patients. Their subjective responses indicated considerable concern and interest about terminal illnesses. Repeated expressions of their personal involvement in the deaths of their patients were offered. There was some indication that older doctors may be more uncomfortable when dealing with terminal patients.[7] In contrast to Oken's study, most physicians questioned were willing to tell patients about their terminal condition, and the majority felt this must be done. In addition, extreme measures to maintain life were rejected, and a majority, at least consciously, did not regard the dying patient as a personal failure. Although this is only one study among many with opposite results, it may indicate that physicians' attitudes are gradually beginning to shift in response to more discussions about death and more patient demands for honesty in communication.

## THE NURSE

The most intense emotional and physical contact with the dying person is usually experienced by nurses. They are responsible for the care of the immediate needs of the patient and, therefore, perform many of the most distasteful functions for the dying and bereaved. They frequently perform these functions, however, without feelings of mastery or the gratification of being appreciated. This is especially true in the nurses's relationship with the physician, who may obligate her to follow and reinforce his decision regardless of the nurse's own opinions, which may be based on superior knowledge of the patient and family.

Quint has reported that nursing students are well prepared for the physical and technical aspects of the care of the dying, but poorly prepared for psychosocial tasks.[8] The fact that nurses as well as physicians have received an inadequate amount of training to equip them to handle the psychosocial aspects of the dying patients has made them vulnerable to learned coping styles based in their own backgrounds. They have frequently been reared in circumstances in which dying has been accepted, but feelings about it have not been pursued. This, in combination with the incorporated roles of self-control and dedication, and direct contact with the most intense affective situations, imposes a real strain on nursing personnel. They usually adapt to this by investing in routines, personal ritual, and the authoritarian structure, but the result is usually guilt and feelings of alienation.

Several studies have indirectly confirmed the above mentioned effects. Leshan reported a study in which he noted nurses' responses to their terminal patients by stop-watching the interval between the sounding of a bedside call and the nurses' responses. Nurses took more time to respond to calls from patients with a terminal prognosis than from patients less seriously ill, and were not aware of the variation in their responses.[9] Kastenbaum asked approximately 200 attendants and licensed practical nurses in a geriatric hospital to describe their usual reaction to a patient's mentioning the subject of death. Only 18 percent indicated they would enter into a discussion of the patient's thoughts and feelings. Lack of inclination to allow patients to talk about their feelings stemmed from desires to see the patient happy, as well as self-protective motives.[10]

Parallel to the trends occurring with physicians, many nurses are now increasingly concerned about helping the patient die in a comfortable and dignified manner, and are frequently hindered by physicians, administrators, or other nurses from performing this role. Consequently, there have been increasing numbers of conferences, seminars, and informal teaching situations to improve the nurse's ability to cope with the dying patient and formulate his role in relation to other health care personnel.

## OTHER MEMBERS OF THE HEALTH CARE TEAM

With the recently increasing emphasis on the dying patient's family, the social worker's role has expanded to a considerable degree. They may take primary responsibility for softening the pain and suffering of the survivors, and, in addition to the resolution of grief, they can act as an advocate for the family in practical matters and as a mediator between them and the members of the health care team.

Other personnel play increasingly important roles in the care of dying patients and their families. Although religion does not play as consistent and unambiguous a role in the lives of most people as it did at one time, it still may be crucial in selected populations. For those who may be comforted by religious involvement, the clergy are an important part of their care. The clergy have been assuming the primary role of caretakers of the dying for centuries, and frequently are able to provide greater comfort than any member of the treatment team. It is important to recognize, however, that the increasingly ambiguous roles played by religion in modern life have also at times created greater anxiety for clergymen.

Other personnel of varied types, including hospital administrators, physicians assistants, nurses aides, dietitians, and funeral directors, have contact with the dying as well as the bereaved. They can, to a considerable degree, reduce the anguish of those with whom they come in contact, as well as provide a responsive support network to relieve the burden of realistic and practical problems. There are no clear-cut lines of demarcation with regard to any discipline. Most of the people mentioned above can provide primary or secondary support for those patients and families who are inclined for whatever reason toward a particular individual, as long as the necessary skills are possessed and roles are clearly defined for a specific situation.

## THE FAMILY

The family of the dying patient will manifest a wide variety of responses to the anticipated or actual loss, and this will depend on the ages of the members, the past, present, and anticipated future relationship between the patient and the bereaved, the internal dynamics of each member of the family, especially in regard to the handling of significant loss and separation, and the family transactional system.

The loss of any child, and especially one who already plays a pivotal role in the family system, is one of the most devastating experiences that any human can endure, and its strain on families is frequently overwhelming. It is especially difficult in marital situations, now increasingly obvious if not more prevalent in our culture, that manifest almost constant discord and turmoil. Whether parents are together or not, preexisting tensions are aggravated by diffuse and displaced feelings of abandonment, anger, and guilt. Reactions such as shock, denial, projection, and displacement impose enormous demands on the most intact marital relationship and overload those characterized by significant denial or disruption. Siblings are frequently ignored, at least temporarily, and suffer lasting feelings of rage, guilt, sadness and a sense of isolation. All members of the family experience a period of turmoil with significant disruptions in routine activities and relationships. Gradually, adaptive patterns become more focused, helping resources are selected and utilized, and active but fluctuant grieving occurs. The possibility always remains, however, that old conflicts will be exacerbated, specific child preferences intensified, maladaptive coping patterns reinforced, and insufficient grief work accomplished. Feelings among all family members of being deprived and irreparably damaged may result, thereby hindering grandparents, parents, and siblings beyond their ability to reconstruct a new family homeostatic process.

The death of a relatively young husband or wife results in a variety of stresses on the survivors. Although there are differences in reactions to expected (usually long-term illness) or unexpected (sudden) death, there is considerable overload on the surviving spouse, not only because of grieving but because of the additional roles to be assumed. Financial, social, and familial difficulties are frequently ongoing and contribute to increased ambivalence toward the deceased during the mourning process. Growing children of deceased parents may evidence immediate or delayed bereavement reactions which interfere with the development of normal phase-related coping mechanisms and may contribute to the development of defensive styles inadequate for optimum growth.

The importance of the loss or impending loss of a spouse, especially in a marriage of long duration, cannot be underestimated no matter how ambivalent the relationship. For some, the loss of a spouse means the loss of the person with whom one has shared most of the gratifications and sorrows of living. For others, it means the loss of one of the major reasons for survival or the loss of an object upon whom one has been extremely dependent. Frequently, as couples grow older, their chief activity is the responsibility for the care of the partner, and the loss of this partner results in helplessness and hopelessness. The remaining spouse often has no one to turn to and may see no reason for living. Some are reluctant to depend on their children, especially if there have been stormy aspects to their relationship or recurrent struggles for control.

Other problems occur in families of middle-aged or elderly which tend to exacerbate accumulated grievances and antagonisms. Disease and disability may have cut into family members' finances, thus providing a nidus for the expression of overt or covert anger. Family systems previously dependent on certain kinds of pattern behaviors on the part of the participants may rupture under overwhelming stress, thus leaving the members confused, frightened, and unable to deal adequately with the feelings and tasks at hand.

Other family members, perhaps ill-prepared for the job, may have to assume some of the roles of the dying patient. If there is conflict over the shifting of roles within the family, threats of disintegration erupt. The concentration of family resources on the ill member may necessitate a change of the established family patterns of gratification. Especially if denial and isolation have been important family coping mechanisms, a grave prognosis may be met with a conspiracy of silence and the loss of the opportunity to deal with anxiety and grief. This may also interfere with realistic planning for both the dying patient and the survivors.

While some report a preference for the care of terminally ill patients at home,[11, 12] there is considerable disagreement over the issue. Some families may accomplish this with great benefit to both the dying and the bereaved, especially if they have facilities for partial hospitalization available to them. Others, however, may attempt to care for very ill family members at home out of guilt or the inability to separate, with disastrous consequences for all concerned. Instead of relative calm, there is turmoil, with resultant unresolved feelings about the dying patient and the dying process.

In some situations, mutual nonsupport and withdrawal reinforces a feeling of abandonment for the dying patient and those around him. This becomes a fertile environment for the expression of hostility and blame, which becomes easily displaced onto other areas. The patient will sense the tension and respond with his own withdrawal or increased complaints and irritability. Those who have intense needs to excercise control may do so in irrational ways, such as not taking even a short break from the patient and neglecting any satisfactory and pleasurable aspects of living. The frustration and anger may then be projected to the caretakers, relatives, and friends. Anger at caretakers may result in a desperate quest for superfluous consultations or unwise treatments resulting in needless expense, frustration, and anguish.

## THE PATIENT

The previously reviewed systems are in continuous transaction with the patient who is dying and are important factors in determining the patient's reactions to dying. Equally and potentially more important determinants, however, are those related to the characteristics of the patient and his belief systems. These occur within the context of recent as well as past experiences. The following are some of those determinants:

1. Stage of the life cycle
2. General physical and mental health
3. Religious orientation
4. Socioeconomic, educational and occupational status
5. Symbolic meaning of death based on experiences with illness, loss, and death
6. Personality characteristics of the patient, including ego strength and predominant coping mechanisms
7. Temporal distance from death
8. Attitudes and fears about death

### Stage of the Life Cycle

The very young child has a developing sense of self and little concern with the abstraction of his own nonbeing. His primary concerns are with the fulfillment of basic needs, usually by others, especially the mother. Therefore, the crucial issues in the experience of dying for the young child are bodily discomforts and separation from parents or parental figures. The increasing sense of self in the older child, as well as increasing cognitive development, stimulates more concerns about death, but the primary issues are still separation and maintenance of immediate physical comfort. There also may be the additional factor of interpreting pain and illness as a punishment for real or imagined transgressions.

Adolescent concerns are identity and autonomy. As he gains greater control over the change in body development, he also strives to integrate this with emotional or moral commitments. Dying removes new-found intellectual, as well as physical abilities and imposes the need for submission to others as part of the process of diagnosis and treatment. This frequently precipitates a struggle between the adolescent, who must insist on some rudimentary autonomy, and his parents and the health care team, who experience their own difficulties coping with especially premature and tragic death.

The young adult tends to be in the position of learning increasing skills and fantasizing about unlimited possibilities. Death is seen as something in the distant future and life is conceived as promising many satisfactions. The development of terminal illness results in severe disappointment, considerable rage, and a struggle with a sense of futility. This is in some contrast with middle adulthood, in which many challenges have been met and the churning of youth tends to mellow with a sense of achievement and competency. There is a great deal of emphasis on the family and the deprivation of present as well as anticipated interpersonal pleasures that death brings. It also stimulates concerns about how others who have been dependent on him will fare without his presence. There is also the feeling of being deprived of some of the pleasures that decades of work have promised either overtly or by implication.

The elderly have found it increasingly difficult to satisfy their basic needs in our present cultural milieu. They are frequently concentrated in relatively segregated living situations that isolate them from the mainstream of modern society and deprived of the opportunity to perform useful services. The decrease in social contact and process of disengagement is further aggravated by their physical decline and repeated interpersonal losses of family and friends. Recognition of the dying process may be more evident to those whose former satisfactions and achievements turn into sorrows and frustrations. The meaning and previous gratifications of one's existence are especially important in determining whether death is viewed relatively calmly or with terror and rage.

## General Physical and Mental Health

The levels of general physical and mental health are important in determining responses to dying. There are considerable differences if one passes quickly from a state of generally good health to severe deterioration than a long period of uncertainty and disability with gradually diminishing function. Physical decline also produces direct and indirect effects on cognitive functions and represents deterioration and disability, which are frightening. The loss of certain functions, especially in the elderly, may lead to diminished communication and contact with others. Loss of vision and hearing may create isolation and distrust. Loss of taste and smell, combined with defective teeth and gums, is depriving of the pleasure and security of certain familiar foods. The decrease of muscle mass or strength can decrease tolerance to exercise or other rehabilitating procedures. Arthritis can limit movement and produce discomfort and pain. Cardiac arrhythmia, infarction, congestive failure, and pulmonary insufficiency can all produce discomfort, fear, and acute and chronic changes in cognitive status. Medical or surgical intervention may increase pain, disability, and sense of helplessness, thus aggravating any other difficulties present. The greater the difference between an individual's present resources and previous capacities, the more difficult coping will be and the more anxious he will become.

Little is known about the effects of long-term cognitive and behavioral dysfunction on the response to dying. It might be assumed that patients with cognitive impairment respond in a more disorganized way, and this appears to be valid in those with significant dementia.

This appears, however, to be less consistent in delirium. In a study by Kastenbaum of 60 patients between the ages of 69 and 96 who were dying, it was found that almost all had retained some ability to observe and interpret their situations just prior to death. One half of the total sample was rated as having consistently been in clear contact, and only 2 out of 60 patients were constantly out of contact during the last days of life. It is also interesting that a corollary finding was that 57 percent of the patients explicitly referred to death, and accepting attitudes were more frequent than negative or regretting ones.[13] In a study reported by Hinton, however, alertness became less common as death became imminent. One third of his patients knew nothing of their last day of existence, and only 6 percent were conscious shortly before they died.[14]

## Religious Orientation

It is commonplace to regard religion as playing a vital role in reactions to death and dying. Traditional teaching expresses the view that the more religious an individual, the more he faces death with equanimity. Although there is certainly some anecdotal evidence for this, it is not consistently seen clinically. Swenson has reported that people with more fundamental religious convictions and more religious activities look forward to death more than do those with less fundamental convictions and activities.[15] In a review of the literature, Lester concludes that results are conflicting but suggests that "religious beliefs do not affect the intensity of the fear of death but channels the fear onto the specific problems that each religion proposes."[16] The questionable effect of religion was also raised by Hinton as part of a study of previous personality on reactions to terminal cancer. He found that the "strength of religious faith and observation had little consistent influence on the patient's response to dying," but added that individual differences may have been lost in group comparisons. He also noted that the one statistically significant finding was in those people with more apparent faith. They were rated by their husband or wife as less depressed.[17]

## Socioeconomic, Educational, and Occupational Status

Riley reported a study in which people were asked what first came to their minds when they thought about death. He found that the lower the socioeconomic status, the greater the concern for the self; the higher the socioeconomic status, the greater the concern for others. He also concluded that a person's age is less directly related than his education to his view of death. In each age category, the higher the education level, the less likely people felt threatened by death, and the more active they were in actions and plans they took in approaching it.[18] In apparent contrast to this, Gorer has reported that, in contemporary Britain, as one ascends the social status scale, the degree of isolation from death and dying is increased. In upper-middle classes, family members were present in 1 out of 8 deaths in contrast to working class families, where they were present in 1 out of 3 deaths.[19]

## Symbolic Meaning of Death

An individual's reaction to death and the process of dying will ultimately depend on what death signifies to him. This will be determined by his assimilation of cultural and family attitudes, personal experiences, and his conceptions of death as it relates to intrapsychic and interpersonal unresolved conflicts, whether concrete or symbolic. Some of the meanings of death and dying in our culture are:

1. Cessation of existence or extinction with loss of identity
2. Indefinite continuation of existence in some type of hereafter or cosmic union based on religious or other beliefs
3. Extreme dependency
4. Extreme disability and/or pain
5. Reunion with a previously lost object
6. Separation from loved ones
7. Total isolation
8. Abandonment
9. Reward or punishment, usually associated with religious beliefs and producing associated changes in guilt and self-esteem
10. Relief of emotional and/or physical pain
11. Defeat of man by nature
12. Ultimate proof of the meaninglessness of life
13. A fear that is representative and symbolic of other more specific fears related to intrapsychic conflicts

It seems evident that a patient will respond to the idea of death differently if he sees it as an opportunity for reunion with a lost object within the context of some type of indefinite continuation of existence rather than a separation from loved ones. In the former, there would be an element of anticipation, while in the latter, sadness would predominate. In actuality, most people accept a variety of meanings, and their reactions will vary.

### Coping Styles and Reactions to Dying

There is very little hard data on the relationship between coping styles or other similar parameters, such as personality patterns or ego strength, and reactions to dying. Wolff attempted to relate personality patterns with reactions to death. He divided 90 patients into different personality pattern types, and then asked questions about aging and death. He felt that his data indicated that adjustment patterns throughout life were predictive of responses to aging and death, and that the older person demonstrates an accentuation of lifelong personality defenses.[20] Methodological limitations, however, preclude any valid generalizations based on the study.

Hinton studied 22 male and 38 female married, terminally ill cancer patients by interviewing the patient, the spouse, and the senior nurse on the patient's ward. Previous information concerning personality, marital patterns, and religious traits was obtained from the patient's spouse. Information about the patient's reactions to his illness came from the patient, the spouse, and the senior nurse. The mean time from the initial assessment interview until death was about 9 weeks. When evaluated, they had been inpatients for at least two weeks, and physical distress had been presumably brought under "reasonable" control. Although assessments were standardized, the patients were in three different hospitals. Those who were seen by the spouse as having coped actively with life's demands seemed to be less depressed, anxious, irritable and withdrawn when using the nurses' ratings. Also, those who faced problems directly in the past were more likely to indicate an awareness that their illness might be fatal. There was a tendency for people who had been regarded as "hypernervous individuals" to reveal to nurses their concern over dying, but there was no statistically significant difference in assessments of anxiety and depression between those judged previously "neurotic" and those judged as "stable." Two factors associated with an easier adjustment to dying were a sense of fulfillment in life and a good marital relationship. With these factors, there seemed to be less emotional distress and less concern about the outcome. Hinton cautions, however, that the results of the correlations were never very high and that, in all probability, "other factors in the situation contributed a major portion of the variance."[17]

In another type of psychosocial analysis, Weisman and Worden[21] used information from psychological autopsies of cancer deaths and attempted to correlate survival with psychosocial findings. They used a series of multiple regression equations from patients who died of more common types of cancers to generate an expected survival score for each individual patient. They compared this with the patient's actual survival, and obtained what they term a survival quotient. In spite of the obvious limitations of this approach, which Weisman and Worden recognized, and the limitations of their psychosocial data-gathering, which at times was open ended and retrospective, some interesting findings emerged. Longevity, as measured by the survival quotient, was positively correlated with patients "who could maintain active and mutually responsive relationships, provided that the intensity of demands was not so extreme as to alienate the people responsible for the patient's care." In contrast to this, shorter survival was found among patients who had a history of long-standing "alienation, depression and destructive relationships." The attitudes of these patients also reflected more despondency, desire to die, and considerable complaining. It was also recognized that the longer-survival patients may at times deny the seriousness of their illness, as well as their progressive weakening. Even if the long survival patients expressed anger, it did not alienate others.[21]

Although much further work needs to be done, some tentative conclusions appear to be warranted. Of the coping styles studied thus far, the ones correlated most consistently with more acceptance and less dysphoric symptoms during the terminal stage of life appear to be a history of active coping with life's stresses, a sense of fulfillment from life, and consistent mutually gratifying relationships with others, especially those closest to them.

## Time Perception and Reactions to Dying

Time and one's perception of it will have considerable effect on reactions to dying. Time perspective changes in accordance with the temporal distance from death, and it affects the patient's and family's perception of their needs. The perception of time remaining is related to the stage of illness that the patient and those around him perceive him to be experiencing. Weisman outlines three stages of fatal illness in which stage one begins with "the onset of symptoms until the diagnosis is made," stage two is "the interval between diagnosis and the onset of terminal decline," and stage three starts when "active treatment is found to have diminishing value."[22]

Pattison[23] also subdivides the process of dying into three clinical phases. The first is the acute phase in which he regards the main force as "the crisis of knowledge of death," in the sense that the crucial task is to adaptively cope with the "peak anxiety" that occurs with the realization that the time remaining is finite in more than an abstract sense. The next phase is the chronic living-dying phase in which there is physical decline and the presence of a variety of fears concerning the process of dying. The terminal phase begins when the "dying person begins to withdraw into himself." Dividing the clinical course is helpful in delineating certain stage-related events, fears, and tasks which must be coped with. It must be emphasized, however, that the fears and tasks are related to the individual's life experiences, feelings, coping techniques, and present relationship, and may vary in presentation and intensity.[23]

No matter what clinical stage patients may be experiencing, they may have a varying sense of time perspective or a sense of acceleration as Kastenbaum and Aisenberg point out.[24] They state that "two people who see themselves as being at the same temporal distance from death may differ markedly in their sense of rate of approach." Their anxiety may be directly related to their sense of imminence. Kastenbaum also feels that time is less fascinating and precious and, therefore, death is less formidable for many old people.[25] The concept of time is also important in the relationship between staff and patient. The sense of time of the staff and of the dying patient may be totally different. The staff may feel that they are keeping the dying patient waiting only a few minutes, but to the patient it may seem like hours.

Verwoerdt and Elmore conducted a year long study of 30 hospitalized patients with fatal illness. As might be expected, those who were closer to death expressed more hopelessness and a greater reduction of expectation of futurity.[26] Lieberman also reported that during the last few months of life there is a sharp rise in focus on the body and a feeling that it is a less adequate instrument. He also reported affective responses indicating an increased sense of hopelessness and shrinking away from future orientation.[27] These studies appear to confirm the thesis that there is awareness of the time remaining, and that emotional reactions will, to some degree, be dependent on that awareness.

### Attitudes and Fears about Death

It is difficult to specifically evaluate the attitude of most people toward death since most studies have focused on direct inquiry which may yield superficial, defensive reactions, or projective testing whose results are almost always inferential. It is likely, however, that some people express attitudes that reflect the kinds of feelings that will predominate even when their dying becomes an immediate reality. It does appear that there are differences between people in regard to how often they think about death and what kinds of affects they have in relation to those thoughts. It is also likely that for the individual it is difficult to separate frequency of death thoughts from the internal, symbolic meanings of death, and at this time there has been little work done to establish whether they are totally interdependent and how other factors including general coping mechanisms affect them.

### Coping with Death and Dying Reactions

The evaluation of which coping mechanisms are being used by a particular patient must include a consideration of how close the patient is to dying, what are the specific threats to life and their symbolic meanings, premorbid adaptive techniques, accumulated life experiences and relationships, and the expectations of those in the immediate environment and the nature of their transactions with the patient. In addition, the health care team must always be aware of the fact that an individual's capacity varies at different times and with different stresses, and should not be viewed as static or immutable.

Coping mechanisms will vary, depending upon the stage of illness and the consequent task to be mastered. For example, when the patient first begins to be aware that something unusual is wrong physically, and that it will not disappear spontaneously, anxiety begins to mount. It continues to rise to intense levels if it becomes even partially clear that the illness has a dreaded name or will not be amenable to treatment. If this is further crystallized into the knowledge that the process of dying will be transferred from an abstract to an immediate reality, the anxiety becomes overwhelming. At this time, it will be necessary for the patient to utilize various kinds of mechanisms which exclude the threat or its significance from awareness in order to cope with the variety of fears which are conscious and unconscious. These include such mechanisms as repression, suppression, rationalization, and denial, which are attempts to minimize the dangerous significance of perceived information. All these mechanisms will continue to play varying roles throughout the patient's course depending on a variety of factors. They should not be construed as "pathological" defenses unless they significantly interfere with the treatment necessary for the management of the specific illness or with the maintenance of previously satisfactory personal relationships other than for limited periods of time. Even denial, which is the repudiation of external reality or its significance, should be considered as adaptive at times, in the sense that it may allow the patient to assimilate painful information within the limits of his tolerance.

There has been much discussion concerning the nature of the coping mechanisms and emotional symptoms of the dying patient. Kubler-Ross, in her extensive work, has identified five stages through which she feels most terminally ill patients pass. The first stage is said to be denial, which allows the patient to gradually assimilate the reality and mobilize other defenses in response to the fact of certain death. This is replaced by anger and resentment toward others, including family and health care personnel. The next stage is bargaining, which is an attempt to postpone pain, disability, and death in return for some promise of good behavior. When the terminally ill patient can no longer deny his illness, he begins to experience a sense of loss and depression. Kubler-Ross feels that when given help in working through these stages, the patient finally reaches a stage of acceptance in which he withdraws from others and awaits his fate with a sense of peace.[12]

Although Kubler-Ross acknowledges that there are overlaps of the stages and that all patients do not demonstrate all stages on an equivalent basis, she implies that, with enough time as well as proper observation and support from treating personnel, these stages are virtually universal. Others, using their own clinical experience or more objective methods, take issue with her results.

Hinton studied 102 patients who were expected to die within six months and a matched control group of seriously ill but not dying patients. Both groups were in the same ward and were seen by the same physician on the same day. He found that only 20 percent of the dying patients were certain they were going to die a week before death. Twenty percent thought death probable in an immediate sense. The dying patients were in more physical distress than the control group and were more depressed and anxious than the controls. They were also more depressed than anxious. Anxiety seemed to be related, especially during the last two weeks of life, to the presence of certain physical symptoms such as dyspnea but did not seem to have much relationship to the patients' awareness of their shortened life expectancy.[28]

Withdrawal is not necessarily the predominant mode of behavior in those who are about to die according to a study by Kastenbaum and Weisman. They studied patterns of behavior occurring just before death and they found that two types predominated. Some patients accepted the prospect of death explicitly, withdrew from social activities and refused medical assistance. Others remained involved in activities and relationships, even though they recognized that death might come at any time. Dramatic expressions of anxiety occurred in patients who were highly disturbed in general or who demonstrated an advanced degree of organic deterioration.[29]

Although it is difficult to compare the work of the different authors, since their samples, methods of data collection, and terminology were not uniform, it is nevertheless clear that opinions are not congruent on the precise sequences of responses in the dying. In addition, much of the data is anecdotal and impressionistic and is, therefore, open to varied interpretations. It should also be noted that one must study the relationships among all the variables mentioned above, especially the precise stage of the patient's illness.

As the illness proceeds and the realization of its potential consequences begins to intrude into consciousness, many fears and tasks must be coped with. These vary depending upon the stage of the life cycle, the quality of the individual's life situation, the types and extent of the disabilities, and the predictability of the course of illness. At first there may be anger at and envy of those around the patient. Concerns about the illness interfering with life's goals, day-to-day satisfactions and responsibilities emerge. A breadwinner may be primarily concerned with the continued sustenance of those who are dependent on him. A person who is responsible for the care of a household and the nurturance of children may be preoccupied with their welfare. When life's roles, which for most people are the primary reinforcers of self-esteem, are interfered with, the results are usually guilt, sadness, and feelings of inadequacy and worthlessness. Some will respond to these emotions with withdrawal, and others will respond by blaming those who are convenient targets for their anger. These may include family, friends, or health care providers.

There are a profusion of responses which occur as the treatment begins to have less effect on the course of the disease or as the process of dying becomes further contemplated. These responses are inconstant, may or may not be conscious, and are frequently expressed in disguised forms. The significance of one's life is reevaluated in the light of previous accomplishments, gratifications, and goals, with a sense of frustration predominating if the fantasied future attainment of certain goals has been vital in the maintenance of self-esteem. The future begins to possess progressively unknown qualities, and all sense of mastery is lost. There are fears of annihilation and nonexistence. These, as with all concerns about dying, may be expressed directly or indirectly.

Patients may express grief over the anticipated loss of family and friends. This may be combined with expressed fears of loneliness or fears of abandonment. The patient may indicate a concern over imposing on the people around him or of losing his importance to those with whom he has been close. At times, these fears are based on realistic expectations, because past experiences with others may have been fraught with conflict and threats of separation. In others, the fears are projections and are based on fantasies nurtured by shame and guilt.

As the terminal illness begins to involve more systems and produce more disability, the above mentioned concerns are heightened and combined with fears of dependency (and helplessness). There is progressive loss of a feeling of control over one's bodily functions, especially if the structures responsible for bladder and bowel control are involved. There are concerns about increasing pain and suffering and fears of being helpless in the face of rampant disease. Fear of loss of control may lead to concerns about symbolic regressions as well as behavioral ones. Some people may even cope with the threat of dissolution by the production of states of altered body awareness, time perception, and mystical reunion fantasies with people or the universe. Although these feelings may at times be adaptive,[30, 31] they can also be frightening and overwhelming.

As death draws closer, adaptive capacities are further taxed. Most patients are aware of their impending deaths, by virtue of their progressive physical decline or the change in attitude or behavior of others toward them, but only make vague references to it or choose not to talk about it at all. Some may talk about it in definite terms on one visit, but only in possibilities on another. Some wait for a cue from another person because of fears of imposing too much burden or grief on those involved with them. At times, religious, socioeconomic, or cultural differences will prevent honest communication between the patient and those around him. There are others who attempt to handle their fears by protecting themselves against the realization of death, and they may present the picture of stoic resignation or even cheerfulness. The picture of stoicism in some, however, may indicate acceptance without denial, especially in those for whom stoicism represents their characteristic adaptational response. Some may displace concerns about death onto specific physical complaints, insomnia, or excessive concern about others. It would seem appropriate to recognize that no one can constantly retain thoughts of their own dying without some respite, and those closest to death are no exception.

In spite of all the difficulties, a measure of acceptance is still the rule for most dying patients, especially the elderly and those who are given an opportunity to mourn their losses. The acceptance may be expressed in withdrawal with an accompanying explanation or in increased concerns with a philosophy of transcendence and a focus on the continuation of progeny. Some are even able to complete practical tasks in relation to business, family, or the disposition of their own body and the accompanying ceremony. While some withdraw without involvement with those around them, others maintain contact and interest until consciousness begins to diminish. Unfortunately, there are a group of patients who are not able to accept the inevitable and whose terminal behavior is marked by intense anger, conflict, unreasonable demands, and refusal to cooperate with those in their immediate environment. They are frequently younger, with a greater sense of unfinished business, a conviction that life has generally been cruel, or a feeling that the reality of death somehow reinforces a chronically low self-esteem. This is especially true if severe pain and dyspnea are present and significantly unresponsive to specific treatments.

## THE PROCESS OF DYING WITHIN INSTITUTIONS

The final responsibility for the care of most dying patients rests in those health care professionals who function in an institutional setting. Strauss and Glaser have studied the interaction between those involved in the process of dying in institutions and have noted what they term "patterns of dying."[32] They have observed that each service in the hospital has its own kinds of deaths and the subsequent development of expectations of appropriate behavior toward patients and families. They also outline a "dying trajectory" which enables certain predictions to be made. When these predictions do not materialize, the staff becomes anxious and develops maladaptive coping patterns of their own. The predictions are attempts to establish patterns which allow the development of feelings of mastery but are frequently too rigid. This contributes to staff disorganization when the sense of mastery is frustrated and patient care is impaired. The staff can usually manage with less anxiety a patient who dies quickly, because the focus of care is on technical aspects. Slow dying presents more problems because the patient and his family must be confronted as human beings, and identifications with their personal characteristics must be made. Slow dying, however, also offers an opportunity for the staff to work through their feelings of significant loss providing the milieu is supportive of it.

The staff's reactions to the death of a particular patient will depend on their conscious and unconscious perception of his social value, likeability, and qualities which may remind them of someone in their own family. The aged tend to have a low social value, since they have lived "long enough," and the young and "successful" have a high social value. The perception of low social value may lead to a lower level of care on the part of the staff and increased hopelessness on the part of the patient.

Strauss and Glaser documented the common practice of placing a dying patient in a room alone during his last days. Although this may be appropriate for some, it increases fears of abandonment, and may lead to more demands on the staff. This tends to result in guilt and mutual recrimination.

Another focus for conflict is what Strauss and Glaser refer to as "manipulation of the trajectory" which involves staff decisions about the timing of death. The decision to prolong or shorten life acts a fulcrum around the issues of who influences those decisons. They also become displacements for intense feelings about the patient, the family, or other staff members. Attempts to resolve these conflicts sometimes result in intensification of negative transactions, with resultant increasing isolation of the patient and helplessness of the staff.

Institutions always have expectations of families in regard to their behavior in the period of anticipatory grief. If the family is perceived by the staff as pleasant, grieving "appropriately," and understanding, support is forthcoming. This may even extend to allowing the family to carry out certain basic nursing tasks. If the family is perceived as exceeding its bound, however, there will be conflict with destructive consequences. This will especially occur if the basic rules of conduct are unclear and unexpected stress occurs. This will provoke disagreement concerning management, as well as unresolved mutual anger.

At the present time, institutions are beginning to emerge which attempt to provide more humane care to the dying patient and his family. Some provide part-time care and some full-time, but most are modeled after St. Christopher's Hospice in London, which has attempted to provide a therapeutic community atmosphere for its patients and staff. [33, 34] The physical setting consists of large open wards, but includes flower-boxed corners for privacy, large windows with bright light, and easy access to spacious gardens. Families are invited to share in the caretaking, and children and pets are welcomed. Staff members are encouraged to touch patients while caring for them. Heroin and gin are used freely with regular around the clock medication established as routine treatment if indicated. It is the impression of patients, family, and staff that the humane care offered at St. Christopher's lends dignity to all involved.

## MANAGEMENT: THE INITIAL STAGE OF TREATMENT

Specific preparation for the care of the terminally ill must begin as soon as a diagnosis has been established and it is clear that survival must be thought of in limited terms. Initially, a thorough evaluation of the patient and his family must be made with attention to the factors mentioned above. This will require interviews with the patient and his family which initially should be done individually and at some point jointly. These can be used to acquire necessary and pertinent information, assess needs, establish a relationship, and make the commitment to provide whatever support is necessary. It is not sufficient to make a series of medical and/or psychiatric diagnoses. The emphasis must be on understanding their feelings, coping styles, concerns, and transactions.

The initial contact will allow the beginnings of an alliance between the patient, family, and members of the health care team. It will also enable those responsible for the treatment to evaluate and explore the pertinent patient and family concerns, as well as their transactions, before any actual treatment is undertaken. It is the time when commitment can be made to the patient and family. Weisman uses the term "safe conduct" to describe the kind of care that must be promised to those patients who will be obliged to surrender their autonomy and control to someone else as their illness progresses.[22] Safe conduct assumes that a physician has made a commitment to control pain and suffering and that he will approach the patient with "acceptance, clarity, candor, compassion, and mutual accessibility."

In any relationship that is considered "therapeutic" or helpful, truth and honesty must be considered as basic ingredients. Nevertheless, they must be consistent with the patient's coping capacities at the moment of the encounter. Within this limitation, the patient's diagnosis and prognosis should be discussed with him, and the information provided gently and gradually while looking for cues to what is needed. Only one issue at a time should be dealt with, since sensory overload confuses and overwhelms, especially in the area of dying. The patient's and the family's ideas about the illness and its care should be actively solicited, since their behavior is frequently a response to fantasies about illness rather than realities. In this situation, however, the realities are frequently harsh and they must be incorporated in stages.

Honesty within reasonable limits will help avoid the tense "conspiracy of silence" atmosphere which tends to increase the patient's isolation and deny him the opportunity to express feelings to family and friends, settle financial affairs, and resolve old interpersonal or religious conflicts. It also allows the patient to control as much of his remaining life as is possible by participation in the determination of the disposition of possessions and the choice of whatever ceremony may follow his death.

The patient should be told the details of his illness and the treatment possibilities in specific, but careful terms without removing hope within the patients definition of the term. Specific time limits of life expectancy should not be discussed unless there are specific issues related to an event occurring in the future. The patient should be provided with some concept of the reasonable expectations and limitations imposed by his disease and the commitment to provide an environment which, as much as possible, will provide auxiliary functions to those limitations.

The discussion of the illness and its consequences must be accomplished even more carefully in those who have an organic brain syndrome. These patients may not be able to assimilate even a moderate amount of information at one time. Nevertheless, the most common organic brain syndrome that is encountered is delirium,[35] and this tends to fluctuate with the amount of acute physical decompensation. If the underlying acute physical process is treated, the patient may resume his previous level of function and may once again participate in decision making as well as exploration of his feelings.

All treatment procedures should be discussed with the patient prior to their implementation and, if he comprehends their nature, he should participate in the decision concerning their use. The withholding of information and decision-making power from a patient who wants to know and participate in his treatment is to deny that individual's right to a personally meaningful autonomous existence. A thorough discussion and clarification of any procedure before it is done will minimize magical expectations or irrational fears of disfigurement or retribution. With each new procedure and possible new disability, the patient must be allowed to express his distress. The patient's active participation should be sought at all times. Although allowances must be made for the disabilities produced, behavioral regression should be discouraged since this usually diminishes self-esteem.

As much as possible, family cohesion must be promoted through the sharing of information and feelings as long as the family indicates verbally and behaviorally that adequate coping devices are available and are being utilized. Denial in the patient or the family should only be challenged aggressively when it interferes with necessary medical treatment, when it threatens to undermine family cohesion, or when family denial undermines the patient's desire for open acknowledgement. At each stage of the illness, real issues such as disruption of households, financial problems, and care of family members must be dealt with in practical terms. The aid of any family member, friend, or helping agency must be enlisted with appropriate intervention from the treatment team. The symbolic meaning of those issued may be pursued after practical help has been provided.

## PHYSICAL MANAGEMENT

During all phases of his illness, the patient's physical needs must be met before they become acute and before the patient must beg for relief. It may be necessary for others to assume increasing responsibility for ordinarily autonomous functions and, as much as possible, the patient should be involved in the timing of when this is to be done.

The adequate relief of pain is a primary function of the health care team. This should involve a concerted attempt to use medication, physical procedures, hypnosis and self-hypnosis, and any other modality available to relieve this most dreaded of all fears. The interpretation of pain as the symbolic representation of punishment should be confronted directly if there is any reason to suspect its presence.

Careful attention must be given to all the patient's physical complaints, even if they appear to be minor and unrelated to his primary disease process. Vigorous treatment should be implemented to combat discomfort, since this will tend to relieve the sense of helplessness felt by the patient and staff, as well as reinforce the patient's sense of personal worth. Attention must also be paid to other complaints that have no obvious relationship to dying but are oblique ways of expressing these fears. These include being alone in a room and fear of the dark and of closed doors. Any reasonable demands made concerning these issues should be fulfilled.

The patient should be physically touched, becaue touch is the most basic mechanism we possess of communicating and giving comfort. This should include frequent back rubs, massages, and holding hands.

The oral care of the dying patient has been discussed at length by Kutscher,[36] and is a particularly important area for concern. As Kutscher points out, the dying patient is unable to satisfactorily experience his once secure environment since it was mediated through tactile, proprioceptive, auditory, and visual senses which have usually become impaired. As physical decline continues, the patient has to rely increasingly on mouth movements for contact with the external world and for a sense of security and gratification. Poor dentition will add to already existing eating problems and will produce difficulties in speaking clearly, which further impairs self-esteem and increases isolation and helplessness. Kutscher also points out that the mouth is an area in which gratification, punishment, and conflict, both actual and symbolic, are expressed. To relieve the patient's distress and to gratify as many basic needs as possible, small frequent feedings of favorite foods and careful attention to hygiene are recommended.

Attention must be given to develop communication and provide comfort to the patient with multiple deficits. Such deficits as hearing, sight, and speech may be present and can be overcome by changing techniques of communication. The patient should still be spoken to and given the opportunity to develop hand and eye signals to respond to the treating person. Once a communication pattern is established, the family can also be taught to incorporate it in their contact with the patient. For patients who are critically ill and on intubation or resuscitative machines, eye or hand contact can be used as well. For patients who are unable to establish meaningful communication, it is still vital that they remain warm, dry, and comfortable and be gently and frequently touched.


**PSYCHOTHERAPY**


Psychotherapeutic work with the dying patient at any stage of his illness is difficult and emotionally threatening to the therapist. In no type of treatment is a person's individuality more important than in those issues surrounding his death. It is especially important here as everywhere else that respect for coping patterns and defensive systems exist. If a patient has a need to exercise denial as a predominant defense during his illness, in spite of ample opportunity to do otherwise, the denial should be supported. However, if a patient wishes to openly acknowledge impending death, explore his fears and concerns, and confront the basic issues of his living and dying with another human being, he should not be denied the opportunity. To do so may produce more isolation and depression.

While approach and management (clearly) must be individualized, the therapist will have to deal with such issues as grief, anger, fear of abandonment and annihilation, as well as concerns about the meaning of the patient's life. These issues should be handled differently depending on the patient's cognitive capacity and his ability to confront and incorporate their implications. There should be no attempt to force or even encourage the patient to talk about feelings simply for the sake of talking. Some people regard the expression of certain feelings as a weakness and a humiliation and this must be respected.

In some patients, there must be concern with the quality of their living, while in others grief and separation are the main problems. During different stages of the illness there may be grief over the loss of the previous body image, role functions, and, ultimately, over family and friends who will be left behind. Although this kind of grief is never totally "worked through," help can be given to achieve acceptance of the separation. There is also the disappointment and grief for what might have been, which is especially prevalent in adolescents and young adults who had conceived of the most gratifying and productive parts of their lives ahead of them both in relationships and accomplishments.

Butler has described the "life review," which he defines as a "naturally occurring universal mental process characterized by the progressive return to consciousness of past experiences and particularly the resurgence of unresolved conflicts; simultaneously and normally these revived experiences and conflicts are surveyed and reintegrated."[37] He feels that the process is prompted by the realization of approaching death. In some patients it is an attempt to create a sense of meaning in their lives, while in others there are lapses into guilt and sadness. Whatever the immediate stimulus, participation of the therapist in a life review might help achieve some resolution of longstanding conflicts including guilt about past misdeeds. The accomplishment of "unfinished business" may include help to achieve one last, but personally meaningful goal which will lead to a greater sense of personal worth before death.

In all situations, the therapist must act as a real person who is not afraid of the encounter although it will stimulate considerable conflict and anxiety. He must demonstrate continual concern and empathy which should be genuine, not feigned. He must be aware of the meanings of death to him, and be willing to share feelings of anger, helplessness, hopelessness, and depression with the patient if it seems to be appropriate to do so. There must be awareness of negative feelings toward the patient and family and the ability to control these feelings without the necessity to resort to overtly hostile behavior. It is important to combine a desire to help with the awareness of the limits of therapeutic and personal grandiosity. This should include the willingness to share responsibility with other members of the health care team.

From the point of view of technique, the patient should determine the subject to be discussed. The patient should be encouraged to express his feelings, and the therapist should adopt a stance of tolerance and respect for those feelings no matter how personally repugnant they may be. At times, there may be the need for reminiscing that is shared, while at other times it may be appropriate to share the patient's agony in silence. The frequency and length of visits must be determined with the patient, but as he grows closer to death, the frequency of visits should increase, and the previous length may be unnecessary. The patient should be made aware of the fact that he has touched the life of the therapist in some way and has added to his knowledge.

## MANAGEMENT OF THE MILIEU

The therapist must also remember that his contact with the patient is not the only one, and there should be communication and general agreement concerning management with all the members of the health care team. The patient's values must be explored and, if desirable, he should be put in contact with someone who shares his religious or philosophical orientation. He may want to talk about or confess something that has been previously concealed, and this accomplishment can produce profound relief as well as acceptance of death.

Throughout all stages of the illness, human contact must be made available and rewarding. Those who have contact with the patient must treat him with respect and anticipate and/or respond to all reasonable demands. The patient's environment must be made as structured and predictable as possible with full preparation for any changes. When the opportunity arises, the patient's past accomplishments and personal qualities must be valued and reinforced. The patient should be surrounded with as many family members and friends as possible (no matter what their ages), as well as personal possessions and opportunities for diversion. This will enhance self-esteem and diminish unnecessary feelings of isolation. For as long as possible, the patient should be offered the opportunity to participate in decisions concerning his care, including, in certain cases, the recognition when active treatment no longer serves his basic needs. Although the latter is a painful and profoundly complicated issue, it can no longer be ignored by our societal institutions, the professionals who are endowed with the responsibility for care, and particularly by those who are or will be the recipients of that care.

## GROUP THERAPY

There have been recent attempts to use the modality of group therapy with the terminally ill, and initial reports indicate that it may be as successful as it is in many other areas. Franzino, Geren, and Meiman described a group which met for a relatively short time, but they felt that the members were able to be helpful to one another.[38] Yalom and Greaves described a pilot study of a four-year experience with a therapy group for patients with metastatic carcinoma.[39] Their once weekly meetings were combined with training in meditation and auto-hypnosis for pain control. Although there were certain limitations, including the exclusion of patients who exhibited "massive denial" of their illness or its implications, their results were quite promising. First of all, patients learned from one another what they realistically could expect from their doctors and how to ask them the questions they wanted answered. While the authors felt that "basic existential loneliness" could not be allayed; only "appreciated," secondary interpersonal loneliness could be dealt with effectively in the group." Patients could share their thoughts concerning almost all the issues confronting them including physical and emotional concerns. The authors felt that the group members could reach out to those who had isolated themselves and could offer constructive advice concerning the treatment of the dying process. Nevertheless, the major focus of the group was on the quality of living rather than on dying, and it is here that patients reported, as they frequently do, that life appeared richer, and focused away from the trivial.

## MANAGEMENT OF STAFF TRANSACTIONS

Support must be available for staff members at all times. This may be mutual or provided by someone outside of the treatment team. No matter where emotional help is available, however, the staff must decide among themselves who is to assume the primary roles in the treatment. This initial decision process should help to minimize covert, as well as overt disagreement. For some patients and families, a team approach with different members assuming different functions, is indicated. Other patients and families, however, can only relate to one primary care provider, and this should be respected as long as undue stress is not placed on that provider.

Communication between members of the health care team must be open when practical considerations and implications of treatment are considered. Any conflicts concerning respective roles must be discussed and worked out. Clinical information must be shared, since each staff member maintains a unique point of view and may interact with the patient and family under different circumstances. The process of communication should include feelings about the patient, the family, the dying process, or the interaction with other staff members. Informal meetings among staff members who are actively involved with a particular patient have the most potential for resolving basic feelings and formulating and implementing specific treatment goals. Formal meetings, conferences, and seminars may be helpful in clarifying some of the didactic issues.

In spite of the rewarding aspects of working with dying patients and families, there are emotional demands which drain and threaten to overwhelm anyone. It is impossible for any person to function at the same level of intensity in this area for long periods of time. It would be helpful if staff members could participate in different levels of services including inpatient, partial hospitalization, and outpatient management in order to obtain the opportunity to work with people who have differing prognoses as well as needs of different urgencies. Results must always be measured in realistic terms, since human behavior is infinitely variable and rarely adheres to the ideal.

## BEREAVEMENT

Bereavement imposes significant tasks on the survivors of the deceased. Anticipatory grief usually follows the notification of the patient's poor prognosis. This includes the feeling of concern for the dying person, the experience of sadness, the rehearsal of the death, and the beginning adaptation to its consequences. If a patient survives for a significant period after the diagnosis, the protracted illness may soften the impact of the actual death, although it does not prevent the experience of stress. At times, the process of anticipatory grief may reduce the overt manifestations of mourning after the death, leading to the mistaken perception by others of a lack of feeling. This may provoke disapproval or rejection by those unfamiliar with the process and may interfere with the necessary care the health care team should provide. Grieving is manifested by a wide variety of responses which are correlated with such factors as cultural, familial, and personal expectations, as well as the precise nature of the feelings about the deceased, the symbolic meaning of the loss, and the personality characteristics of the mourners.

The personality characteristics of the bereaved are important indicators of their style in dealing with the loss. If denial is a strong part of the individual's coping system, it may interfere with acceptance of the loss which is a necessary prelude to the turning to others. If excessive helplessness and dependency exist in the bereaved, they may make unreasonable demands on others, which will alienate them and prevent appropriate support. This will lead to mutual suspicion and anger, thus reinforcing feelings of helplessness in the bereaved. The bereaved who complain and blame others as a coping style will also provoke the anger of those who are being asked for sympathy. An excessive display of exaggerated guilt or shame will provoke a punitive response which reinforces the vicious circle.

## Bereavement and the Development of Subsequent Illness

The issue of bereavement and subsequent illness has received much attention in recent years and is still being investigated by increasingly more sophisticated research studies. Thus far, most of the studies have been done with bereaved older widows, and it is only recently that men and women of different age groups, socioeconomic backgrounds, and life styles have been studied.

Parkes and his colleagues originally examined the relationship between cardiovascular disease and the increased mortality of elderly widowers as compared with married men of the same age group. They found that widowers over the age of 55 had a 40 percent higher mortality in the six months following their wives' death, and that the significant increase in mortality was because of cardiovascular disease.[40] Rees and Lutkins extended these findings to a bereaved close relative group, apparently indicating that the relationship is not restricted to husbands and wives. They found a significantly higher mortality in the first year of bereavement among the close relatives. In addition, they noted that the risk of close relatives dying during the first year of bereavement was doubled when the death occurred in the street or highway rather than at a hospital or home.[41] Another earlier study reported similar findings in young widowers, especially with death rates compared to control groups tending to decrease with increasing age.[42]

Although there is some disagreement about the evidence of death following bereavement, there seems to be increasing evidence for the occurrence of increasing physical symptomatology, especially based on self reports and increasing numbers of physician visits.[42, 44, 45] Parkes has also noted a relationship between psychiatric illness with hospitalization and the death of a spouse.[46] Lindemann reported agitated depression as a result of grief, but standardized instruments were lacking and criteria for diagnosis were unclear.[47] Other effects of grief that have been reported are increased alcohol and sedative drug intake in a widowed group.[44]

Parkes, in a recently reported study, attempted to define some of the specific factors which might predict which of the bereaved would do poorly. He studied 68 young widows and widowers for a year, and a subgroup for three years after that. The factors present at the initial interview which predicted poor outcome at one year included low socioeconomic status, short terminal illness with little warning of impending death, multiple life crises, and reactions such as severe distress, yearning, anger, or self-reproach. In addition, the bereaved whose spouses died with little warning after a short terminal illness and who evidenced intense yearning for the spouse, as well as possessing a relationship described as clinging, did poorly. They manifested "aimless depression with idealization of the dead and preoccupation with his memory." Other factors which may influence outcome are cultural and social factors which reinforce the inability to separate from the deceased.[48]

## The Stresses on the Bereaved

Other tasks await the bereaved, including the social isolation and loneliness following widowhood. The isolation is not only imposed internally, but also occurs because married friends tend to be rejecting. Those widows or widowers with young children are frequently preoccupied with their welfare and overwhelmed by their realistic and unrealistic needs and demands. Financial problems frequently add an increasing emotional burden. There are changes in family relationships as well, especially among the elderly who may be faced with the highly ambivalent choice of living with children who have already created their own lives and who resent the intrusion. Work and sexual adjustment also present considerable problems.

Another potential sequel of the death of a significant family member which may or may not be related to bereavement has been described by Bowen, who calls it the "emotional shock wave."[49] By this he means severe physical illnesses or social dysfunctions that occur as major life events in multiple members of the extended family. He attempts to delineate which family member deaths might precipitate such a wave and mentions the deaths of either parent when the family is young, an important child, and the "head of the clan." Although there is anecdotal evidence of "the emotional shock wave" in certain families, Bowen lacks carefully controlled studies to support his contention. Nevertheless, it may be an important factor to assess in any evaluation of a bereaved family.

### Clinical Features of Bereavement

The clinical features of bereavement are an initial period of shock and disbelief followed by a tearfulness, restlessness, and subjective physical distress. There may be a sense of increased distance from others, with feelings of unreality sometimes extending to misperceptions of the deceased's presence. There is usually crying, bitterness, and anger, even at times toward the deceased. There may be anorexia, difficult sleeping, and withdrawal from all previous areas of interest, combined with poor concentration and anhedonia. There may be frequent feelings of guilt which are powerful and difficult to suppress no matter how irrational. Much activity is spent thinking about and pining for the deceased, with an inability to terminate the process even when consciously desired. The dividing line between normal mourning and pathological bereavement is very difficult to define, but most observers would regard the pathological as prolonged or sustained sadness and anhedonia combined with an inability to assume age-appropriate roles or separate emotionally from the deceased and become invested in new relationships. Although grief may be a growth experience for some, the general expectation should be a functioning level consistent with coping capacities in the pregrief state.

## TREATMENT OF THE FAMILY

Before and after the patient's death, the family must be an object of intensive and sustained therapeutic activity. Failure to respond to a family's need during the patient's illness may produce barriers to the resolution of the grieving process and make the family's survival more disabling. The family must be encouraged to ventilate their feelings, including those that consist of anger toward the health care team. There should be no prohibitions against the expression of the powerful emotions because these feelings may then be displaced toward scapegoating behavior. The individual process of grieving should not be defined by anyone other than the griever. Questions by family or close friends should be answered directly and with an appreciation that advice may not be followed. The family must be helped to progress through their own stages of grief with the awareness of the meaning of the dying individual for the family system. At times it may be indicated to meet jointly with the patient and family to clarify their communications and allow them to grieve together. The institution should flexibly allow visits of family members of all ages as long as this does not substantially interfere with medical care. Minor interferences with routine should not be used as an excuse and a rationalization for the staff to avoid an emotionally difficult situation. Nevertheless, the patient and family should be encouraged to avoid interfering with the other's coping.

Before and after the death, the family members must be helped with their realistic legal, household, and financial matters, not only because these are important in themselves, but they also provide interfering displacements from grief.

The staff must be sensitive to the family's feelings about the patient's body and their concerns over its ultimate disposition. Insensitive attempts to demand autopsies and provoke more guilt will be met with justified anger and communication breakdown.

Working with the bereaved is a necessary part of the treatment of the dying. They must be encouraged to express the pain of the loss, as well as to gradually accept the finality of it. As much as possible, ambivalent feelings toward the deceased, as well as guilt and anger at abandonment, should be discussed. Gradually, the bereaved should be encouraged to give up old emotional and physical ties with the deceased, as well as understand the reasons why the relinquishing process is so difficult. This may include the transitional objects which come to represent the continued presence of the deceased and make separation very difficult. Over a period of time, the bereaved must be encouraged to reinforce old and seek new social, vocational, and sexual outlets. It may be necessary to offer practical help in establishing those outlets, including the use of contacts with the patient's family and friends. As with any other therapeutic situation, the bereaved's coping style will determine the timing and the force of any interventions. Defenses must be respected, although it may, at times, be necessary to interpret the reluctance to experience certain emotional states or grasp certain intrapsychic or interpersonal dynamic connections. In any supportive relationship, some dependency will develop, but this can be dealt with by stressing the nature of the specific tasks and allowing for periodic contact, as well as the expression of feelings of separation and loss. At times, treatment responsibilities can be shared by varied members of the treatment team, thus allowing the individual who is grieving to experience the impact of different people and utilizing those experiences to establish other relationships. For those who have a need to express their grief in physical complaints, careful support within the context of a medical setting should be provided. A group experience may also be helpful in providing support, whether it is in a therapeutic or self-help setting.

## PHARMACOTHERAPY FOR THE TERMINALLY ILL
## AND BEREAVED

A variety of psychopharmacological agents are commonly used in the management of the terminally ill and the bereaved, but their use is frequently based on inadequately documented evidence and wishful thinking. On the basis of the available evidence, the final acceptance of death by the dying individual and the final resolution of loss by the bereaved are psychosocial processes which in the majority of situations should be resolved by psychosocial treatment, with drugs being used only as temporary adjuncts. This does not include those situations in which standard psychopharmacological indications are present.

The reduction of pain is the primary indication for the use of medication in dying patients. The narcotic analgesics in appropriate pharmacological dosage and at appropriate pharmacological intervals are necessary, and to withhold them is antitherapeutic. Mixtures of alcohol, narcotics, analgesics, and psychotropic medications (cocktails) have been found to be effective. Patients should never have to beg for medication, and they should have the right to refuse it if they believe it benefits them to do so. Unless the patient indicates in some way that he desires it, pain medication should not be used to diminish the patient's awareness of his psychological state. It may also be necessary to use other methods of reducing pain, including acupuncture or surgical techniques. The recent discovery of endorphins, which are endogenous polypeptides whose biological actions resemble opiate agonists, may in time provide more help for those in significant pain, but their specific utilization is as yet unknown.[50]

Phenothiazines, among their other effects, potentiate the action of analgesic drugs, thereby producing a state in which the patient requires less of a dose of analgesics. This can be helpful to a patient who needs the antiemetic effect of the phenothiazines and requires that his high dose of narcotic analgesics be reduced because of untoward side effects. Although it is widely believed that phenothiazines reduce the patient's anxiety in regard to death, there is no conclusive evidence that this effect has been primary rather than adjunctive to pain relief. The primary effect of phenothiazines is antipsychotic with considerable effect on agitation. Some indications for their use are patients with organic brain syndromes who are out of contact with reality, extremely agitated, unresponsive to soothing personal contact, and interfering with medical care designed to improve their status. Another indication is a patient who develops a paranoid psychosis and presents a danger to the continuation of medical treatment, the rational settling of his affairs, or is threatening the family resolution of grief.

Hypnotic drugs may be used when sleeping is difficult for the patient, and antianxiety drugs may be indicated if there is apprehension and anxiety that are severe and unresponsive to psychosocial treatment methods; one must be careful, however, not to withdraw emotional support prematurely because ordering a drug may be easier than persevering to establish contact.

Hollister raises the issue of the use of tricyclic antidepressants for more severe symptoms of depression, especially if these are marked by a "loss of interest in daily activities and feelings of complete hopelessness."[51] There is, however, little hard data to support this contention and, in addition, tricyclics have significant side effects which may contribute to physical and emotional distress. The incidence of side effects including delirium is an issue for the use of all psychotropic medication in dying patients, especially with their physical deterioration which alters the dose levels they can tolerate. Definite answers in this area must await further controlled studies.

## PSYCHEDELIC COMPOUND THERAPY

Pahnke et al. have reported the use of LSD in dying patients as an attempt to induce feelings of serenity and euphoria.[51] Grof et al. have reported a clinical study in which two psychedelic compounds were used as an adjunct to a brief course of intensive psychotherapy.[52] Although they reported global improvement in emotional and physical distress, other parameters measured demonstrated no statistically significant differences and the roles of different variables were difficult to define. The role of these drugs may be to allow certain people to achieve states of altered body awareness, time perception, and mystical reunion fantasies which are important to their acceptance of death. At the present time, however, this technique must be considered experimental, although it seems to have been helpful for certain people in allowing them to feel more at peace with themselves and their families.

## USE OF PSYCHOTROPIC DRUGS IN BEREAVEMENT

Bereavement is also a state that should be dealt with primarily psychosocially rather than pharmacologically, although pharmacotherapy may be adjunctive. This may be especially true for those who experience the dispensing of drugs as nurturance. The dispersing of hypnotic or antianxiety medication as a routine way to decrease the mourner's responses to his losses should be a thoroughly condemned practice, however. Its only effect is to spare those around the mourner from being confronted with intense affect. These drugs should be used only when suffering is so intense that the process of bereavement is blocked or when agitation is so extreme that nothing constructive can be accomplished in its presence.

The antidepressants are of questionable value, with their effects in the majority of cases limited to the production of anticholinergic side effects. Until further definitive indications are established, their use should be limited to those in whom the loss precipitates an endogenomorphic process; however, at the present time, little is known concerning its early identification before the clinical picture becomes full blown. What is needed is a controlled double blind study of mourners to determine the efficacy of the antidepressants and the specific subgroup of those who develop a state responsive to them.

Some bereaved individuals will need medication for sleep if other necessary activities are compromised because of its absence, but the prescription of drugs in these circumstances should always be temporary.

Any standard psychiatric condition known previously to respond to pharmacotherapy and precipitated by bereavement should be treated accordingly.

## IMPLICATIONS FOR FUTURE RESEARCH

More rigorous studies in the area of death and dying need to be done in order to clarify some of the issues mentioned previously. The individual characteristics and the specific interactions of the variables need to be defined more precisely.

The questions that have been raised by the work done with dying patients are many and varied. Do certain kinds of people with characteristic coping styles respond in predictable ways to dying and, if so, can their treatment be oriented to those pivotal factors influencing their responses? What are the roles of different types of family systems in the reactions to chronic illness, death, and bereavement, and what can be extrapolated from them to help with the management of those states? What are the specific effects of different styles of religious commitment and socioeconomic, educational, and occupational status on reactions to death and bereavement? What is the role of such factors as previous illness, hospitalization, or the death of someone close? How can the separation process be eased for people with meaningful relationships, and how can it be resolved for those with intensely ambivalent ones? What are the long-term effects of bereavement on physical and psychiatric illness? If these exist, are they subject to different types of psychosocial interventions at the time of the stress or afterward.

What of the providers of care, and who will provide for them? How can they be helped to cope with their own feelings about dying and the intense feelings raised by frequent contacts with tragedy and death? What is the role of the social structure in promoting adaptive, rather than maladaptive responses to the dying and the bereaved? How can established institutions be changed if humane care dictates their alteration? These are some of an almost endless variety of questions that must be pursued if the quality of care is to be proportionate to the needs of those that require it. Precise definition of terms, as well as advanced statistically valid techniques, are necessary to evaluate, measure, and compare variables. Only then will we have the necessary data to compare treatment techniques and determine their effects on outcome.

In spite of the quest for hard data, our primary concern must rest with the individual and his unique experiences and responses to dying and bereavement. We must continue to search for better methods of communicating support, providing comfort, maintaining self-esteem, and promoting a sense of meaning.

### References

1.  Becker E: The Denial of Death. New York, The Free Press, 1973

2.  Garrity TF, Wyss J: Death, funeral and bereavement practices in Appalachian and non-Appalachian Kentucky. Omega 7:209–229, 1976.

3.  Freeman H, Brim OG, Williams G: New dimensions of dying. In Brim OG, Freeman H, Levine S, Scotch NA (Eds.), The Dying Patient. New York, Russell Sage Foundation, 1970, p. 17

4.  Feifel H, Hanson S, Edwards L: Physicians consider death. Proceedings of the 75th Annual Convention, American Psychological Association, Washington, D.C., 1967

5.  Krant M: Dying and Dignity: The Meaning and Control of a Personal Death. Springfield, Illinois, Charles C. Thomas, 1974, p. 53

6.  Oken D: What to tell cancer patients. JAMA 175:86–94, 1961

7.  Rea MP, Greenspoon S, Spilka B: Physicians and the terminal patient: some selected attitudes and behavior. Omega 6(4):291–302, 1975

8.  Quint J: The Nurse and the Dying Patient. New York, MacMillian, 1967

9.  Leshan L: In Bowers M, Jackson E, Knight J, Leshan L (Eds.): Counseling the Dying. New York, Thomas Nelson, 1964, p. 6–7

10. Kastenbaum R: Multiple perspectives on a geriatric death valley. Community Ment Health J 3:21–29, 1967

11. Wilkes E: Terminal cancer at home. Lancet, 1:799, 1965

12. Kubler-Ross E: On Death and Dying. Toronto, MacMillian, 1969

13. Kastenbaum R: The mental life of dying geriatric patients. Gerontology 7:97–100, 1967

14. Hinton JM: The physical and mental distress of the dying. Q J Med 32:1, 1963

15. Swenson WM: Attitudes toward death in an aged population. J Gerontol 16:49–52, 1961

16. Lester D: Religious behavior and the fear of death. Omega 1:181–188, 1970

17. Hinton J: The influence of previous personality on reactions to having terminal cancer. Omega 6(2):95–111, 1975

18. Riley J: What people think about death. In Brim OG, Freeman H, Levine S, Scotch NA (Eds.), The Dying Patient. New York, Russell Sage Foundation, 1970, p. 30–41

19. Gorer C: Death, Grief and Mourning. New York, Doubleday, 1965

20. Wolff K: Personality type and reaction toward aging and death. Geriatrics 21:189–192, 1966

21. Weisman AD, Worden JW: Psychosocial analysis of cancer deaths. Omega 6:61–75, 1975

22. Weisman A: Care and comfort for the dying. In Troup S, Greene W (Eds.), The Patient, Death and the Family. New York, Scribner's, 1974, p. 97–111

23. Pattison EM: The experience of dying. In Pattison EM (Ed.), The Experience of Dying. Englewood Cliffs, NJ, Prentice-Hall, 1977, p. 43–60

24. Kastenbaum R, Aisenberg R: The Psychology of Death. New York, Springer-Verlag, 1972, p. 223

25. Kastenbaum R: As the clock runs out. Ment Hyg 50:322–326, 1966

26. Verwoerdt A, Elmore J: Awareness of death. J Am Geriatr Soc 15:9–19, 1967

27. Lieberman M: Observations on death and dying. Gerontologist, 2:70–72, 1966

28. Hinton J: The physical and mental distress of the dying. Q J Med 32:1–21, 1963

29. Kastenbaum R, Weisman AD: The psychological autopsy as a research procedure in gerontology. In Kent DP, Kastenbaum R, Sherwood S (Eds.), Research, Planning and Action for the Aged: The Power and Potential of the Social Sciences. New York, Behavioral Publications, 1969

30. Noyes R, Jr., Kletti R: Depersonalization in the face of life threatening danger: a description. Psychiatry. 39:19–27, 1976

31. Noyes R, Jr., Kletti R: Depersonalization in the face of life threatening danger: an interpretation. Omega 7:103–114, 1976

32. Strauss AL, Glaser BG: Patterns of dying. In Brim OG, Freeman H, Levine S, Scotch NA (Eds.), The Dying Patient, New Patient. New York, Russell Sage Foundation, 1970, p. 129–156

33. Saunders C: Care of the Dying. London, MacMillian, 1960

34. Saunders C: A therapeutic community, St. Christopher's hospice. In Schoenberg B, Carr AC, Peretz D, Kutscher AH (Eds.), Psychological Aspects of Terminal Care. New York, Columbia University Press, 1972, p. 275–290

35. Lipowski LJ: Organic brain syndromes. In Benson DF, Blumer D (Eds.), Overview and Classification in Psychiatric Aspect of Neurological Disease. New York, Grune and Stratton, 1975, p. 11–34

36. Kutscher AH: The psychological aspects of the oral care of the dying patient. In Schoenberg B, Carr AC, Peretz D, Kutscher AH (Eds.), Psychosocial Aspects of Terminal Care. New York, Columbia University Press, 1972, p. 126–145

37. Butler RN: The life review: an interpretation of reminiscence in the aged. Psychiatry 26:65–76, 1963

38. Franzino M, Geren JJ, Meiman GL: Group discussion among the terminally ill. Int J Group Psychother 26:45–48, 1976

39. Yalom ID, Greaves C: Group therapy with the terminally ill. Am J Psychiatry 134: 396–400, 1977

40. Parkes CM, Benjamin B, Fitzgerald RG: Broken heart: a statistical study of increased mortality among widowers. Br Med J, 1: 740, 1969

41. Rees WD, Lutkins SG: Mortality of bereavement. Br Med J, 4:13, 1967

42. Kraus A, Lilienfeld A: Some epidemiological aspects of the high mortality rate in the young widowed group. J Chron Dis 10:207, 1959

43. Parkes C: Effects of bereavement on physical and mental health: a study of the medical records of widows. Br Med J 2:274, 1964

44. Maddison D, Viola A: The health of widows in the year following bereavement. J Psychosom Res 12:297, 1968

45. Wiener A, Gerber I, Battin D, Arkin A: The

process and phenomenology of bereavement. In Schoenberg B, Gerder I, Wiener A, et al. (Eds.), Bereavement, Its Psychosocial Aspects. New York, Columbia University Press, 1975, p. 53–65

46. Parkes CN: Recent bereavement as a cause of mental illness. Br J Psychiatry 110:198, 1964

47. Lindenmann E: Symptomatology and management of acute grief. Am J Psychiatry 101:141–148, 1944

48. Parkes CM: Determinants of outcome following bereavement. Omega 6:303–324, 1975

49. Bowen M: Family reaction to death. In Guerin PJ (Ed.), Family Therapy, Theory and Practice. New York, Gardner Press, 1976, p. 335–349

50. Goldstein A: Opiod peptides (endorphins). Pituitary & Brain Science 193:1081–1086, 1976

51. Hollister LE: Psychotherapeutic drugs in the dying and bereaved. In Goldberg IK, Malitz S, Kutscher AH (Eds.), Psychopharmacologic Agents for the Terminally Ill and Bereaved. New York, Columbia University Press, 1973, p. 65–72

52. Pahnke WN, Kurland A, Unger S, Savage R, Grof S: Psychedelic therapy with cancer patients. J Psychedelic Drugs 3:63–75, 1970

53. Grof S, Pahnke WN, Goodman L, Kurland A: Psychedelic drug assisted psychotherapy. In Goldberg IK, Malitz S, Kutscher AH (Eds.), Psychopharmacologic Agents for the Terminally Ill and Bereaved. New York, Columbia University Press, 1973, p. 91–134

54. Klein DF: Endogenomorphic depression. Arch Gen Psychiatry 314:447–454, 1974

Toksoz B. Karasu
Marc Hertzman

# 14
# Therapeutic Milieu and Medical Care: A Systems Approach

The idea that the treatment environment is a major influence upon health outcomes for the patient is as old as recorded medicine itself. Ancient accounts of the live-in clinic run by Hippocrates confirm that the Father of Medicine himself believed firmly in the efficacy of sunshine, open air, and—most important—the supportive relationship of the healer toward the suppliant.[1] At the opposite extreme, during the great plagues of Medieval and Rennaissance times, the hospital often came to be feared as the place to go to die. It was popularly recognized that there was some relationship between the house of disease and the horrors of dying away from the home among strangers. In this century, it is well-known that tuberculosis began to decline in prevalence with the advent of improved housing, lessened crowding of living space, better nutrition, and general preventive health measures before the advent of antibiotics.[2]

Nevertheless, the question remains: how much influence does the therapeutic environment, especially including the people and how they relate to each other, exert on the patient's health? Considering the centuries of interest in environmental variables, it is astounding that only recently has some attention been given to studying them systematically. This singular failure to research such matters is itself worthy of contemplation.

In this chapter we will attempt to draw upon some lessons learned about the therapeutic milieu in psychiatry since World War II in an effort to suggest where medicine might profitably benefit from psychiatry's experiences with manipulating the environment of health care both for better and for worse. We would like to know what maximizes the likelihood that patients will engage in behavior that promotes good health. In order to understand this, we need to undertake an examination of the factors that have impact upon the patient within the health care system.

After elaborating the concepts of "open and closed systems," we will try to sort out, in a medical context, what may probably lead to success or failure; and, most importantly, what attitudes have to change in order for the medical care to be humanistically therapeutic. Most of our remarks are addressed to institutional practice, both because we are more familiar with it and because we believe that the practice of medicine will continue to center in a major way upon organized institutions of care for decades to come.

## SOME "SYSTEMS" CONCEPTS FOR UNDERSTANDING THE THERAPEUTIC CONTEXT

The "environment," by definition, consists of all of those factors surrounding and/or including an individual organism. Most definitions of "environment," "milieu," or "context" are necessarily couched in a language at such a level of abstraction that they are abstruse and anything but clear about their implications. For this reason, we choose to take an approach which defines matters operationally. Since the distinguished physicist, Bridgman, originally proposed them as an alternative to formal but often tortuous all-encompassing verbalizations, operational definitions have obtained a reputable place in science.[3]

We shall start out by suggesting that all such words—"environment," "milieu," "context"—have certain operational characteristics in common, namely:

1.  They all suggest that a *system* of interrelated variables exist.
2.  The system has *boundaries,* or limits. Where these limits are taken to be, or seen to exist, however, is one of the major problems for understanding a given system.
3.  In general, if one variable within a system changes, multiple other variables are altered as well, both directly or indirectly.
4.  The system is capable of entering discrete states over time.

### "Open" Verses "Closed" Systems

In a "closed" system, all the dependent variables change only within the boundaries of the system. In an "open" system, information and matter (and even people) pass freely across the boundaries of the system (i.e., there is a steady-state of the system at any one given moment, but this may be achieved by constant influx and outflow of matter and energy).[4] We thus need to add to our operational definition as follows:

For purposes of definition, consider a community to be a group of people interacting within a definite living space. Functionally, a ward is a community, a circumscribed system of people. People and information move freely across its borders. But, although personae may change rapidly, roles are quite stable over time. It is this relatively agreed upon set of caregiver roles—doctor, nurse, aide—that lends structure to the community. The medical ward is a "quasi-open" community because its culture is transmitted from one generation of personnel to the next. Particular doctors come and go, but the role of the doctor varies little. Permanency and continuity are characteristics of what can be termed the "Primary Caregiver" roles, for this is how the culture-bearers, the doctors and nurses, and the aides look upon themselves. All those who are outside this circle of Primary Caregivers impinge upon the Primary Caregivers' role conceptualizations.

Who is "in" the system and who "out?" Although belonging is to some extent a matter of degree, it is generally clear-cut. Nurses and doctors are most clearly "in." Nursing aides and LPNs are usually "in." Social workers may be "in" or "out," depending on how they are accepted by the Primary Caregivers, but usually are treated as outsiders. Cleaning and maintenance staff are clearly "out." This brief tabulation of the cast of characters of the community should serve to emphasize that certain people fill roles that are clearly beyond the boundaries of the community even when they are physically present in it. Both the patient and the consultant, and usually even the ward attending, are looked upon by members of the ward community as belonging to that space beyond the circle of the ward staff.[5]

## Some Implications of Operationally Defining the Therapeutic Context as an Open Social System

Our operational definition and its emphasis on the "open social System" nature of therapeutics in a medical context deserves some comment. First, we have spoken of the "boundaries" or limits of the system. When we are speaking of a single organism, it may be considerably clearer what the limits are. The "open system" concept was originally invented to describe biological phenomena.[4] For example, at a casual glance, it might seem that the definition of the endocrine system could be focused fairly sharply upon the secretory glands and their target effect on organs. As we have gotten deeper into the understanding of this relatively hard scientific system, however, we have discovered that the boundaries of the system are much fuzzier than originally conceived. The influence of the brain is considerable, and it now seems that psychological and even social influences exert considerable control over the internal secretory glands via the cerebral cortex and the hypothalmic mediators.[6]

The point is that where we choose to draw the boundaries of the "system" may be crucial in how well we understand how the system is functioning. If this is true for a single organism, it is even more vitally true for an elaborate social system. Consider, let us say, the medical ward where the treatment takes place; the hospital, or the community, including where and with whom the patient is during follow-up care; the setting (office, ward, etc); human interactions (How is he treated by nurses, physicians, other patients, handymen, etc.? How do they relate to each other?). How do various kinds of distresses and/or complications influence the patient's illness and treatment of his physical condition: e.g., casts, operations, radiation therapy, ICUs, etc; psychological, social, and familiar variables in illness (conflicts in the family, problems at work, the psychological make-up of the patient, his defenses and strengths, etc.)?

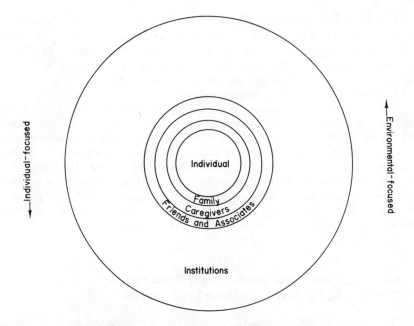

**Fig. 1.**  A person-centered viewpoint.

Illness does not happen in isolation. It occurs within the context of an individual's environment, within or outside of institutions. Whether it is considered of sufficient seriousness to be a "disease" is a question of psychosocial factors, as much as medical ones. We all know that the vast bulk of "illness" never reaches a doctor or other caregiver. This is, in fact, the problem precisely for early prevention-detection: how to identify serious illness early enough to enhance the likelihood of help without creating undue strain on the health care system from false alarms.[7]

Figure 14-1, "A Person-Centered Viewpoint," expresses diagrammatically some of the concepts we are attempting to convey. The individual, in this case, the patient, is central to our thinking. As we move outward, the concentric circles represent the individual's world as it appears to him. Much of this chapter is devoted to the idea that the caregivers, the physicians, and other health workers often can do both the individual patient and themselves a service by broadening their focus to include factors in the environment. To do this, they must look at the world from the patient's perspective.

Although the circles are drawn concentrically, for convenience of notation, more often they are probably better represented as overlapping circles (Fig. 14-2). The caregiver may, for instance, assume the role of mediator, interpreting the individual's behavior to his family and their responses back again. For many professionals, beginning in this kind of in-between position is quite uncomfortable and unaccustomed, something for which training may not have been adequate. Nevertheless, it may be an essential role for the patient's well-being.

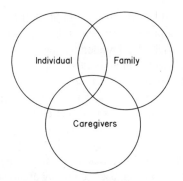

**Fig. 2.**   Person-centered relationships.

Although health care delivery is supposedly organized along the direction in which the "individual-focused" arrow goes, in Figure 14-1 much of the system appears to function so as to satisfy institutional requirements rather than patient needs.

Let us consider an example to illustrate how a social system viewpoint may be applied. Suppose we are dealing with an intensive care unit. The patients are extremely well-attended. Two trained nurses are on duty 24 hours a day. All patients are on cardiac monitors. Adequate and appropriate medications are given and reviewed frequently. The patients, however, are scared to death to leave the unit. Mr. Jones, a 55-year-old businessman having his first MI, develops angina every time he is taken out onto the main medical floor, and there is no known cause for his pain. It has become increasingly frustrating for the CCU staff, who realize that their unit is no longer necessary for him. And, if we view the "system" as being the CCU, they are quite right.

Suppose, however, we look at the totality of the medical service as the "system." We discover that there are four staff nurses during the daytime hours; two in the evening; and one nurse, an LPN, at night for 35 patients. It's about all the one nurse can do to get the medications distributed and physical treatments done in an eight-hour shift. It should not surprise us that the patient with a fresh MI is worried about being out on the floor. Although Mr. Jones' particular ways of coping with these fears should be of concern to us to understand, we also need to understand the patient's interactions with the larger medical context.

Let us now expand the horizons of our "system" to include a world—of Mr. Jones—outside the hospital altogether. His wife and married daughters are quite concerned about him. Mr. Jones' internist, Dr. Wise, after huddling with the family, goes to consult with Mr. Headley Grant, the hospital director. Mr. Grant, who is a well-trained hospital administrator, has studied and recognized the value of live-in arrangements in hospital care. With his blessing, Dr. Wise arranges for a family member to attend Mr. Jones at night in the hospital. The evening and night nurses are relieved not to be buzzed every half-hour by Mr. Jones to meet inconsequential demands.

The problem presented by Mr. Jones might well have been insoluble had it been seen *only* as his problem; or a problem of the CCU alone; or even a problem of the nurses of medical service. By broadening the scope of "systems" about and around the patient through which interventions might be made, however, Dr. Wise found a creative solution to problems at several system levels. These were the patient's, the physician's, the CCU's, and the medical service's. The family as a system was also certainly altered in the direction of involving family members constructively in the patient's care. While these things were going on, Dr. Wise was also discovering that it was getting easier for Mr. Jones to begin to understand his own fears of death, and of being a cardiac cripple after being discharged from the hospital. Although Dr. Wise was not used to talking about such things with patients, and even doubted the wisdom of doing so, the patient seemed quite relieved to talk. Gradually, Mr. Jones seemed to be relaxing.

Sometimes a creative solution to a problem in patient care can de designed at one level of a system where none existed by defining the system's limits more broadly. In this case, the family and community were brought into the hospital. In other cases, it may be necessary to consider narrowing the focus when a problem is defined too globally to be amenable to amelioration.

## Boundary Phenomena

In speaking of systems, we are often borrowing an analogous term from physics. One of these is the concept that "turbulence" tends to increase at boundaries between or among systems (or subunits of systems). A system may maintain its own steady state quite uneventfully, until it comes up against information about another organism or another system at its peripherae, which impinge upon it in some way. Often this requires integrating new information or new organisms or new people into the system.

The term "boundaries" itself may be confusing. Sometimes we mean physical limits. This is certainly the case when we speak of a particular ward location. But it is misleading to think of boundaries solely in this way, because they frequently include other elements, especially in a health or social system. When a person's job functions are unclear (e.g., role definitions around their work is blurred), so may the boundaries of the system in which they work be quite fuzzy. Under these circumstances, there is often a ready-made battleground for conflict near the system boundaries.

First, however, consider the physical boundaries of the traditional nursing station. It is constructed as a small enclave where the staff can congregate, and to which they often retreat when, for one reason or another, they wish to be away from the patients. Now, there are many ostensible reasons for such an arrangement, but almost all the explanations have to do with limiting access to charts and creating a particular sanctum for professionals.

Suffice it to say for present purposes that the staff feel free to discuss patients under such circumstances in their most intimate case history details. This is true even when the station is quite open to hearing lines to the outside world, whether one stands on one side of the nursing station desk or the other. We must conclude that the artificial boundaries serve other purposes than the professed ones of limiting access to the records and work space. Indeed, in some jurisdictions, the official rationale has been made a sham of by right-to-privacy laws, which make all records the property of the patient instead of the hospital or the professional.

More recent hospital design has tended to stress circular rather than long-corridor ward arrangements. Here, the nursing staff has more access to and sight lines of the patient's quarters. This does seem to be a decided improvement in accessibility. Curiously, the enclosed nursing area has remained.

Now, let us consider other nonphysical types of boundaries. In particular, how does the professional role isolate ward staff from the patients? It has been shown that, on some general hospital services, the amount of time spent with a patient is inversely proportional to the socioeconomic status of the persons working on the ward: doctors spend the least time, social workers and other allied health professionals the next most; then nurses; and finally, the cleaning help may actually spend more time talking with patients than any other single group.[8] Some hospital services take advantage of this by recognizing the important part patients take in caring for other patients. The sickest patients are put with other patients who can serve as their advocates when they cannot catch the nurses' or doctors' attention. In general, this is probably therapeutic for the advocate patient as well, although one can well conceive of people who would do better to be by themselves, no matter what their state of health or illness.

Boundaries, as we have indicated, are more than just physical limits. They are also created by tradition, cultural norms, and role definition. The most central social rules of relevance to our discussion are those of the respective professions.

It is at the boundaries of well-delineated roles that professionals come into conflict. Certain work functions are clearly those of doctors, or, equally, clearly those of nurses.

Consider the task in drawing blood. Many nurses are clearly more skilled at the technology than doctors. Once again, at the boundaries of roles, where either person could fulfill the function required, conflict and negotiation are the order of the day.

Often there is an implicit *quid pro quo*. It tends to take the form of, "You treat me well and I might do a favor for you." When the ward is working well, it may be because, when things are not very busy, the doctors and nurses sit around and engage in friendly banter. Sometimes, this has sexual teasing overtones. In such instances, the implicitly sexual content may, in fact, be a way of putting off getting more cohesion among a working group.

In this regard, a small investment of time by the physicians in authority can yield large dividends in cooperation by the nursing staff, anticipating problems while they are still small, and preserving good relations. One way of doing this is to include the head nurse, and preferably some staff nurses, in on rounds, as well as decision-making. This serves a number of functions. The nurses may know things about the patients which the doctors do not but may need to. In addition, it serves to educate the nurses about the medical problems of their patients. In many hospitals, the nursing staff receives little inservice training, and they may have few incentives to perform well on their jobs. Rounding can make at least a modest contribution to making them feel more a part of the team on the ward.

It is also worth pointing out that there are three nursing shifts during the day, constituted of different types of people. Some attention needs to be devoted to the evening and night shifts. It has been found that on psychiatric services where much time and effort is devoted to achieving strong consensus around the patient treatment plans, the evening and night shift nurses still tend to have quite a different view of the patient. In part, this is because there are simply far fewer professionals around at night. More importantly, the evening and night shifts have far fewer chances of participating in the decision-making processes around patients and are, therefore, much more likely to be alienated from the whole process. In many hospitals, the socioeconomic status, and sometimes the race, of the night shift is quite different from the day shift. This is another potential source of conflict.

A relatively efficient way to bring evening and night shift staffs into the fold of the ward culture is to hold group meetings around the change of shift several times a week. Thus, if the meeting extends the night shift by half an hour one day a week, and similarly in the evening, it is not an overwhelming time demand on anyone.

The meetings need not focus on staff problems, but the physician and the nurse in charge do need to be alert to problems and aware of them when they arise. Probably the most productive and least threatening way to conduct such meetings is to structure them specifically around patient care. If they focus on the patients whom the staff feel the most need to know about, staff conflicts can be handled in a constructive, nonpunitive way simply by discussing what needs to be done for the patients. The reason this is so is that "problem patients" are those around whose care the staff is often in the greatest disagreement among themselves. After the members of such a group get comfortable with each other, they usually will feel freer to share mutual gripes and talk about ways in which these can be handled so as not to interfere with the work of patient care, but, in fact, to improve it.

Let us now step back from our suggestions about strengthening the functioning of working groups on a medical ward, and consider what these procedures mean in "system" terms. Basically, we may consider them changes which sharpen the definition of the boundaries of the ward. They do this by: (1) strengthening the group spirit and the pleasure of working together on the ward—experts on groups refer to this as "cohesion"; (2) including in the team everyone who works on the ward, some of whom might ordinarily be on the peripherae and feel isolated from the rest of the personnel. Thus, it becomes clearer to the people working in the context of the ward that they are part of a "system" which is not faceless, but one where the staff actually cares about patients and other staff members as individuals.

## THE THERAPEUTIC COMMUNITY

So far, we have been discussing medical treatment, particularly in-hospital, as taking place within the context of an "open system." There is a more comprehensive way of viewing the ward situation and the entire environment surrounding it. This world-view is referred to as the "therapeutic community" (TC).

We shall attempt to restate the principles of the TC as practiced in general psychiatric hospitals, and then point out both their strengths and limitations for adaptation in practice.

1. Everyone who lives and works on the ward participates in decision-making about himself to the maximum extent possible.
2. Patient treatment plans are determined individually for each patient.
3. Every activity of staff, patients, families, and significant others should contribute directly or indirectly to furthering individuals' taking responsibility for themselves.
4. Every activity engaged in by patients, staff, and others should be understood in terms of the contribution it makes toward making them independent and responsible decision-makers for themselves.
5. Certain activities are necessary to the survival and maintenance of the ward community, even though they may be incompatible at times with the principles of the "TC." These inconsistencies should be recognized and dealt with so as to keep their interference to a minimum.

As elaborated by Maxwell Jones[9] and others, the ideas of the TC are much more all-encompassing than the principles we have enumerated above. Some of them are worth elaborating, because they shed light upon what we think is realistic, and what we feel either does not work in practice or is unreasonable and inconsistent with the open social system of medical practice. For one thing, the TC eventually came to be viewed as a great leveller and democratizer. In this view, the ideal would be to have all participants in the system—patients, professionals, allied health workers, nonprofessionals, family members, and others—share equally in the community. Although certain members of the community would be recognized as leaders for a particular function, this recognition would be based upon competence for that function only. It would not extend to other functions.[10] Thus, for example, if a nurse or aide were recognized as the best *de facto* team leader, she or he might be designated to carry out this function. In point of fact, this is done in a number of psychiatric settings, and often appears to work quite well as gauged by the participants themselves.

There are certain limitations to this ideal and its practice. For one, it is quite unacceptable to many physicians, who consider themselves to be in control in medical situations. This is generally a realistic view. Even when this perception sometimes is inaccurate on their parts, it is an attitude that cannot be ignored.

Aside from attitudes, there are also genuine supervisory and fiscal considerations. If a supervisor is responsible for, let us say, an aide's behavior and performance, it is not easy to reconcile this function with having the aide in charge of a group for certain tasks where the supervisor is only a group member. This is one extreme variant of a type of organizational structure dubbed the "Oak Tree" arrangement, where each person is the servant of several masters. Once again, these barriers of sharing of power and authority are not unconquerable in certain situations, but probably impractical or extremely difficult to realize in most.

What is undoubtedly more important is that participatory democracy represents a set of values. In fact, most of the ideas of the therapeutic community are grounded in certain assumptions that tend to be associated with other value sets. Gilbert and Levinson have demonstrated that ideas about authority, and the degree of personal flexibility or rigidity on political matters, also provide considerable predictive power towards how people will view ward situations, including the concepts of the TC.[11]

In our observations, it was certainly no accident that the TC seemed to reach the pinnacle of its vogue in the United States in the mid 1960s. The general tenor of the country was one of recognizing disparities of income, status, race, creed, and other differences, and also of "doing something" to make these differences less. The ideals of the TC, in its fullblown form, came along at the right time to fit into this climate. The community health movement was in need of a philosophy, and TC was one such competing philosophy, parts of which were adapted wholesale when they seemed to fit the situation.

Another basic problem with the comprehensive TC philosophy also related to its origins. We have stated that the idea that an environment should be made more healthy for humanitarian reasons came to be replaced by the notion that the environment could be the sole healing agent. It is at this extreme that the TC breaks down. For, in order to make this argument stand up, it is necessary to test rigorously the TC as total healer versus other combinations of healing agents. And, when this was done, it was found that even a salutory environment had little healing power for the mentally ill taken by itself.[12]

Even making allowances for difficulties in the methodology of the study, and the problem of whether the TC is set up to handle it, it seems unlikely that the TC by itself can substitute for conventional psychiatric care. The same is obvious in general medicine. What it can do is add an important dimension that is all too often missing in patient care. It is important to point out that a number of practices developed in TCs have been proven to be useful, even if the total concept requires close examination. For instance, Fairweather et al. have shown that wards can be structured so as to require patients to take maximum responsibility for themselves.[13] This has made it possible for the previously long-term care psychiatric patients to move out of the hospital as a group and to live in less-than-total care "lodges" in the community. Self-help groups in medical care are another constructive offspring of the TC ideal.[14]

In what ways are the more realistic principles of the TC, which we believe we have reformulated, applicable to the medical/surgical wards? How might they conceivably improve patient care?

The elements of a healthful setting are nonspecific. Indeed, a medical care delivery system should feel free to borrow and copy the best of all possible worlds that help make for the feeling of well-being.

### Principles of "TC" Applied to a
### General Medical Context

If a total cure is possible for a given illness, our present system of care can deal with it. Medicine has, however, increasingly tended to become the lessening of pain and disability for chronic diseases. Moreover, for chronic relapsing illnesses, the system of care, including its financing, often militates against those very values of maximizing patient independence and self-care which most physicians seem to cherish. In this regard, psychiatry's contribution is, perhaps, to have had to cope with massive numbers of chronically ill persons, whose course was often likely to be one of recurrence, if not gradual downhill progression. TC may be conceived as a form of adaptation to the problems of chronic illness, with acute exacerbations. This is a medical model in the best sense.

Let us consider the course of a patient from the time the patient first enters the hospital. In order to make a diagnosis, a good history is required. This is the first postulate of medicine. The exchange with a patient that creates this history can be thought of, among other things, as a negotiation. The patient feels certain needs, usually pain among others, that he thinks the doctor may be able to help meet. The history is the patient's subjective articulation of these needs, subject to what interests the physician, what the physician will accept, and his skill in encouraging the articulation of needs.

It is possible to develop a much higher degree of reproductibility of interpretations of histories among independent observers, than of many common laboratory tests. This will seem strange to many people in medicine, accustomed as we are to poring over and relying heavily upon our own physician's examination findings, and our often quite sophisticated technological diagnostics.

That the interpretation of histories should be more reliable in terms of reproductibility may not be so counterintuitive, however, if one thinks about it for a minute. In the case of history-taking, two observers have direct reference to symptoms from their source, the patient. Whereas when laboratory or physical examination tests are at issue, there frequently are multiple instrumentations, as well as technologists, that stand between the performance and the interpretation of the test. This is why histories, even psychiatric, can be quite reliably consistent,[15] and our usual diagnostic aids, such as x-rays, may very well be subject to interpretation. In fact, in the absence of history, radiologists may do only moderately better than chance in interpreting routine chest films.[16]

If this is the case, why then, has the subjective become so subordinate in the practice of medicine? Why do we so mistrust our own judgments and rely on increasingly complex, expensive, and often more remote technologies with such faith? Clearly, Ivan Illich, for all his vituperation and exaggeration has made his point—as alienation has increased, so has medicine become estranged from the very people it is supposed to help, as well as the professionals themselves who are accredited to do the helping.[17]

In medical care, continuity is important to maintain, i.e., the least displacement of the patient from his environment. In this sense, treatment rendered in an out-patient setting by a family physician, or in the small community hospital where access by family and friends is facilitated and the workers are well-known to the patients, is least disruptive. Larger hospitals, with rotating staffs who commute from distances, have an impersonal quality of interactions. Therefore, they are less conducive to creating therapeutic communities.

There are intrinsic healing powers in the hospital setting. Some of this is nonspecific, such as conditions conducive to getting the patient well: a place for rest, comfort, allowable regression, and stress-reduced atmosphere; and staff who generate high esteem for the patient, and convey caring and tenderness with a sense of being accepted and respected. A healing institution should increase one's hopes for getting better by the creation of a realistic, optimistic environment. An open, trusting relationship should be established between the patient and the institution. Every day's experience should be well anticipated. There should be few surprises, little undue anxiety from the unexpected. One should not underestimate the physical setting, such as lighting, cleanliness, colors, and the functional aspect of the unit, which can help to dispel the patient's loneliness and depression related to displacement.

Once a treatment begins to be formulated, the doctor must come back continually to the patient to renegotiate what the two of them and everyone else involved will do in order to meet the patient's needs. This becomes a constantly modifiable contract, in which the roles of doctor and patient are more implicit than otherwise.

Staff should make every attempt to prevent immobility and the development of nonadaptive defenses. Efforts should be made for the patients to feel useful while they are in the hospital, to create object constancy and provide three therapeutic elements which are more specific:

1. *Knowing*—about the illness, the institution, the staff, the program;
2. *Experiencing*—the illness itself, removable from the daily routines and other feelings that are associated with being in the hospital;
3. *Sharing the power*—allowing the patient to participate in decision-making areas, from food and pain killers, to even minor details of the hospital routine.

One can state that the absence of these, such as the patient's not knowing where he is, what disease he is suffering from, not being allowed to experience what he is going through; and being at a complete loss of control regarding his fate, may be the most antitherapeutic situation imaginable. Some nursing homes reach this extreme in depersonalization.

In general, the small extra investment in time and energy explaining the treatment to the patient and his family is often rewarded by greater cooperation and likelihood of the patient's following through in a meaningful way. This may seem trivial, but it is surprisingly consequential. For example, a significant percentage of people on antibiotics for streptococcus infections will stop them after three or four days when they feel well, despite the fact that the bacteria are not dead. A minimum reinforcement of their understanding of the significance of this act, by patient education reminders, may greatly increase the likelihood of follow-through.

In addition, patients tend to be more satisfied when they feel that they have been given adequate explanations.[18] Although medicine is not generally thought of as a business, it is often practiced in settings where repeat business and personal referrals of patients by other patients are essential business practice. To put it even more crassly, it is the dissatisfied patients who sue for malpractice. In fact, it is probably not practitioners in the community who may have a low standard of actual practice who are sued for the largest amounts successfully, but, rather, the sophisticated, highly trained, highly specialized practitioners in large referral centers who are doing complicated procedures. Why? One answer may be that the former have a cordial relationship with their patients, and tend to value it. The latter may have little or no relationship, except by referral, and may be more enamoured of their technology than of the pleasures of dealing with the patient.

TC emphasizes independence, responsibility, and individualized decision-making. Are these only statements of our own values, or do they have a contribution to make to the practice of medicine? We would like to suggest, given our own biases, that they do matter.

Hospital services concerned with chronic diseases are natural cousins of the psychiatric situations we have discussed above. One of the earliest of medical services to adapt the TC enthusiastically was the rehabilitation unit. The goals of rehabilitation are outstandingly consonant with the salient purpose of TC, mainly to make it possible for the patient to care for himself independently to the greatest extent possible. It was also clear that much reinforcement to this process could be created by making use of the naturally cohesive groups which form on a rehabilitation unit. The patients in many hospitals sit around feeling bored a good part of the day.

In other areas of medicine, specific approaches suggested by the TC ideology might well be useful, but have been slow to be adapted in this country. Live-in arrangements have been known for sometime in Europe on both obstetrical and pediatric services. Here, arrangements are made for parents, particularly mothers, to take charge of much of the care of their newborns or their sick children on pediatric wards.

As with the TC in other areas, there is much resistance by doctors and nurses to doing this. The resistance seems to center mainly around two concerns: first, that the parents will interfere significantly in the care; and, second, that the parents will be critical of the care being rendered, perhaps even to the point of proving litigious. Neither of these fears appears likely to be borne out in practice.

Latterly, the movement to deliver one's own baby at home has taken hold to a limited extent. Obstetricians are quite critical of the women's movement for risking the lives of mothers and newborn infants by encouraging home delivery without medical care. So far, however, obstetrical services have failed to respond to the telling criticisms that have been made of them, which are reflected in reactions by the movement toward home delivery. Many obstetrical services still overmedicate women in labor, despite the well-known danger to the fetus. In most hospitals, even if fathers are allowed in the labor or delivery rooms, they are only permitted a limited role in the birth process. Fathers feel impotent and helpless at a time of great stress to themselves.

Similarly, although newborn nurseries may be more efficient for nurses, there is no particular evidence that they are healthier for babies than having the babies in the rooms with their mothers. Quite the contrary, the newborn nursery is a frequent source of life-threatening epidemics. Moreover, mothers are often treated as sick invalids in the hospital, rather than as responsible women recovering from an exhausting, painful, but normal life process.

It is quite plausible to organize such services differently and more therapeutically. For instance, many hospitals give some instruction in newborn baby care. Few, however, capitalize on the presence of women with major and realistic concerns, who could share with each other both their hopes and fears, and even suggestions about how to manage when they leave the hospital. No program with which we are familiar does anything of this kind for fathers, despite the fact that postpartum depression in fathers is a well-documented and widespread phenomenon that may be preventable.

Finally, there are the hospitals which openly devote themselves to the treatment of the dying patient. They function quite differently from a conventional medical ward. The nurses and doctors make a point of spending time with the patients, and explicitly discuss the impending death and its implications. Patients seem to respond quite satisfactorily to this, given their situation. Families are also well-informed and welcomed to the hospital, and, indeed, are worked with by staff concerning the meaning of the family member's death to them. Such services are also unafraid to give the requisite pain medication to the dying patient.

The primary reason why the TC has been implemented only in the modest ways we have outlined, then, has to do with the doctors' and other health professionals' self-images. Recognizing the validity of the TC constructs implies that we also accept our own limitations; that others are much like us, and that mutual assistance and frankness can make each of us more satisfactorily self-reliant.

## CONCLUSION

Throughout this chapter, we have attempted to suggest a patient-centered approach to medical care. This approach is as old as the art of medicine itself, yet, curiously, in practice observed largely in the breach. Referring to Figures 14-1 and 14-2 we recommend expanding the health care-giver's view of the patient outward to include the entire environment around the patient. Broadening the horizons for intervention can make critical differences in the patient's well-being.

In addition to the nonspecific factors which promote health, we have described a model of "Therapeutic Community" for medical settings which may help to improve the psychosocial environment for patient care.

**References**

1. Sigerist HE: The Great Doctors, New York, Doubleday-Anchor, 1958
2. Dubos T, Dubos J: The White Plague: Tuberculosis, Man and Society. Boston, Little Brown and Company, 1952
3. Bridgman PW: Logic of Modern Physics, New York, MacMillan, 1927
4. von Bertalanffy L: An outline of general systems theory, Br J Phil Sci 1:134–163, 1950

5.  Karasu TB, Hertzman M: Notes on a contextual approach to medical ward consultation: the importance of social system mythology, Int J Psychiatry Med 5(1):41–49, 1974

6.  Mason JW: Review of psychoendocrine research on pituitary-adrenal-cortical system. Psychosom Med 30:576–607, 1968

7.  Mechanic D: Medical Sociology: A Selective View, London, The Free Press, 1968

8.  Coser RL: Life in the Ward, East Lansing, Michigan State University Press, 1972

9.  Jones M: Beyond the Therapeutic Community: Social Learning and Social Psychiatry. New Haven and London, Yale University Press, 1968

10. Signell KA: Following the Blackfoot Indians: toward a democratic administration of a community mental health center, Community Ment Health J, 11(4):430–449, 1975

11. Gilbert DC, Levinson DJ: Custodialism and 'humanism' in mental hospital structure and in staff ideology. In Greenblatt M, Levinson DL, Williams RH (Eds.), The Patient and the Mental Hospital, Glencoe, Illinois, The Free Press, p. 20-35

12. May PRA: Schizophrenia: evaluation of treatment methods. In Freedman AM, Kaplan HI, Sadlock BJ (Eds.), Comprehensive Textbook of Psychiatry I. Baltimore, Williams and Watkins, 1975, p. 955–982

13. Fairweather GW, Sanders DH, Maynard H, Cressler DL, Bleck DS: Community Life for the Mentally Ill. Chicago, Aldine Pub., Co., 1969

14. Hurvitz N: Peer self help psychotherapy groups: psychotherapy without psychotherapists, In Roman PM, Trice NM, (Eds.), The Sociology of Psychotherapy, New York, Jason Aronson, 1974

15. Ley P: Reliability of psychiatric diagnosis: some new thoughts. Br J Psychiatry 121:41–43, 1972

16. Little JC: Objectivity in clinical psychiatric research, Lancet 2:1072–1075, 1968

17. Illich I: Medical Nemesis: The Expropriation of Health. New York, Pantheon Books, 1975

18. Jolly C, Held B, Caraway A, Prystowsky H: Research in the delivery of female health care: recipient's reaction, Am J Obstet Gynecol 110:291, 1971

Toksoz B. Karasu
Robert Plutchik

# 15

# Research Problems in Psychosomatic Medicine and Psychotherapy of Somatic Disorders*

The concepts used in psychosomatic research reflect the historical origins of the discipline. In the 1920s and 30s, a number of physicians with psychoanalytic training began to speculate about the relations between emotional states or unconscious conflicts and medical conditions. Most such speculations were based upon case histories or summaries of groups of cases; seldom were comparison groups used.

By 1935, Flanders Dunbar summarized much of this growing literature in her book, *Emotion and Bodily Changes*. It was enthusiastically received, and stimulated interest in psychosomatic medicine, so that the new journal *Psychosomatic Medicine* came into existence in 1939.

In the first 20 years of its existence as a separate discipline with its own journal (1939–'1959), the major emphasis in psychosomatic medicine was on theoretical formulations. Research consisted mostly of anamnestic and therapeutic studies at first, but gradually, clinical and laboratory studies began to appear, with most such studies initiated by psychoanalysts and psychiatrists. By the late 1950s, internists had largely turned away from psychosomatic research, but psychologists had increasingly begun to enter the field. According to Wittkower,

> The focus turned from clinical observations to basic research. Areas covered during this research period include: (1) the role of the hypothalamus as part of a feedback system which mediates and regulates neural impulses concerned with emotions and neuroendocrine activity; (2) the limbic system which according to MacLean, mediates visceral rather than ideational

*The authors wish to thank Dr. Herbert Weiner for his most invaluable critique of this chapter.

311

functions; (3) the differentiation of noradrenaline from epinephrine; (4) the role of the adrenals and importance of corticoids in the defense against trauma; (5) the effect of adrenergic hormones in mobilizing those defenses, and (6) last, but certainly not least, the relevance of emotional factors to the etiology of so-called psychosomatic disorders.[1]

In the period between 1959 and 1973 psychosomatic research broadened considerably. A great deal of attention was paid to such issues as the psychobiology of separation and loss, the epidemiology of psychosomatic disorders, doctor-patient relations, and psychopharmacology. It became evident that the various efforts that had been made to validate psychoanalytic concepts had not been particularly successful, probably because of the many methodological research problems that existed. More work became directed toward isolating and quantifying both biological and psychological variables. In addition, animal research dealing with these variables became more fashionable, and efforts were made to develop animal models of illness.[2]

## MAJOR INFLUENCES ON THE DEVELOPMENT OF PSYCHOSOMATIC RESEARCH

Although many individuals contributed to the development of concepts related to psychosomatic medicine, it is possible to identify four major influences on the thinking of most contemporary researchers in the field. These influences stem from the work of Freud, Cannon, Pavlov, and Selye.

### Freud

Although Freud had little to say directly about psychosomatic issues, many psychoanalysts have presented theories of mind-body interaction based upon psychoanalytic concepts. Notable among these contributors are Alexander,[3] Dunbar,[4] and Grinker.[5] Their major preoccupation has been with personality patterns, defensive styles, and unconscious conflicts that are associated with medical illnesses. For example, Dunbar reported that there were similarities in the personalities of those individuals who were suffering from the same illness. She went on to describe a "typical" ulcer personality, coronary personality, arthritic personality, as well as others.

Some recent work has tended to support these ideas of typical personality types. For example, cancer patients have been reported to be relatively undemanding,[6] unaggressive, self-sacrificing, and self-effacing,[7] and often filled with feelings of hopelessness and helplessness even prior to the development of the neoplasm.[8]

A major difficulty with these kinds of studies, however, is that they are often not consistent with one another. In addition, the same constellations are identified in different types of medical illnesses. Colitis patients are reported to have an aggressive, dominating mother with much ambivalence in the mother-child interaction.[9] A similar constellation has been reported for cancer patients.[7] Such disagreements have made the concept of particular personality types for particular illnesses less acceptable than it once was.

Another key psychoanalytic concept is based on the concept of regression. If an individual is placed in a situation which he cannot master, regression to an earlier stage of development is likely to occur. Only parts of the organism regress, however, and only to various degrees. From this point of view, psychosomatic symptoms are interpreted as a stress-induced physiological regression associated with a psychological regression.[10]

Verwoerdt has developed this idea in more detail.[11] He suggests that there are three classes of defense mechanisms that deal with threats and that influence the development of pathophysiological reactions. The first type of defense is a form of retreat from the threat. It implies regression revealed by hypochondriasis, depndency, and self-centeredness. The second class of defense is an attempt to exclude the threat from awareness. This includes denial, suppression, rationalization, projection, and introjection. The third way to deal with threat is to overcome it. According to Verwoerdt this is done by intellectualization, isolation, counterphobic reactions, obsessive-compulsive styles, and sublimation. According to this model, a combination of these defensive maneuvers, with emotional responses to particular stresses, produce the highly varied combinations of affective response actually seen plus physiological syndromes. Although these ideas sound generally plausible, they tend to remain vague in detail, and no one has shown how they can be used to predict the type of illness any particular individual has. A later section of this chapter will deal with this problem in more detail from a research point of view.

The third major psychoanalytic concept that has provided a basis for psychosomatic researches, deals with the problem of symptom specificity. When it became apparent that there was little association between specific diseases and specific personality types, an alternative interpretation was proposed by Graham et al.[12] They suggested that each major psychosomatic disease has a certain characteristic attitude associated with it. The "attitude" is a combination of how a patient feels and what he wants to do about his feelings. Some research by these authors appears to support this idea, but there has been no independent verification. In any case, these authors do not suggest that the attitude is responsible for the development of the disease, but only that it is part of the disease process.

Other psychoanalytic concepts such as unconscious conflicts, dynamics, regression to lower psychosexual stages, etc., have become part of the language of psychosomatic medicine. They are, however, difficult to define, difficult to measure, and difficult to use in a predictive research design.

### Cannon

Cannon's researches on the physiological changes associated with emotional states were in part an extension of William James' theory, and in part, a reaction against it. His work, early in the 20th century, tried to identify the autonomic, as well as central neural structures and changes associated with emergency reactions, particularly fight or flight reactions. Cannon concluded that emotions were energizers that produced total body reactions that modified the homeostatic balances of the body. These emergency reactions affected the interacting mechanisms through which an organism maintains a dynamic equilibrium despite changes in the environment.

These views stimulated a good deal of research of the more narrow laboratory variety (e.g., studies of autonomic changes in college students exposed to electric shocks, loud noises, or dirty pictures). By 1964, this type of research had expanded sufficiently to justify the appearance of a new journal, *Psychophysiology,* which has maintained this same direction of inquiry.

An important issue which this type of research has been concerned with is that of specificity versus generality. Many psychoanalysts working in the area of psychosomatic medicine have assumed that particular diseases such as asthma or ulcers tend to be associated with particular emotions, conflicts, or personality traits. In contrast, Cannon and many researchers who work within his tradition, have tended to assume that emotions or conflicts create a generalized arousal or activation condition of the organism, and that symptom formation reflects a kind of overflow reaction of congenitally "weak" or predisposed organs. "Controversy between the adherents of the specificity concept on the one hand and the adherents of the activation concept on the other, arose early and has continued to the present, with the debate sometimes assuming the proportions of the earlier 'nature-nurture' controversy, and, like that controversy, often characterized by considerable acrimony."[13]

One attempt at clarification of this issue has been presented by Roessler and Engel.[13] They distinguish between stimulus-response (SR) specificity and individual-response (IR) specificity. By the former, they mean a consistent response by most subjects in a group to a particular stimulus (e.g., tachycardia elicited from most persons by immersion of the hand in ice water). IR specificity refers to the fact that some people react most strongly with one type of response (e.g, increased blood pressure) to a wide variety of stimuli. Such individuals are more likely to become hypertensive patients than others.

Roessler and Engel suggest that an individual's personality traits and his cognitive appraisals influence, if not determine, whether SR specificity or IR specificity is to be found. At the present time, however, this is more speculation than fact. They emphasize the need to assess each individual's appraisals in all psychosomatic research.

## Pavlov

The identification of the conditioned reflex, and the exploration of its properties by Pavlov and many others, led to new insights into autonomic physiology, as well as new research strategies. The conditioning of salivation and other involuntary responses led researchers to the conclusion that visceral behavior could be manipulated only by respondent conditioning paradigms. In addition, it was believed that such conditioning could be considered to be the basis for most emotional reactions seen in animals and in humans. Pavlov also came to the conclusion that all so-called higher mental activities were elaborations of simple conditioned reflexes, and were subject to the laws of inhibition and enhancement. He even tried to develop a schema of basic personality types that influenced the degree and nature of the conditioning each type was exposed to.

The relation of Pavlovian conditioning to psychosomatic medicine became increasingly evident as evidence accumulated that a large variety of physiological processes could be conditioned. For example, it was shown that heart rate, blood pressure, pupillary reflex, and hormone secretions could all be conditioned. Thus, psychosomatic syndromes such as hypertension could conceivably be the result of a conditioning process.

By the early 1960s, research showed that the so-called "involuntary" autonomic responses such as skin resistance changes, heart rate, and even EEG changes could be conditioned by operant paradigms. Researchers both in America and Russia enthusiastically began to explore these possibilities, and this research became one of the sources of the current interest in biofeedback. Recent proponents of conditioning strategies in psychosomatic medicine have claimed that a new method of treatment of psychosomatic illness is becoming available as a result of these developments. They write:

[Psychosomatics] has emphasized relations between emotion and illness, relying on the personality of the patient as a source of the problem and the focus of therapy. This approach to disease is akin to psychodynamic methods of dealing with behavioral disorders, and it tends to invoke ambiguous hypothetical constructs between the stimuli confronting that patient and the disorder. This results in a treatment plan aimed more at a vaguely defined cause than at the critical behavioral and physiological problem occurring in a social context. In contrast, a psychophysiological model employing operant conditioning techniques sees as its target for therapy the environment rather than the personality of the individual and its capabilities for enhancing self-control.[14]

There are two major differences between this view of psychosomatic medicine and the more traditional one. First, instead of focusing attention on inner psychic conflicts, it focuses on a specific physiological dysfunction (e.g., hypertension), largely in isolation. Second, it tries to use conditioning procedures, both operant and respondent, as methods of modifying the disturbed physiology. Research problems center around the issue of the extent to which these goals can be successfully reached.

One important research implication of this behavioral, conditioning approach to psychosomatic medicine, is the new emphasis it has given to an exploration and understanding of environmental variables. This concern with the environment is now referred to as social ecology.

In a review of the literature on social ecology, Moos has pointed out that there are a number of variables that have been identified for conceptualizing and describing social environments, and that some correlations have been established between such dimensions and physiological changes or medical illnesses.[15] Moos suggests that there are three basic categories of social environment dimensions: relationship dimensions, personal development dimensions, and system maintenance and change dimensions. Examples of the first category include the variables of affiliation, peer cohesion, staff support, and expressiveness. Illustrations of the second category include autonomy, practical orientation, and competition. The third category is exemplified by the dimensions of order and organization, clarity, control, and work pressure.

Evidence is cited to support the idea that high levels of involvement in group activities are associated with increases in cardiovascular responses, and that cohesive groups are less subject to the effects of stress than noncohesive groups. Other studies have shown that individuals given major responsibility over others (e.g., pilots of military aircraft) show greater corticosteroid responses than do the less responsible members of the group. In the same vein, it has been demonstrated that air traffic controllers have higher risks and earlier onsets of hypertension and peptic ulcers than do members of a control group. This is interpreted as a result of the operation of the environmental variable of work pressure. Moos concludes that this way of describing the environment in terms of discrete variables is more meaningful, useful, and predictive than is the use of a single global term such as stress.

### Selye

The fourth major figure who has influenced research in psychosomatic medicine is Hans Selye. From the 1930s to the present time, he has singlemindedly pursued the problem of measuring the effects of stress on the body. His major contribution was the concept of a "general adaptation syndrome" which consists of three stages: alarm, resistance, and exhaustion. If a stress persists beyond the initial alarm reaction, then tissue damage could eventually occur during the stage of resistance. Such damage could be thought of as "diseases of adaptation." Continued presence of a major stressor would lead eventually to exhaustion of defensive resources and death.

Despite the emphasis by Selye on the general adaptation syndrome as a nonspecific reaction to all stressors, he does point out that every stimulus produces both specific as well as nonspecific effects. This point is important since a perennial problem of psychosomatics is that of symptom specificity; i.e., why does a particular individual develop a particular symptom or illness at a particular time in his life? One approach is to assume that differences in the type of disorder individuals develop are due to particular weaknesses or vulnerabilities in particular organ systems, rather than in differences in the nature of the stresses an individual is exposed to. This view is emphasized most strongly by Holmes and Rahe, who have obtained evidence that stresses associated with any kinds of life changes (divorce, marriage, deaths, births, etc.) are linearly cumulative, whether the changes are desirable or not.[16] Persons with high life change scores over a one-year period have a considerably higher risk of illness than those with low scores.

An alternate position argued by Lazarus is that the effects of stressors depend on several factors: "(1) the formal characteristics of the environmental demands; (2) the quality of the emotional response generated by the demands, or in particular individuals facing these demands; and (3) the processes of coping mobilized by the stressful commerce."[17] The major point of this view is that individuals differ in their cognitive appraisals of particular stressors and, as a result, experience different emotional reactions to them. A person who reacts to stresses with feelings of anxiety, depression, and helplessness is likely to exhibit different bodily reactions than one who reacts to life events with anger, resentment, or hostility. From a research point of view, detailed evidence is needed on the possibility of such differential emotional reactions and their special effects.

One parallel version of this view of stress is described by Wolff.[18] He proposed that psychosomatic illness can be interpreted as the effects of long-term reactions of normal, adaptive biological responses to symbolic threats rather than physical stressors of the kind typically studied by Selye. Under conditions of symbolic threat, the body reacts with such normal defenses as swelling, hyperemia, hypersecretion, and hypermotility. No clear explanation is given, however, for the appearance of medical symptoms in one organ system rather than another.

Although Selye was instrumental in directing the attention of researchers to the problems of stress, there has developed a considerable difference of opinion concerning the meaning and significance of the term. For example, Patkai,[19] as well as others, have pointed out that in laboratory research on stress using human subjects, there is no *a priori* way of knowing, or to what degree, the experimental conditions will be stressful. Researchers such as Holmes and Rahe, who prefer situational definitions of stress, assume that certain events mean pretty much the same thing to most people. They tend to assume that stressors are linearly additive, even though there is little or no evidence on the statistical properties of environmental stress events. In actual laboratory practice, three types of stressors are typically used for such research. One involves the use of stimuli productive of pain (e.g., electric shock, cold pressor test, or pain produced by a pressure cuff). The second involves the use of conditions which threaten the individual's view of himself. Criticisms of task performance or criticism of personal values are examples of this type of stress. The third type of laboratory-environmental stress is based on poor performance related to the reality of difficult tasks. If an individual is required to work under time pressures or distractors, stress is usually produced.

More often, stress is measured by responses rather than by stimuli. In such cases, the investigator obtains self-reports of emotional reactions (e.g., anxiety or anger), or uses adjective check lists. Sometimes behavioral measures such as facial expressions, speech changes, or changes in work performance are used. Most widely used in stress studies are physiological indices such as heart rate, blood pressure, GSR, or EMG changes. Occasionally, biochemical measures of blood chemistry or hormone excretion are measured.

Problems exist with these various response measures aside from the problem of the reliability of the indices. Self-report measures are subject to distortions, denial, and suppression, as well as the problem of excessive compliance with the "demand characteristics'' of the situation. Behavioral measures are not always adequate, since individuals often learn to compensate for increased work demands by improving their effort and hence their output. With physiological indices, a major problem is the well-known lack of correlation between arousal indices in different organ systems. Stimulus and response specificities often make physiological measures difficult to interpret.

The only solution to these problems that has been seriously proposed is the gathering of multiple indices so that all types of response measures and all types of body systems are simultaneously measured. Since it is manifestly impossible to measure everything, however, various approximations become necessary. Some of the differences in research results reflect the different decisions made by investigators in what they are willing to sample.

One important point should be made in this context. It is probably true that almost any event will have some effect on any individual. Most such effects are probably quite minor, however, and hardly worthy of note, given the body's capacity to make constant dynamic adjustments at all times. What is important is the need to order the different life events or stressors in terms of their likelihood of making a significant impact on life functioning. As Ader has said, ''Multicausality remains an empty concept if no attempt is made to accurately describe and order the diverse causes . . .''[20]

The contributions of Selye and others to the concept of stress are noteworthy, but they have also engendered a counterreaction. Hinkle, for example, has raised some issues about the concept of stress, and has questioned the usefulness of the construct.[21]

In his paper, he describes the origin of the term. In the 17th century, the word meant "hardship or adversity." By the 19th century, the term had been adopted by scientists to mean "force, pressure, strain, or strong effort." By the early 20th century, "stress and strain" had been adopted by psychiatry as a cause of ill health or mental disease, and in 1925, Cannon used the term stress in relation to homeostasis; i.e., the tendency of the body to "resist distortion" caused by an external force. In the late 1930s, Selye introduced the concept of a general adaptation syndrome as a state of stress consisting of all the changes produced in common (in the pituitary, adrenals, thymus, and intestinal tract) by a variety of physical stressors (heat, cold, immobilization, toxic substances, etc.). In the 1968 revision of *Stress and Disease,* stress is described as "a dynamic state within an organism in response to a demand for adaptation, and since life itself entails constant adaptation, living creatures are continually in a state of more or less stress."[22]

Hinkle then points out that neurohumoral changes brought about by changes in the social environment can have intense and long-lasting effects on all body systems. But the problem remains: what is the nature of the stimulus needed to produce profound changes in organ functions? His answer is that, although a few reactions are genetically programed (e.g., reactions to loud noises or pain), most are based upon information exchange with the environment. And in a fundamental sense the most important aspect of the environment of higher social animals is the existence of other social animals of the same group. The major activities within a social group are: food gathering, defense, courtship, sexual relationships, and the care of the young; and the major function of social behavior is to help the individual maintain his role relationships within the group. "Any information that implies to an animal that the appearance of another animal might lead to a change in its role relationship within the social group is highly meaningful to the animal that receives it, and is liable to be associated with pronounced behavioral or physiological changes."[21]

In the light of these considerations, Hinkle concludes that any biological process within the organism, including disease processes, can be influenced by the neural and hormonal reactions of the individual to his social environment. There is, in fact, no difference between a state of stress and a state of being alive, and therefore, there is no need for a special term ("stress") to describe this condtion. Hinkle also points out that, although some challenges to the integrity of the organism produce biologic reactions that have something in common, a fundamental feature of living systems is the ability to produce responses that are specifically directed toward counteracting the effects of specific threats. "An animal that responded to a bacterial invasion of its lung by creating inflammation and new bone in its left ankle would not survive very long" (p. 361).[21]

In his critique, Hinkle then goes on to ask: are there events within the social environment which are inherently stressful or disease producing? He cites studies of soldiers, of concentration camp victims, and others which appear to indicate that people who are suffering prolonged hardships not only do not develop psychosomatic diseases, but often lose those they had before the hardship occurred. The consistencies reported by Holmes and others in "stress ratings" of certain life events probably reflect the importance of certain social relationships in Western societies; but in other societies quite different ratings might be expected. Hinkle's answer to his question is therefore "No." His concluding note is that, just as there is no single explanation or single cause for any biologic event, so too there is no interpersonal relation or life event that can be the sole cause of any psychosomatic illness.

Hinkle's erudite critique of the concept of stress raises several important questions: (1) if all biologic reactions are attempts to maintain a dynamic equilibrium, is there such a thing as "stress diseases"? (2) if all biologic events can be affected by one's interpretations of social events, is it meaningful to talk about a separate branch of medicine called "psychosomatic medicine"? Let us consider these questions.

## WHAT IS A PSYCHOSOMATIC DISORDER?

Weiss has reviewed the psychosomatic literature and, as a consequence, suggested that there seem to be at least three characteristics that define a psychosomatic disorder.[23] The first one, which he names "the psychogenic proposition," is that the appearance of a medical illness is caused by some antecedent psychological characteristic of the patient, such as a particular dynamic conflict. Weiss rejects this proposition on the grounds of limited evidence obtained by correlational and not causal studies.

A second characteristic of a psychosomatic illness is that the course of the illness can be noticeably affected by psychological factors (the "precipitant/aggravant proposition"). Evidence on this point is clear and supportive. It may be said, however, that all illness, of whatever type, can be affected to some degree by psychological events. To the extent that this is true, it implies that either all medical illnesses are "psychosomatic" or that there is no special class of such illnesses.

A third feature of psychosomatic illnesses that has been proposed is that there is a specific connection between a particular type of psychological event and a particular type of symptom (the "specificity proposition"). Three versions of this proposition have been advanced. Dunbar has suggested that particular personality profiles correlate with particular disorders.[4] Alexander has substituted particular unconscious conflicts for the personality traits.[3] Graham et al. have proposed that certain attitudes are specifically related to certain illnesses.[12] Although these views seem plausible, the actual research data that has been advanced to support them are limited and subject to criticism on various methodological grounds (e.g., lack of a control group, experimenter bias, overlap of profiles, or weak effects).

Do these conclusions of Weiss' imply that one should simply drop the concept of psychosomatic illness? Weiss does not take this position, but instead argues that the research questions should be stated in a different way than is traditional. The basic research questions should be: "Who are the patients within a given illness population for whom psychological variables are of primary significance?", or "Which variables are relevant for which patients?" What Weiss appears to be calling for is a rank-ordering of the most important variables that affect the appearance or change in various medically defined disorders. This is useful, but it hardly resolves the issues raised by him.

Another way to look at the matter is to recognize that the actual conduct of research in the area of psychosomatic medicine is quite difficult, partly because of the interdisciplinary nature of the research, partly because of a lack of adequate measuring techniques for the important dimensions, and partly for other reasons. In other words, it is possible that all three of the propositions that Weiss criticizes are in fact true, but that the evidence is simply not yet available to make definitive statements about them. Therefore, if the field is to continue advancing, increased attention should be given to the various methodological research issues that exist. With that end in mind, the remainder of this paper will discuss in some detail the more important research problems that exist when psychosomatic research is undertaken.

## PROBLEMS OF RESEARCH IN
## PSYCHOSOMATIC MEDICINE

The basis for many of the research problems that exist is to be found in the fact that psychosomatic medicine is a complex, interdisciplinary field with inputs from many sources. Not only should the researcher or research team be expert in terms of a traditional medical education, but other specialties are also necessary. The fact that psychoanalysis was a central source for psychosomatic thinking implies that more than a superficial acquaintance with it is necessary. The contributions of Pavlov suggest that a knowledge of learning and conditioning concepts is extremely useful. Cannon's influence implies the need for some expertise in neural mechanisms and in psychophysiological instrumentation. The contributions of Selye and others on the neuroendocrine effects of stress imply the need for more than a casual knowledge of biochemistry. And last, but certainly not least, the fact that the term psychosomatic implies a relation between mind and body, means that the researcher must have detailed knowledge of psychological tests and of psychometric test construction.

These demands on the investigator of psychosomatic problems are obviously great, and there are few if any persons, who can meet them. This is why most such research must be conducted by teams, or must be so narrow in scope that one or two people can carry it out. As a not unimportant aside, it should be mentioned that most psychosomatic research has to be conducted with medical patients, which means that the whole institutional structure of clinics, hospitals, and review boards must become involved at some point. These various complexities make for slow overall progress and there is little reason to believe that the future will be any different. With this framework in mind, let us examine the research problems.

### The Problem of Biochemical Measurement

A number of studies have been interpreted as indicating that certain groups of psychosomatic patients (e.g., hypertensives) have abnormal levels of various biogenic amines,[24] but the reports are conflicting.[25] Such observations have led investigators to attempt to relate catecholamine secretions to various organic diseases, mental illnesses, and temporary states. In order to adequately interpret such studies, however, it is necessary to have precise measurements of the biochemical parameters being investigated.

Over the years, increasingly precise methods have been developed for measuring the major biogenic amines serotonin, norepinephrine, and dopamine. A problem remains, however, in the interpretation of such measurements, since most depend upon the evaluation of peripheral urinary metabolites of these amines. Such peripheral metabolites sometimes bear no simple relation to brain neurotransmitters, and they can be affected by a number of essentially extraneous variables. For example, it is well known that dietary catechols have frequently contaminated the endogenous metabolite pools. Bananas, oranges, legumes, caffein, and alcoholic beverages will all affect release of norepinephrine, dopamine, or serotonin.[26] In addition, it is also known that the phenothiazines used widely as tranquilizers, and antidepressants such as imipramine also affect the secretion of the metabolites of norepinephrine. Even such a common variable as exercise will increase the secretion of catecholamines. These observations, therefore, indicate the need for vigorous controls over such variables when attempts are made to relate catecholamine secretions to stress or disease.

## The Problem of Physiological Measurement

In a good deal of psychosomatic research, particularly within the Cannon tradition, efforts are made to relate environmental or subjective stresses to transient physiological changes. For example, electric shocks are given to volunteers, and their skin resistance (GSR), blood pressure, or heart rate are measured. Although this is widely done, many investigators are not sufficiently sensitive to the many sources of error that can affect the results of such research. This may be illustrated by reference to work on the galvanic skin response, which is a widely used index of sweating and resistance change of the skin.

Any adequate system for measuring the electrical properties of the skin for use in psychosomatic research should meet at least two requirements. It should: (1) be relatively free from artifacts due to the apparatus—such artifacts as electrode polarization and uncontrolled variations in current; and (2) give results that are unambiguous and meaningful within the standard body of electrical theory. The d-c systems which are commonly used for studying galvanic skin responses do not generally meet these requirements in that polarization effects are difficult to control, the levels of current applied are often unspecified or subject to uncontrolled variation, and the assumption is sometimes made implicitly that the body acts as a simple linear resistor.

In one study dealing with these issues, Plutchik and Hirsch investigated skin impedance and phase angle as a function of frequency of a-c and current levels, using "dry" silver electrodes without paste.[27] It was demonstrated that skin impedance and phase angle both decrease as frequency goes up in the range of 1–1000 Hz. The magnitude of the impedance and phase angles were invariant with changes in the level of current used, although this is not true when d-c is used. It thus appeared that the use of a low-frequency a-c sine wave input avoids some of the artifacts often associated with research on the GSR; despite this, most researchers have continued to use the d-c system mainly because of its simplicity.

That this simplicity can be misleading can be illustrated by a number of facts. In a 1953 paper, Schlosberg and Stanley stated: "We question the widespread use of EKG or EEG electrode pastes designed to minimize skin resistance when one wishes to measure resistance."[28] Several years before that, Burns had shown that by vigorous rubbing of the skin combined with the use of electrode paste, the basal resistance could be reduced from about 100,000 ohms to as little as a few hundred ohms.[29] This is important in light of the fact that several investigators have reported racial and sex differences in average skin resistance. It is possible that indiscriminate use of pastes and skin rubbing techniques may have washed out real differences that exist.

Edelberg and Burch have shown that GSR changes and basal resistance were greatly affected by both the type and concentration of electrode paste used.[30] Other problems concern polarization effects, constant current versus constant voltage issues, and location of electrodes. In one study of electrode location effects, Plutchik compared seven different electrode placements in terms of sex differences and stability over time.[31] It was found that women consistently have a higher average impedance than men, and that certain placements maximized sex differences while others minimized them.

These examples were given to illustrate the fact that many sources of error exist that affect the results of physiological measures of autonomic function. The fact that numbers can be obtained from an instrument does not necessary imply that the number truly measures a biological phenomenon.

## The Problem of Psychological Measures

Fundamentally, psychosomatic research is concerned with the relations between mind and body. In order to establish such relations, it is necessary to have reliable measures of *both* mind and body. From the point of view of the body, this requires the availability of measures of biochemical functioning, electrical activity of the nervous system, and measures of mechanical or hydrolic activity of organ systems. Such measures are generally available, although caution must be exercised to avoid the many sources of error that can occur. From the point of view of the mind, it is necessary that measures of affect, personality, dynamic conflicts, and coping styles be available. That they are available only to a limited degree is unfortunately a truism of psychosomatic research, and this fact is one of the major reasons for difficulty in replicating research.

Because of the historic origins of psychosomatics, there was an initial heavy emphasis on "dynamic interviewing" of patients to try to establish connections between personality styles and medical conditions. Such interviews were usually conducted by one person—the investigator—and were subject to all his biases and expectations. That these are often important is illustrated by Barber,[32] and discussed in detail by Plutchik.[33]

When psychological tests began to be used, they were usually limited to projective tests such as the Rorschach, the TAT, or figure drawings. Although such tests are useful in the hands of a skilled clinician, they do not meet the requirements of psychometric reliability, and are of questionable validity as research tools. As these problems became recognized, attempts were made to use standardized diagnostic tests such as the MMPI, or standardized personality tests such as the Cattell 16PF. These instruments were long and tedious to take, were academic in content, and did little to further psychosomatic research.

During the course of time, new measuring instruments have been developed that appear to have more promise for research, but there is still a dearth of relevant clinical instruments for measuring affect states, personality, ego defenses, and conflicts. Among the more promising measures are those developed by Plutchik to measure moods,[34] affects,[35] personality,[36] and ego defenses.[37]

An alternative measuring technique that holds promise for research has been developed by Gottschalk.[38] He points out that there are three major methods that have been used for providing indices of psychological variables: self-report inventories, psychiatric rating scales, and content analysis of verbal behavior. In describing these methods, he notes that self-reports reflect subjective states well, but are subject to two kinds of biases—malingering and lack of awareness of one's own states. Psychiatric rating scales are useful in that a trained observer can utilize both verbal and nonverbal cues to make judgments about psychological variables. Different observers may elicit different information from the same person, however, and, in addition, personal rater biases may still operate.

Objective content analysis of verbal behavior works with transcripts of tape recordings of interviews or dreams. Raters make evaluations of the degree of presence of various dimensions. A major problem with the method is the large amount of time and training needed to make reliable judgments, as well as the high level of inference required of the raters. It is thus obvious that there is no panacea for the problems of reliable and valid measurement of psychological variables, but progress has been made and will undoubtedly continue. What is of central importance is for the investigator of psychosomatic phenomena to devote as much time and concern to the measurement of psychological variables as to the measurement of biological ones. It should no longer be possible to say what White said in a 1956 symposium on *Research in Psychosomatic Medicine:* "What seems to happen in a number of studies is that the physiological data is extremely refined while the psychological data is trivial or of little significance" (p. 21).[39]

### The Problem of Control Groups

The problem of establishing appropriate control groups is always a problem in research, but it is of special importance in psychosomatic research. The issue always arises: suppose that a particular group of ulcer patients or hypertensives or cardiac patients are found to have a certain average personality profile or average defense style. What does this tell us about possible origins of each particular illness? Can we even state that these traits or defenses are correlated with the presence of each particular medical illness?

Given only the information cited above, the obvious answer to the questions is "No." Without an appropriate control group, it is possible that the characteristics found in the ulcer or hypertensive patients are also found in everyone else. This problem is particularly acute if the sample size is small and if the sample is not selected on the basis of some kind of random sampling plan.

In other words, if the sample being evaluated consists of half a dozen patients obtained through a physician's private practice, it is highly probable that sampling artifacts are present. If the sample being evaluated consists of 50 consecutive patients seen in a medical clinic, the likelihood that they will represent a larger population is much greater. Sample sizes of *one,* although frequently useful in helping develop hypotheses about relevant variables, are usually anecdotal reports, and have little value in the process of documentation or validation of hypotheses.

An interesting example of this problem is found in the work that has been done on patients with a gastric fistula. In the 1940s, Wolf and Wolff had an opportunity to make careful and extensive observations on the stomach of a hospital employee named "Tom," who had had a gastric fistula since he was a child.[40] The investigators measured various stomach functions such as motility, secretion, and engorgement, during regular work hours, and at times, during artifically contrived situations designed to create emotional disturbances in Tom. The results indicated that periods of resentment were associated with high acid secretion and high motility of the stomach, while periods of depression were associated with flaccidity and low secretion.

A short time later, Margolin and his associates were able to study a young black woman with a similar gastric fistula.[10] She, however, was seen while an inpatient at Mount Sinai Hospital; and in addition, observations were made on her stomach mucosa while she was in concommitant psychoanalytic therapy. Observations were made by nurses on her overt behavior, while inferences about her dynamic underlying conflicts were made by a psychoanalyst on the basis of her dreams, free associations, and other verbal materials. The results of this study apparently showed that stomach activity could not be correlated with conscious overt behavior, but could be correlated with unconscious motives and conflicts. When unconscious needs were "pressing for expression," gastric secretions and other stomach activities tended to be high; when the patient was in psychic equilibrium, stomach activity was low. When there was strong unconscious conflicts as inferred by the psychoanalyst, however, the different stomach activities acted in asynchronous ways; for example, hypermotility might be associated with hyposecretion.

The observations of Wolf and Wolff[40] and those of Margolin are in apparent contradiction. There is no way of knowing whether the differences in the conclusions are due to a sex difference, an age difference, a personality difference, or a methodological difference. It is obvious that larger numbers of patients must be evaluated, and that controls for these other possible variables must be introduced.

This raises the further questions: what is a control group and what is being controlled? In a general sense, we recognize that all experiments are performed in order to answer specific questions. When doing experiments, sources of error or bias arise. These biases may be thought of as factors that make for an erroneous conclusion or that make a conclusion ambiguous. Another way of describing error is to define it as any unspecified factor which affects one condition or one group differently from others. Errors may occur in connection with the overlooking of relevant variables, through inadequate analysis of data, through inadequate sampling procedures, through experimenter expectancies, and for other reasons.[41]

In research, the word "control" actually has three different meanings: (1) it can refer to a reference point or reference group against which something is compared; (2) it is used in the sense of the control or manipulation of independent variables; and (3) it is used in the sense of restraint or the keeping constant of variables that are not being investigated. As an example of the last use of the term, if age or sex is considered important as variables, then the groups being compared are made up of individuals of the same sex, and of the same average age.

In psychosomatic research, the major question that arises concerns the first use of the term: to what extent are the results of the observations the same or different from those obtained from a reference or comparison group. In specific terms: to what extent are the ambitiousness, drive, and repressed dependency needs found in ulcer patients also found in nonulcer patients.

Conceptually, this is a simple idea, but practically it is often very difficult to obtain an appropriate comparison group. The major reason for this is the funadmental difference between laboratory research and clinical research. In the typical laboratory setting, a group of animals or normal subjects are randomly divided into two groups. One, arbitrarily called the experimental group, is exposed to some experimental condition or stress. The other, arbitrarily called the control group, is not exposed to the stress, or is given a placebo of some sort.

In contrast, typical psychosomatic research begins with observations of naturally occurring groups which are not created by the investigator, and which have characteristics not usually specifiable in advance. Thus, psychosomatic patient groups of interest might be: all ulcer patients treated as inpatients at a general hospital during a certain period of time; a random sample of essential hypertension patients attending an outpatient clinic; a group of diabetic adolescents seen for an initial evaluation at a clinic; etc. Although these groups are sometimes referred to as "experimental groups," the term is clearly a misnomer, since they were not created by the experimenter and since they do not have an equivalent randomly selected control group.

The usual procedure that is followed in trying to establish control groups for patient groups is to try to identify a naturally occurring comparison group that can *reasonably* provide a reference point. Control groups of this type that are frequently used include: other patients who have illnesses not defined as psychosomatic; emergency room patients; medical student volunteers; college students; siblings of the identified patient; etc.

Now, although this is the typical procedure for selecting control groups, it is obvious that the method has certain problems connected with it. Although the control group may be similar to the "experimental" group in some respects, it obviously differs from it in a number of other ways. For example, if the control group consists of patients with nonpsychosomatic illnesses (e.g., hernia or appendicitis), they may differ from the experimental group on age or sex distribution, social class or background, type of recent stresses, and, perhaps most importantly, in type of reaction to the illness itself.

A good example of this problem is given by West.[42] Fifty cases of chronic ulcerative colitis were selected as the "experimental group." The control groups consisted of hospital patients without psychosomatic disorders and other types of psychosomatic patients. West writes:

Despite all of our control groups, we are unable to provide certain critical controls. For example, what psychological effect is produced in an individual, what regression occurs, what defenses of denial are mobilized when he is tormented with 20 or 30 or 40 stools a day? If we were truly to control this "somatopsychic" effect, we'd be required to produce an artifical colitis in people who are otherwise psychologically "normal," have them defecating 30 times a day for many months, with psychological measurements before and after to define what changes they had undergone. So far, no one has stepped forward to volunteer for such an experiment . . .[42]

This example points up the fact that it is very difficult to obtain closely similar control groups for an existing patient sample of whatever type. It means that, at best, the results of psychosomatic research will have a relatively large area of uncertainty surrounding them. It also means that a great deal of emphasis must be placed upon the replication of results by independent investigators.

This last point may be highlighted by referring to the work of Cohen.[43] He was interested in comparing personality patterns in patients with asthma or hypertension. He obtained some evidence of statistically significant differences in coping styles among these patients. He then tried to replicate the findings with new comparable groups of patients, but was unable to do so. "Two consecutive studies (by the same investigators) showed entirely different findings and both studies were statistically reliable." Cohen concludes by recommending that every experiment should include an attempt at replication in the original plan.

These problems that have been cited are related to the general question of the degree of similarity or comparability of the experimental and control groups. It has probably occurred to the reader that one way of dealing with this problem is by the use of matching of subjects. Since this is an important issue, the following section will deal with it.

## The Problem of Matched Groups

First of all, it should be clear that matching of subjects is a technique designed to exclude variables and to eliminate their possible influence. It has nothing to say about which variables are causal variables for the people involved. For example, if an experimental and a control group are matched for age and sex, then, presumably, any differences that remain between the two groups are related to other variables than age and sex. Matching does not tell the investigator which other variables are relevant.

At the same time, matching of subjects creates a number of other problems. The simplest and most obvious is that one cannot study the operation of variables if they are kept equal. In other words, if age of patients is a relevant factor in (say) the types of conflicts they have, then by matching on age, we are unable to learn whether or not age is relevant. Only if age is permitted to vary can we determine if people of different ages have different conflicts.

A second problem created by matching is that we often do not know what we should match on. As a result, most investigators who use this technique, match on a few obvious (if not necessarily relevant) variables such as age and sex. Since any two groups will differ on a large number of variables, however (e.g., education, IQ, income, family size, religion, type of residence, neighborhood, etc.), matching on only two or three of them hardly is likely to make the groups equivalent. If we then try to match on more than two or three variables, our ability to locate equivalent persons decreases, and the number of subjects in the matched groups gets smaller and smaller. For example, in order to find 40 schizophrenics who were matched on age, sex, IQ, and family income, over 500 records had to be examined in one state hospital study.[44] The question then arises: if 90 percent of possible patients are discarded from the study because they cannot be matched, how representative can the results be? Therefore, the attempt to match on many variables creates the problem of the unrepresentativeness of the samples. Matching on only a few variables does not make the groups comparable.

A third problem that results from attempts at matching is another kind of sampling bias. For example, suppose that asthma patients are, in fact, more intelligent than colitis patients. If we then match patients from these two groups on IQ, we will be implicitly selecting the relatively duller asthma patients and matching them to the relatively brighter colitis patients. Neither group will then be particularly representative of its larger population.[45]

These problems created by matching are not trivial. Their presence may be among the reasons for difficulty in replicating results of investigations. Despite these problems, there are several methods that are useful in minimizing their effects.

One method is to rely on true random sampling procedures as much as possible. For example, if there is a clinic that handles 200 colitis patients a year than a random sample of (say) 30 cases might be selected for intensive research study. If they are to be compared with a control group of other medical patients on a ward, then a random sample of these other patients should be selected. In general, whenever possible random sampling procedures should be used.

The other method that may be helpful in dealing with some of the problems of control groups is called the "implicit scaling of multiple control groups."[46] This may be illustrated in the following way. Suppose we were interested in identifying the presence of certain personality traits in hypertensive patients. The usual approach would be to compare a group of such patients with a "normal" control group, possibly matched on two or three variables. An alternative plan would be to try to identify several groups of hypertensive patients who vary systematically in the degree of hypertension that they exhibit. Thus, one group might consist of extreme hypertensives, a second group could be moderate hypertensives, and a third group could be comprised of minimal hypertensives. We might then try to determine if these groups also vary in a regular way in the degree to which repressed hostility or some other trait of interest was present.

The general idea in this approach is to obtain control groups that are implicitly scaled on the dimension of interest. We then consider whether the dependent variable(s) being studied also vary in a parallel way.

## SPECIAL PROBLEMS IN THE MEASUREMENT OF AFFECT

The point has already been made that a major problem in psychosomatic research concerns the inadequacies in the measurement of psychological variables in contrast to physiological ones. This issue is of particular importance with regard to the measurement of affect. In all explanatory schemas in this field, strong emphasis is given to emotional states such as anxiety, depression, and hostility and to their interactions and conflicts. Despite this emphasis, the description and understanding of emotions is relatively limited. The present section will therefore discuss the problems of affect in more detail. It will describe some of the important factors that have made the study of emotion so difficult, and will conclude with a description of recent attempts that have been made to measure emotions and their interactions in more precise ways.

The major disagreements about the nature of emotions have arisen through lack of recognition or concern with the evaluation or measurement of the *intensity, persistence,* and *purity* of the emotions studied, and through a misunderstanding of the role *individual differences, introspection,* and the *definition* have in the results obtained from studies. This section will attempt a clarification and analysis of these problems and is based upon an analysis first developed by Plutchik.[47]

### The Problem of Intensity

Emotions may differ qualitatively, but a given emotion may also exist in varying degrees. Thus, in every day conversation one distinguishes between startle, fright, fear, anxiety, panic, and horror, or contentment, pleasure, happiness, joy, and ecstasy. Two different studies designed to produce fear may produce it to different extents, and the resulting overt or physiological measures may be quite different.

The basic need is therefore to be able to study the physical, the physiological, and the subjective concomitants of emotional states as a function of the intensity of the emotion. In connection with this, it is necessary that adequate scaling procedures be developed so that the magnitude or intensity of the emotional state can be unequivocally specified.

### The Problem of Persistence

In general, the data concerning the emotions have been gathered from two sources: experimental laboratory work on animals and humans and clinical experience with human beings suffering emotional disorders. Cannon's work is the former approach, while Dunbar's book is typical of the latter approach.

The laboratory studies of emotion generally take a "normal" subject and induce some kind of emotion by using disturbing stimuli such as electrical shocks, loud noises, or certain kinds of pictures. Introspective reports are then related to overt behavior and/or physiological changes. Conclusions are then drawn concerning the physiological basis of "fear" or "anger" or "startle" or "joy."

On the other hand, the clinical studies usually examine a patient who has been suffering anxiety or depression or resentment for a long time, often for years, and then try to determine the physiological changes which have taken place, or those which take place when stressful aspects of the patient's life situation are discussed.[18]

Obviously, the kinds of events being called by the same name, anger or fear, in the two kinds of subjects, and in the two kinds of situations, are not identical. Anger which is induced in a normal subject, and which is expressed and over in a few minutes or less, is not the same thing as the chronic resentment which Wolff's peptic ulcer patient showed, and it is to be expected that the results of such studies will not, in general, be found identical. Mahl has provided some evidence to indicate at least one difference between acute and chronic fear.[48, 49] He reports that, in dogs and monkeys, hydrochloric acid secretion increases only during chronic fear and not during acute fear.

The work of Selye on the "general adaptation syndrome" has provided evidence to indicate that the particular character of the physiological changes which occur as a consequence of stress depends upon the amount of time during which any stress-provoking agent is applied.

The implication to be drawn is that some estimate of the degree of persistence of the emotional state be obtained if experiments are to be comparable.

## The Problem of Purity

In the laboratory study using normal persons, the emotions produced are usually quickly over and relative-pure (e.g., the *anger* will be expressed without much *fear* of punishment). On the other hand, in the clinical situation, many patients have conflicts about the expression of their emotions. For an emotion to persist implies in all likelihood that an opposite emotion is acting to prevent complete overt expression of either one. A person suffering chronic resentment certainly has anger, but he also feels fear over the expression of anger. Psychotherapy of depressed patients almost invariably uncovers much aggression which has been directed against the self, through fear of punishment or fear of loss of love. Thus it is clear that studies done with patients must of necessity be dealing, in most circumstances, with mixed rather than pure emotions; the many disagreements in the clinical area suggest that mixed emotions may have different characteristics than pure ones.

Here again, the experimental study of emotions in the clinical framework should include some statement of the kinds of emotions which are acting simultaneously in the subject. One direction of advance would involve developing an empirical typology of "emotion mixture," just as the study of "color mixture" has led to laws describing how pure colors interact to produce the complex qualities of everyday experience.

## The Problem of Individual Differences

There is good reason to believe that subjects in the laboratory stress situation fall into discrete classes or types. A study by Funkenstein et al. has shown that randomly selected college students subjected to a stress situation respond in at least two characteristic ways with regard to the expression of anger, some directing it outward, and others toward themselves, with a development of anxiety.[49a] There exist corresponding decreases in heart rate for one group and increases for the other. Some subjects or patients show marked anxiety to injection of adrenalin and some show none. Lacey et al. have also demonstrated that different subjects tend to respond by the activation of different major physiological response systems, and that within any large group of subjects there always exists several general types of responders.[50] This implies that a simple average of the responses for a group of subjects has no meaning, but that the response measures must be sorted according to the consistent subclasses which will very likely appear.

## The Problem of Introspection

There has been a great deal of concern in theories of emotion with the problem of introspective reports, or what might be called the "feeling" of emotion. The early controversies over the James-Lange theory were mostly concerned with where the *feeling* of the emotion was to be placed when the whole sequence of events is considered which might be related to emotions.

There are two important things to be said about this view. First, the evidence on which this kind of theory is based stems largely from the laboratory studies of "pure," momentary emotions and not from the persistent "mixed" emotions of clinical experience.

The second major problem in this area is that many emotional states are not conscious. If repression is a fact, and there is good reason to believe it is, what is repressed generally is exactly this feeling of whatever emotion the individual is experiencing. This is a commonplace in clinical practice. Often a fair amount of treatment is required before the patient recognizes the feelings he may have of hostility, anxiety, sadness, longing, and so on. If this is the case, then the subjective feelings of an emotion should not be a necessary part of the definition of an emotion.

There is also another reason for not regarding introspection as essential to a definition of emotion. This is the fact that many studies are done with lower animals. If these experiments are to be considered as valid studies of emotion, then introspections cannot be crucial. How then are these problems to be met? This concerns, at least in part, the question of definition.

## The Problem of Definition

Somehow, the necessary and sufficient conditions for application of the term emotion have to be determined such that (1) they do not require introspections, (2) they can be applied to lower animals, (3) they can be applied to mixed or pure emotions, (4) they can be applied to emotions of varying intensity, and (5) they can be applied to individuals of different personalities or modes of reacting.

"Pure" emotions in this ideal sense may be defined by various properties which can be approached experimentally only by a series of successive approximations, as the different variables which affect the measurement of the emotion are eliminated or kept constant. It is only through a recognition of what these variables are that an effective experimental program can be instituted.

## The Measurement of Emotions

A number of different methods have been developed for the measurement of emotions. These are described in some detail by Plutchik, so that only a summary will be presented here.[51]

Of the four general ways that exist for measuring emotions, the most common is self-report. Some self-report tests are designed to measure immediate moods, while others are designed to measure emotions or feelings which are characteristic of the person over a long period of time. Mood scales usually present the subject or patient with a list of emotion adjectives such as cheerful, sad, bored, and angry, and ask him to check those that describe his present mood. Sometimes brief sentences are used that reflect certain feelings (e.g., "I worry about making mistakes"; "I am shy"; etc.). A version of this procedure was developed by Plutchik and Kellerman, and is one which asks the patient to choose one out of each of a series of pairs of adjectives, as descriptive of himself.[36] For example, he is asked whether he is:

Affectionate or Adventurous
Resentful or Shy
Quarrelsome or Obedient

Based on his answer to each question, his emotional disposition or emotional profile is determined. Such self-report scales have been used to identify the effects of psychotropic drugs, to predict suicide potential, and to study group interactions, among other things.

A second method of measuring emotions is by means of behavior rating scales. Such scales have been used mainly with four types of populations: psychiatric patients, mentally retarded patients, children and infants, and lower animals. Behavior rating scales usually provide a brief description of an emotional event and ask an observer to rate the presence or absence of that event, or the degree to which it has occurred. For example, when studying children the observer (usually a parent, or a teacher) will be asked to rate the following kinds of items:

Is restless and unable to sit still.
Has temper tantrums.
Picks on other children.

The analysis helps to determine the influence of different variables upon children's behavior and affective states.

A third way to measure emotions is by indirect evidence. For example, the Rorschach projective test and the Thematic Apperception Test (TAT) provide indirect measures of emotional states on the basis of fantasy and perceptions. Free associations, dreams, and slips of the tongue observed in psychoanalytic therapy sessions are also indirect indices of emotional states in the patient. So, too, are facial expressions. Although important avenues of contact with underlying emotional states, these methods are often difficult to quantify.

The fourth method used to study emotion is based on the frequently observed fact that a heightened state of emotion is typically associated with changes in body physiology. The lie detector test is based on this association. Many experiments have been done which show widespread biochemical and physiological changes in the body at times of emotion and stress. There is little evidence of a single emotion being associated with one particular pattern of physiological changes, however; so that at present, we cannot use bodily changes as direct measures of specific emotions.

## RESEARCH ON THE TREATMENT OF
## PSYCHOSOMATIC DISORDERS

In order to treat psychosomatic disorders, some acceptable definition of the term must be available. In 1965, Hambling suggested that a psychosomatic illness could be defined in terms of the following criteria: (1) its origin is related to a period of crisis; (2) it gets worse with the appearance of additional stresses; and (3) it disappears when the stress situation is relieved.[52] Unfortunately, no one has demonstrated that these criteria apply in any unequivocal way to any illness. An alternative schema was suggested by Ramsey, Wittkower and Warner.[53] They suggest that psychosomatic illnesses are based on (1) inherited or early acquired organ vulnerability; (2) chronic arousal leading to damage of the organ system; (3) personality patterns of conflict and defense; and (4) precipitating life stresses. There is also little direct evidence of this schema.

In the absence of appropriate general criteria for defining a psychosomatic illness, it is necessary to define simply by enumeration. In the 1930s, seven illnesses were considered to be psychosomatic: bronchial asthma, rheumatoid arthritis, ulcerative colitis, essential hypertension, neurodermatitis, thyrotoxicosis, and peptic ulcer. Gradually, many other illnesses were added to the list (e.g., diabetes mellitus, migraine, coronary artery disease and cancer). It now appears that just about any medical illness can be exacerbated by life stresses, or has an increased probability of appearing after life stresses, and can therefore be called "psychosomatic." Most physicians would consider such usage much too broad, but no satisfactory set of delimiting criteria have been proposed.

Despite this existing vagueness of definition, there have been many attempts to treat "psychosomatic" illnesses by both psychiatrists and physicians of other specialties. Unfortunately, many such attempts at treatment have been carried out without the benefit of any appropriate control groups. The typical study of this type simply lists the number of patients who have been "cured," the number improved, and the number unchanged. For example, Daniels et al. reported a followup of 57 patients with ulcerative colitis who underwent psychoanalytic psychotherapy.[54] About 9 percent had excellent results, 55 percent good results, 30 percent had little or no change, and 6 percent got worse.

Another example of an uncontrolled study of psychosomatic patients was reported by Weisman.[55] Six duodenal ulcer patients were treated by means of psychoanalytic psychotherapy over a period of several years. All patients were found to have intermittent recurrences of symptomatology, and no therapy variables were believed to account either for the frequency or duration of exacerbations of the ulcer. The major conclusion the author reached was that larger groups of patients need to be evaluated.

There are several problems with studies of this sort from a research point of view. First, there is no control group of colitis patients to compare these results against. The basic question is: if no therapy had been offered these or similar patients, how many would be cured, how many would improve, and how many would get worse?

A second problem in this kind of research relates to the problem of experimenter biases or expectancies. Too often, the investigator has a stake in a favorable outcome, and since the judgment of outcome is usually based on interviews and is usually made by the investigator, there is a possibility that the list of changes is an overestimate of what has really happened.

For example, Weinstock reported a questionnaire survey of the results of 25 ulcerative colitis patients by experienced analysts.[56] The therapists reported that 80 percent of their patients were symptom-free for many years. These findings, which appear quite good, are better than those reported by Daniels et al., and may possibly reflect biased reporting. Since there was no independent evidence for the correctness of the descriptions, it is possible that the therapists overestimated their successes.

Another example of possible bias in research may be seen in the report by Daniels et al.[54] They examined the records of six ulcerative colitis patients who had completed their analyses, and found that the number of years the patients were in treatment and the number of sessions per week did not correlate with either improvement or worsening of the condition. More important was the fact that the group studied represented less than 10 percent of the total sample of patients. There was no way to estimate the degree of bias contributed by the nonrandom sampling method used to select patients for evaluation.

A third problem in research of this kind is related to the fact that the very process of psychotherapy is often unstructured and difficult to specify. For example, in a study by Ripley, Wolf, and Wolff of over 800 patients who had attended a clinic, a description was given of the types of psychotherapeutic procedures that were used.[57] They included reassurance and emotional support, free expression of conflicts and feelings, advice about attitudes and behavior, explanation of psychophysiological events, symptomatic drug treatments, dream analysis, and help by social workers, among other things. With such a pot pourri of procedures which overlap different schools of psychotherapy, it is difficult, if not impossible, to attribute changes in patients to *one* particular psychotherapeutic approach.

Another illustration of the problem of specifying what psychotherapy is all about can be seen in the work of Karush et al.[58] They reported that hopeful, active patients did better regardless of the type of therapy offered, and the "psychoanalysis is . . . contraindicated even during a remission . . . in symbiotic (patients)." They also concluded that supportive and cathartic approaches were often more helpful than long-term analyses. O'Connor concluded that the effects of psychotherapy on psychosomatic illnesses are still not well understood.[59]

Finally, there is evidence that many psychosomatic patients show transient improvement associated with entrance into a hospital, or with beginning of treatment;[60, 61] followup over time shows a deterioration in functioning, or lack of maintenance of improvement.

These problems that have been briefly described imply that research on the outcome of therapy is difficult to do, and is particularly difficult in the area of psychosomatic medicine. Despite this reality, several studies have been reported in which different types of psychological treatment, ranging from didactic lectures to individual psychoanalysis, have produced positive results as compared to some sort of control groups.[62] These reports are optimistic about the value of psychotherapy with psychosomatic patients, but they can hardly be considered definitive in view of the many problems of research that have already been cited.

## A CONCLUDING NOTE

Psychosomatic medicine is a complex, interdisciplinary field conceptually abstruse and demanding. Research in psychosomatics requires the skills of a physician, epidemiologist, biochemist, psychoanalyst, and psychologist in order to deal with the challenging problems that exist. This chapter has discussed these various problems. It has shown that the historical origins of the field are diverse, and that theories of mind-body relations (or more specifically, personality-illness relations) are multiple and varied. Research in the field has often been inconsistent.

These inconsistencies are due to a host of factors, most of which have been described here. They include: problems in defining an illness; problems in measuring personality, or affects, or psychotherapy; problems in establishing appropriate control groups; problems of drawing conclusions from retrospective research; problems of measuring stress; and problems of matching groups; to name a few. Many of these problems are not limited to psychosomatic research, but are inherent in most kinds of clinical research undertakings.

One point that has not been sufficiently emphasized in the foregoing pages is the problem created by heterogeneity in the origins and symptoms of various medical illnesses. On this issue Weiner has written:

> In the past 25 to 30 years, psychosomatic investigation and theory has (often) consisted of a dialectic between proponents and opponents of the opinion that certain diseases are characterized by specific, unconscious psychological conflicts. In retrospect, this heated debate obscured the fact that the diseases under study were not uniform—different subforms of the disease exist. . . . Progress in psychosomatic investigation might be enhanced in the future by carefully characterizing patient groups according to the subforms of the disease from which they suffer. The subforms of the disease might then be compared socially and psychologically with each other.[63]

The value of a critique of research issues of the kind presented here is that it brings attention to problems that need to be solved. Only when we are clearly aware of the problems can progress be made in dealing with them.

## References

1. Wittkower ED: Historical perspective of contemporary psychosomatic medicine. Int J Psychiatry Med 5:309–319, 1974
2. Startsev VG: Primate Models of Human Neurogenic Disorders. Hillside, New Jersey, Laurence Erlbaum, 1976
3. Alexander F: Psychosomatic Medicine: Its Principles and Applications. New York, WW Norton, 1950
4. Dunbar F: Emotions and Bodily Changes (4th ed.). New York, Columbia University Press, 1954
5. Grinker RR: Psychosomatic Research. New York, WW Norton, 1953
6. Renneker RE: Countertransference reactions to cancer. Psychosom Med 19:409–418, 1957
7. Perrin GM, Pierce IR: Psychosomatic aspects of cancer: a review. Psychosom Med 21:397–421, 1959
8. Goldfarb C, Driesen J, Cole D: Psychophysiological aspects of malignancy. Am J Psychiatry 123:1545–1552, 1967
9. Lidz T, Rubenstein R: Psychology of gastrointestinal disorders. In Arieti S (Ed.): American Handbook of Psychiatry, I. New York, Basic Books, 1959
10. Margolin SG: Genetic and dynamic psychophysiological determinants of pathophysiological process. In Deutsch F (Ed.), The Psychosomatic Concept in Psychoanalysis. New York, International University Press, 1953
11. Verwoerdt A: Psychopathological responses to the stress of physical illness. In Lipowski ZJ (Ed.), Psychosocial Aspects of Physical Illness, Advances in Psychosomatic Medicine, 8. Basel, Karger, 1972
12. Graham DT, Lundy RM, Benjamin LS: Specific attitudes in initial interviews with patients having different "psychosomatic" disease. Psychosom Med 24:257–266, 1962
13. Roessler R, Engel BT: The current status of the concepts of physiological response specificity and activation. Int J Psychiatry Med 5:359–366, 1974

14. Shapiro D, Surwit RS: Operant conditioning: a new theoretical approach in psychosomatic medicine. Int J Psychiatry Med 5:377–387, 1974

15. Moos R: Conceptualizations of human environments. Amer Psychol 28:652–665, 1973

16. Holmes TH, Rahe RH: The social readjustment rating scale. J Psychosom Res 11: 213–218, 1967

17. Lazarus RS: Stress and coping in adaptation and illness. Int J Psychiatry Med 5:321–333, 1974

18. Wolff HG: Life Stress and Bodily Disease. Baltimore, Williams & Wilkins, 1950

19. Patkai P: Laboratory studies of psychological stress. Int J Psychiatry Med 5:575–585, 1974

20. Ader R: The role of developmental factors in susceptibility to disease. Int J Psychiatry Med 5:367–376, 1974

21. Hinkle LE, Jr: The concept of "stress" in the biological and social sciences. Int J Psychiatry Med 5:335–358, 1974

22. Wolff HG: Stress and Disease. Revised by Wolf S, Goodell H. Boston, Little Brown, 1968

23. Weiss JH: The current state of the concept of a psychosomatic disorder. Int J Psychiatry Med 5:473–482, 1974

24. Euler US, Hellner S, Purkhold A: Excretion of noradrenalin in urine in hypertension. Scand J Clin Lab Invest 6:54–61, 1954

25. Brunes S: Catecholamine metabolism in essential hypertension. N Engl J Med 271: 120–124, 1964

26. Hoeldtke R: Catecholamine metabolism in health and disease. Metabolism 23:663–686, 1974

27. Plutchik R, Hirsch HR: Skin impedance and phase angle as a function of frequency and current. Science 141:927–928, 1963

28. Schlosberg H, Stanley WC: A simple test of the normality of 24 distributions of electrical skin conductance. Science 117:35–37, 1953

29. Burns RC: Study of skin impedance. Electronics 23:190–196, 1950

30. Edelberg R, Burch NR: Skin resistance and galvanic skin response. Arch Gen Psychiatry 7:163–169, 1962

31. Plutchik R: Effect of electrode placement of skin impedance-related measures. Psychol Record 14:145–151, 1964

32. Barber TX: Pitfalls in Human Research: Ten Pivotal Points. New York, Pergamon, 1976

33. Plutchik R: Foundations of Experimental Research (2nd edition). New York, Harper & Row, 1974

34. Plutchik R: Multiple rating scales for the measurement of affective states. J Clin Psychol 22:423–425, 1966

35. Plutchik R, Platman SR, Fieve RR: Repeated measurements in the manic-depressive illness: some methodological problems. J Psychol 70:131–137, 1968

36. Plutchik R, Kellerman H: Emotions Profile Index Manual. Los Angeles, Western Psychological Services, 1974

37. Plutchik R, Kellerman H, Conte HR: A structural theory of ego-defenses. In Izard C (Ed.), Emotions and Psychopathology, New York, Plenum, 1978

38. Gottschalk LA: Quantification and psychological indicators of emotions: the content analysis of speech and other objective measures of psychological states. Int J Psychiatry Med 5:587–610, 1974

39. White KL: Interdisciplinary research, with special reference to cardiovascular research. In Research in Psychosomatic Medicine. APA Psychiatric Research Reports, 3, 1956

40. Wolf S, Wolff HG: Human Gastric Function (2nd ed.). New York, Oxford University Press, 1947

41. Plutchik R: Foundations of Experimental Research (2nd ed.). New York, Harper & Row, 1974

42. West LJ: Psychodynamic causality in psychosomatic research: problems of experimental design. In Research in Psychosomatic Medicine. APA Psychiatric Research Reports, 3, 1956

43. Cohen LD: A note on the repetition of experiments. In Research in Psychosomatic Medicine. APA Psychiatric Research Reports, 3, 1956

44. Kellerman H: The development of a forced-choice personality index and its relation to degree of maladjustment. PhD Dissertation. New York, Yeshiva University, 1964

45. Plutchik R, Climent C, Ervin F: Research strategies for the study of human violence. In Smith WL, Kling A (Eds.), Issues in Brain/Behavior Control. New York, Spectrum, 1976

46. Plutchik R: Problems of multidimensional evaluation. Ann NY Acad Sci 218:78–86, 1973

47. Plutchik R: Some problems for a theory of emotions. Psychosom Med 17:306–310, 1955

48. Mahl GF: The relationship between acute and chronic fear and the gastric acidity and blood sugar levels in Macaca rhesus monkeys. Psychosom Med 14:182, 1952

49. Mahl GF: Physiological changes during chronic fear. Ann NY Acad Sci 56:240, 1953

49a. Funkenstein DH, King SH, Drolette ME: Mastery of Stress. Cambridge, Harvard University Press, 1957

50. Lacey JI, Bateman DE, Van Lenn R: Autonomic response specificity: an experimental study. Psychosom Med 15:8, 1953

51. Plutchik R: Emotion. Homewood, Illinois, Learning Systems, 1975

52. Hambling J: The psychosomatic patient. In Wisdom JO, Wolff, H (Eds.), The Role of Psychosomatic Disorders In Adult Life. Oxford, Pergamon, 1965, p. 53–62

53. Ramsey RA, Wittkower ED, Warner H: Treatment of psychosomatic disorders. In Wolman B (Ed.), Therapists Handbook: Treatment of Mental Disorders. New York, Van Nostrand, Reinhold, 1975

54. Daniels GE, O'Connor JF, Karush A, et al.: Three decades in the observation and treatment of ulcerative colitis. Psychosom Med 24:85–93, 1962

55. Weisman A: A study of the psychodynamics of duodenal ulcer exacerbations. Psychosom Med 18:2–40, 1956

56. Weinstock H: Successful treatment of ulcerative colitis by psychoanalysts: a survey of 28 cases, with follow-up. J Psychosom Res 6:243–249, 1962

57. Ripley HS, Wolf S, Wolff HG: Treatment in a psychosomatic clinic. JAMA 138:949–951, 1948

58. Karush A, Daniels G, O'Connor J, et al.: The response to psychotherapy in chronic ulcerative colitis II. Factors arising from the therapeutic situation. Psychosom Med 31:201–226, 1969

59. O'Connor J: A comprehensive approach to the treatment of ulcerative colitis. In Hill OW (Ed.): Modern Trends in Psychosomatic Medicine, 2. New York, Appleton-Century-Crofts, 1970

60. Nemiah JC: The psychological management and treatment of patients with peptic ulcer. In Weiner H (Ed.), Advances in Psychosomatic Medicine, 6. Duodenal Ulcer. Basel, Karger, 1971, p. 169–185

61. Chappell MN, Stefano JJ, Rogerson JS, et al.: The value of group psychological procedures in the treatment of peptic ulcer. Am J Dig Dis 3:813–817, 1936

62. Malan DH: The outcome problem in psychotherapy research: a historical review. Arch Gen Psychiatry 29:719–729, 1973

63. Weiner H: The heterogeneity of "psychosomatic" disease. Psychosom Med 38:371–372, 1976

# Index